Rights at Stake and the COVID-19 Pandemic

The COVID-19 pandemic has reshaped life across the world, placing people at risk as our responses to it alter not only health and well-being but also governance, economies, social relations, and our interaction with the natural environment. This volume draws globally recognized human rights scholars and practitioners into dialogue over the costs and consequences of the pandemic. With insights and data from fields as diverse as medicine, anthropology, political science, social work, business, and law, these contributors help us make sense of the pandemic's ongoing effects and its potential impact on future systems and processes. Drawn from two special issues of the *Journal of Human Rights*—one published within eight months of the first lockdowns and the other published almost two years into the pandemic—this book offers one of the most comprehensive collections of such research available. It will be of interest to researchers and advanced students of Politics, Sociology, Social Work, Economics, Anthropology, Social and Political Geography, and Public Policy.

Shareen Hertel is a Professor of Political Science at the University of Connecticut, USA, jointly appointed with the UConn Human Rights Institute. She is the Editor of the *Journal of Human Rights* and has worked with United Nations agencies, foundations, and nongovernmental organizations in the United States, Latin America, and South Asia.

Catherine Buerger is the Director of Research at the Dangerous Speech Project (DSP). She is the Managing Editor of the *Journal of Human Rights* and has published widely in academic and policy outlets. She holds a PhD in Anthropology from the University of Connecticut, USA.

Rights at Stake and the COVID-19 Pandemic

Two Special Issues of the *Journal of Human Rights*

Edited by
Shareen Hertel and Catherine Buerger

Routledge
Taylor & Francis Group
LONDON AND NEW YORK

First published 2023
by Routledge
4 Park Square, Milton Park, Abingdon, Oxon, OX14 4RN

and by Routledge
605 Third Avenue, New York, NY 10158

Routledge is an imprint of the Taylor & Francis Group, an informa business

British Library Cataloguing-in-Publication Data
A catalogue record for this book is available from the British Library

ISBN13: 978-1-032-21825-0 (hbk)
ISBN13: 978-1-032-21826-7 (pbk)
ISBN13: 978-1-003-27019-5 (ebk)

DOI: 10.4324/9781003270195

Typeset in Minion Pro
by codeMantra

Publisher's Note
The publisher accepts responsibility for any inconsistencies that may have arisen during the conversion of this book from journal articles to book chapters, namely the inclusion of journal terminology.

Contents

Citation Information viii
Notes on Contributors xi

Part I
Early views and analysis of the pandemic 1

Introduction—Human rights in the time of COVID-19 3
Shareen Hertel, Catherine Buerger, and Benjamin C. Carbonetti

Centering rights-based theory and praxis 4

1 Revisiting interdependence in times and terms of crisis 5
Michael Goodhart

2 A forecasted failure: Intersectionality, COVID-19, and the perfect storm 13
Kimberly Theidon

3 Solidarity in times of crisis 22
Kathryn Libal and Prakash Kashwan

Re-examining health 32

4 Global health and human rights in the time of COVID-19: Response, restrictions, and legitimacy 33
Lisa Forman and Jillian Clare Kohler

5 Human rights obligations of drug companies 43
Michael Santoro and Robert Shanklin

6 What COVID-19 revealed about health, human rights, and the WHO 54
Wendy H. Wong and Eileen A. Wong

Contesting power and control 68

7 Legal empowerment approaches in the context of COVID-19 69
Sukti Dhital and Tyler Walton

8 Freedom of movement, migration, and borders 80
Jaya Ramji-Nogales and Iris Goldner Lang

9 State surveillance and the COVID-19 crisis 90
Kristine Eck and Sophia Hatz

10 Hazardous confinement during the COVID-19 pandemic: The fate of migrants detained yet nondeportable 100
Didier Fassin

Part II
Ongoing debates 113

Introduction—Beyond complacency and acrimony: Studying human rights in a post-COVID-19 world 115
Giacomo Chiozza and Jeffrey King

11 The state of human rights in a (post) COVID-19 world 116
Giacomo Chiozza and Jeffrey King

Windows of opportunity to worsen human rights 133

12 Can nonviolent resistance survive COVID-19? 134
Erica Chenoweth

13 The COVID-19 pandemic and authoritarian consolidation in North Africa 147
Sammy Z. Badran and Brian Turnbull

Fighting COVID-19, maintain human rights: Challenges and tradeoffs 167

14 Pandemic patriarchy: The impact of a global health crisis on women's rights 168
Alison Brysk

15 The effect of the COVID-19 pandemic on human rights practices: Findings from the Human Rights Measurement Initiative's 2021 Practitioner Survey 189
K. Chad Clay, Mennah Abdelwahab, Stephen Bagwell, Morgan Barney, Eduardo Burkle, Tori Hawley, Thalia Kehoe Rowden, Meridith LaVelle, Asia Parker, and Matthew Rains

16 Global perceptions of South Korea's COVID-19 policy responses: Topic modeling with tweets 206
Jeong-Woo Koo

Lessons learned for the future 226

17 Hindsight is 2020: Lessons from the COVID-19 pandemic for future human rights research 227
Amanda Murdie

Index 239

Citation Information

The chapters in this book were originally published in the *Journal of Human Rights*, volume 19, issue 5 (2020) and volume 21, issue 3 (2022). When citing this material, please use the original page numbering for each article, as follows:

Introduction
Human rights in the time of COVID-19
Shareen Hertel, Catherine Buerger, and Benjamin Carbonetti
Journal of Human Rights, volume 19, issue 5 (2020) pp. 519

Chapter 1
Revisiting interdependence in times and terms of crisis
Michael Goodhart
Journal of Human Rights, volume 19, issue 5 (2020) pp. 520–527

Chapter 2
A forecasted failure: Intersectionality, COVID-19, and the perfect storm
Kimberly Theidon
Journal of Human Rights, volume 19, issue 5 (2020) pp. 528–536

Chapter 3
Solidarity in times of crisis
Kathryn Libal and Prakash Kashwan
Journal of Human Rights, volume 19, issue 5 (2020) pp. 537–546

Chapter 4
Global health and human rights in the time of COVID-19: Response, restrictions, legitimacy
Lisa Forman and Jillian Clare Kohler
Journal of Human Rights, volume 19, issue 5 (2020) pp. 547–556

Chapter 5
Human rights obligations of drug companies
Michael Santoro and Robert Shanklin
Journal of Human Rights, volume 19, issue 5 (2020) pp. 557–567

Chapter 6
What COVID-19 revealed about health, human rights, and the WHO
Wendy H. Wong and Eileen A. Wong
Journal of Human Rights, volume 19, issue 5 (2020) pp. 568–581

Chapter 7
Legal empowerment approaches in the context of COVID-19
Sukti Dhital and Tyler Walton
Journal of Human Rights, volume 19, issue 5 (2020) pp. 582–592

Chapter 8
Freedom of movement, migration, and borders
Jaya Ramji-Nogales and Iris Goldner Lang
Journal of Human Rights, volume 19, issue 5 (2020) pp. 593–602

Chapter 9
State surveillance and the COVID-19 crisis
Kristine Eck and Sophia Hatz
Journal of Human Rights, volume 19, issue 5 (2020) pp. 603–612

Chapter 10
Hazardous confinement during the COVID-19 pandemic: The fate of migrants detained yet nondeportable
Didier Fassin
Journal of Human Rights, volume 19, issue 5 (2020) pp. 613–623

Introduction
Beyond complacency and acrimony: Studying human rights in a post-COVID-19 world
Giacomo Chiozza and Jeffrey King
Journal of Human Rights, volume 21, issue 3 (2022) pp. 245

Chapter 11
The state of human rights in a (post) COVID-19 world
Giacomo Chiozza and Jeffrey King
Journal of Human Rights, volume 21, issue 3 (2022) pp. 246–262

Chapter 12
Can nonviolent resistance survive COVID-19?
Erica Chenoweth
Journal of Human Rights, volume 21, issue 3 (2022) pp. 304–316

Chapter 13
The COVID-19 pandemic and authoritarian consolidation in North Africa
Sammy Z. Badran and Brian Turnbull
Journal of Human Rights, volume 21, issue 3 (2022) pp. 263–282

Chapter 14

Pandemic patriarchy: The impact of a global health crisis on women's rights
Alison Brysk
Journal of Human Rights, volume 21, issue 3 (2022) pp. 283–303

Chapter 15

The effect of the COVID-19 pandemic on human rights practices: Findings from the Human Rights Measurement Initiative's 2021 Practitioner Survey
K. Chad Clay, Mennah Abdelwahab, Stephen Bagwell, Morgan Barney,Eduardo Burkle, Tori Hawley, Thalia Kehoe Rowden, Meridith LaVelle, Asia Parker, and Matthew Rains
Journal of Human Rights, volume 21, issue 3 (2022) pp. 317–333

Chapter 16

Global perceptions of South Korea's COVID-19 policy responses: Topic modeling with tweets
Jeong-Woo Koo
Journal of Human Rights, volume 21, issue 3 (2022) pp. 334–353

Chapter 17

Hindsight is 2020: Lessons from the COVID-19 pandemic for future human rights research
Amanda Murdie
Journal of Human Rights, volume 21, issue 3 (2022) pp. 354–364

Notes on Contributors

Mennah Abdelwahab is a recent Graduate of the University of Georgia, USA, obtaining degrees in International Affairs and Journalism. Her research interests include human rights, political repression, and the Middle East region.

Sammy Z. Badran is an Assistant Professor of International Studies at the American University of Sharjah, UAE. His research focuses on Middle East and North African (MENA) politics. He has published articles in the *British Journal of Middle East Studies*, *Journal of North African Studies*, and *Journal of International Women's Studies.*

Stephen Bagwell is an Assistant Professor at the Department of Political Science at the University of Missouri, St. Louis, USA. His research focuses on the economic consequences of governments behaving badly, development, and statistical methodology.

Morgan Barney is a PhD Candidate in Political Science and International Affairs at the University of Georgia, USA. Her research focuses on human rights, international NGOs, discourse shift, and issue framing among international actors.

Alison Brysk is the Distinguished Mellichamp Professor of Global Governance at the University of California, Santa Barbara USA. She is the author or editor of 15 volumes on international human rights, including *The Struggle for Freedom from Fear: Contesting Violence Against Women at the Frontiers of Globalization.*

Catherine Buerger is the Director of Research at the Dangerous Speech Project (DSP). She is the Managing Editor of the *Journal of Human Rights* and has published widely in academic and policy outlets. She holds a PhD in Anthropology from the University of Connecticut, USA.

Eduardo Burkle is a Research Analyst at the Human Rights Measurement Initiative and holds an MA in Human Rights and Democratization from the Global Campus of Human Rights. His research interests include transitional justice, human rights, and far-right populism in contemporary politics.

Benjamin C. Carbonetti is the Director of the Human Rights Program and a Lecturer in Human Rights at Trinity College, USA. He is the Data Editor of the *Journal of Human Rights.*

Erica Chenoweth is the Frank Stanton Professor of the First Amendment at the John F. Kennedy School of Government and the Susan S. and Kenneth L. Wallach Professor at the Radcliffe Institute for Advanced Study at Harvard University, Cambridge, USA. They study political violence and its alternatives. Chenoweth has authored or edited nine books and dozens of articles on mass movements, nonviolent resistance, terrorism, political violence, revolutions, and state repression.

Giacomo Chiozza is the Sir Easa Saleh Al-Gurg Professor of International Studies at the American University of Sharjah, UAE. His research primarily focuses on US foreign policy, anti-Americanism, and international security.

K. Chad Clay is the Director of the GLOBIS Center and an Associate Professor of International Affairs at the University of Georgia, USA. He is also the Co-Founder and Methodology Research and Design Lead of HRMI. His research focuses on the measurements, causes, and consequences of human rights practices and conditions.

Sukti Dhital is the Executive Director of the Bernstein Institute for Human Rights at the New York University School of Law, USA, and the Co-Founder of Nazdeek. She is a frequent Speaker at institutions and conferences concerning issues of social and economic rights, gender equality, clinical legal education, and legal empowerment.

Kristine Eck is a Professor at the Department of Peace and Conflict Research at Uppsala University, Sweden. Her research interests concern state coercion and policing.

Didier Fassin is the James D. Wolfensohn Professor at the Institute for Advanced Study and a Director of Studies at the École des Hautes Études en Sciences Sociales, France. An anthropologist, sociologist, and physician, he studies moral and political issues in contemporary societies.

Lisa Forman is an Associate Professor at the Dalla Lana School of Public Health at the University of Toronto, Canada. She is an International Human Rights Law Scholar whose research has explored how the right to health may contribute to reducing global health inequities. She holds a Canada Research Chair Tier 2 in Human Rights and Global Health Equity.

Michael Goodhart is a Professor of Political Science and of Gender, Sexuality, and Women's Studies at the University of Pittsburgh, USA, and the Director of its Global Studies Center. His core research interests include democracy, human rights, (in)justice, and emancipatory political struggles.

Sophia Hatz is a Associate Senior Lecturer at the Department of Peace and Conflict Research at Uppsala University, Sweden. Her research interests relate to state-led human rights violations and restrictions on civil liberties, particularly civilian responses to state coercion and repression.

Tori Hawley is an LLB student at the University of Liverpool, USA. She received a BA in International Relations from Western University, London, Canada, in 2020. Her research interests include human rights and international criminal law.

Shareen Hertel is a Professor of Political Science at the University of Connecticut, USA, jointly appointed with the UConn Human Rights Institute. She is the Editor of the *Journal of Human Rights* and has worked with United Nations agencies, foundations, and nongovernmental organizations in the United States, Latin America, and South Asia.

Prakash Kashwan is an Associate Professor of Environmental Studies at Brandeis University, Waltham, USA. His teaching, research, and scholarship address questions about the intersecting pursuits of socioeconomic development, environmental conservation, and radical climate action.

Thalia Kehoe Rowden is Strategy and Communication Lead with the Human Rights Measurement Initiative. She holds a BA in Linguistics and LLB(Hons) from the Victoria University of Wellington, New Zealand.

Jeffrey King is an Assistant Professor of Political Science at the Department of International Studies at the American University of Sharjah, UAE. His research mainly focuses on the intersection between political economy and human rights.

Jillian Clare Kohler is a Professor at the Leslie Dan Faculty of Pharmacy, the Dalla Lana School of Public Health, and the Munk School of Global Affairs at the University of Toronto, Canada. She is also the Director of the WHO Collaborating Centre for Governance, Transparency, and Accountability in the Pharmaceutical Sector. Her research focuses on global access to essential medicines.

Jeong-Woo Koo is a Professor of Sociology at Sungkyunkwan University, Seoul, South Korea. His research examines how world cultural processes shape state, organizational, and individual outcomes. His recent focus lies in the use of topic models to show the dynamic evolution of human rights norms and online users' attitudes toward rights.

Iris Goldner Lang is a Jean Monnet Professor of EU Law and the UNESCO Chair on Free Movement of People, Migration and Inter-Cultural Dialogue at the Department of European Public Law at the Faculty of Law at the University of Zagreb, Croatia. She is the Editor-in-Chief of the *Croatian Yearbook of European Law and Policy (CYELP).*

Meridith LaVelle is a PhD Candidate in Political Science and International Affairs and the Director of the GLOBIS Human Rights Research Lab at the University of Georgia, USA. Her research interests include human rights, international human rights law, political violence, contentious politics, political economy, and quantitative methodology.

Kathryn Libal is an Associate Professor of Social Work and Human Rights and the Director of the Human Rights Institute at the University of Connecticut, USA. Her scholarship has focused on the Middle East and United States. Libal has published on women's and children's rights movements in Turkey and on the advocacy of international non-governmental organizations on behalf of Iraqi refugees.

Amanda Murdie is the Georgia Athletic Association Professor of International Affairs and the Head of the Department of International Affairs at the University of Georgia, USA. She studies international relations, specializing in the behavior of international nongovernmental organizations and their interactions with states, local populations, and intergovernmental organizations.

Asia Parker is a PhD Student in Political Science and International Affairs at the University of Georgia, USA. Her research focuses on human rights, women's rights, advocacy, foreign aid, feminist theory, and qualitative methods.

Matthew Rains is a PhD Candidate at the School of Public and International Affairs at the University of Georgia, USA. He is also HRMI's CPR Metrics Lead. His research focuses on oppression, human rights, political violence, and measurement.

Jaya Ramji-Nogales is an Associate Dean for Academic Affairs and the I. Herman Stern Research Professor at Beasley School of Law at Temple University, USA. Her current research examines refugee law under the Trump Administration and global migration law, described further in a symposium in the *American Journal of International Law Unbound.*

Michael Santoro is a Professor of Management and Entrepreneurship at the Leavey School of Business at Santa Clara University, USA. He is a founding Co-Editor of the *Business and*

Human Rights Journal and founding President of the Global Business and Human Rights Scholars Association.

Robert Shanklin is a Lecturer at the Philosophy Department at Santa Clara University, USA, where he teaches business ethics and Chinese philosophy. His teaching and research focus on ethics and human language.

Kimberly Theidon is the Henry J. Leir Professor in International Humanitarian Studies at The Fletcher School at Tufts University, USA. Her research interests include political violence, transitional justice, humanitarian and post-conflict interventions, gender studies, and drug policy.

Brian Turnbull is an Assistant Professor of Instruction at the Department of Sociology at the University of South Florida, USA, with interdisciplinary interests in social change, political sociology, and qualitative methodology.

Tyler Walton is the Tuttleman Legal Empowerment Fellow at the Bernstein Institute for Human Rights at the New York University School of Law, USA. As a Fellow, he works on legal empowerment, researching and co-developing strategies with affected community members to access and exercise their rights and shift power paradigms back towards communities and individuals.

Eileen A. Wong completed her PhD in Molecular Virology and Microbiology at the University of Pittsburgh, USA, researching immunology of tuberculosis.

Wendy H. Wong is a Professor of Political Science and Principal's Research Chair on the Irving K. Barber Faculty of Arts & Social Science, University of British Columbia, Canada, and is also a member of the Royal Society of Canada's College of New Scholars, Artists & Scientists. She is particularly interested in human rights and emerging technologies, the role NGOs play in global human rights norms, and corporate obligations in human rights.

Part I: Early views and analysis of the pandemic

Introduction—Human rights in the time of COVID-19

The urgent need to create a special issue on the human rights impact of the COVID-19 pandemic became apparent as soon as it began to unfold in early spring 2020. As an editorial team, we are deeply grateful to our Editorial Board for its support in composing this issue. Board members themselves either agreed to author contributions, or quickly suggested scholars and practitioners working directly on related research, policy or grassroots efforts aimed at safeguarding rights as the pandemic deepened. The ten articles that follow draw on some of the most up-to-the-moment ethnographic and scientific data available to assess the scope and depth of underlying inequities, emergent hazards, and future impact of the pandemic. However, we recognize that it is only a first step. We need more articles, drawing on an even wider range of voices across more disciplines and lived experiences if we are to accurately convey the state of human rights in a world that is ailing on multiple levels. We hope this special issue paves the way for those conversations across multiple volumes of JHR.

Shareen Hertel

Catherine Buerger

Benjamin C. Carbonetti

Centering rights-based theory and praxis

Revisiting interdependence in times and terms of crisis

Michael Goodhart

ABSTRACT
Scholars and lawyers have long debated the meaning of the interdependence of human rights. Revisiting that question in the context of the COVID-19 pandemic demonstrates both that the substantive enjoyment of many human rights is *practically* interdependent and that that relationship is neither logically nor functionally *necessary*, as much of the literature imagines. This article introduces the idea of *negative interdependence*, a term that highlights how crises can trigger chain reactions of rights violations and deprivations that disproportionately affect oppressed and vulnerable people. It argues that negative interdependence provides a crucial analytical and critical framework for the political project of securing the equal enjoyment of human rights for everyone.

> The right to health is closely related to and dependent upon the realization of other human rights, as contained in the International Bill of Rights, including the rights to food, housing, work, education, human dignity, life, non-discrimination, equality, the prohibition against torture, privacy, access to information, and the freedoms of association, assembly and movement. These and other rights and freedoms address integral components of the right to health. (UN Office of the High Commissioner for Human Rights 2000: [3])

Rights in crisis

In recent months, governments around the world have imposed varying restrictions on social and economic activity to slow the spread of the SARS-CoV-2 virus that causes COVID-19, and sometimes for more nefarious reasons as well (Gupta 2020). As the pandemic rages, the multidimensional crisis triggered by the disease and by governmental responses to it has led to widespread and systematic human rights deprivations and violations.

Frequently, these lapses are not isolated: Rather than a single boulder falling from a cliff face, the process resembles the erosion or collapse of a hillside. In the United States, the triggering event might be the loss of employment, which can often precipitate a loss of health insurance—for those fortunate enough to have had it to begin with—as well as food and housing insecurity, educational disruption for children, and other related problems (Despard, Grinstein-Weiss, Chun, and Roll 2020). Maintaining employment can also be a trigger: Low-wage workers whose jobs have been labeled "essential" but whose conditions of work remain deplorable may be compelled by economic necessity to accept heightened risks of exposure on the job in hopes of avoiding the kind of collapse just outlined. People who have been asked to stay at or return to work, often in unsafe conditions, have been threatened with furloughs, or with the loss of unemployment and other benefits if they refuse to return (Johnson 2020). Some who have organized to demand improved health and safety conditions have been terminated (O'Donovan 2020). If people work or return to work and become sick, they may lose their jobs anyway, infect their families, and endure a similar cycle of rights erosion (Schulze 2020).

The destabilization of rights "in the background" accelerates and exacerbates these collapses. School closures have limited access to nutritional food sources for many struggling families and created broader childcare challenges; in some instances, these challenges can jeopardize parental employment (Dunn, Kenney, Fleischhacker, and Bleich 2020). Fear of visiting hospitals and emergency rooms aggravates health issues for older people, people with chronic illnesses, and for the uninsured and underinsured (Rosenbaum 2020). Sheltering at home exposes women and children to increased risk of domestic violence, a problem worsened by the strains on emergency services and by limited mobility, both physical and economic (Abalaka 2020). Reduced transit ridership and reduced driving, attributable to shelter-at-home orders and economic recession, conspire to undermine funding for public transportation (Duncan 2020), leading to cuts that make it harder for many workers to get to and from their jobs and threatening to strand older, poorer, and sicker people far from grocery stores, healthcare centers, and other vital facilities. Moreover, the very restrictions designed to protect public health—such as curbs on assembly, movement, worship, and social and economic activity of various kinds—themselves result in derogations of rights, albeit potentially within the scope of the temporary curtailments permitted under international law.

In short, people's lived experiences of the COVID-19 pandemic seem to verify the interdependence of human rights. Certainly, the present crisis dramatizes the very practical ways in which the enjoyment of some rights is intertwined with the enjoyment of others. It would be a mistake, however, to treat this practical interconnection as confirmation of the doctrine of interdependence as most scholars and practitioners understand it, as the crisis also reveals. Revisiting interdependence in times and terms of crisis provides an opportunity to reconsider what interdependence means and what analytical and political work it can do for human rights advocates.

Revisiting interdependence

As Daniel Whelan (2010: 1) observed, the tripartite formulation that human rights are indivisible, interdependent, and interrelated is taken by scholars and practitioners as given. The terms are often used interchangeably, but Whelan's comprehensive history of their evolution showed that each had a distinct meaning in the changing political contexts of the twentieth century, although each was initially shaped in the crucible of Cold War debates about the two categories of rights introduced by the creation of two international covenants (on civil and political rights and on economic, social, and cultural rights; Whelan 2010: 207).

Each term is used to describe or explain something about the nature of rights and to characterize the relationship between the two categories of rights. Historically, *indivisibility* was a way of insisting on the equal status and priority of economic, social, and cultural rights with civil and political rights, most famously in the 1968 *Proclamation of Teheran* (International Conference on Human Rights 1968, 3[13]),[1] whereas *interrelatedness* was invoked to show that the supposedly different kinds of rights in each category shared common (conceptual or philosophical) characteristics (Whelan 2010: 3–8). *Interdependence*, Whelan argued, referred to the idea that "despite their distinctiveness as particular rights … the enjoyment of any right or group of rights requires the enjoyment of others," an idea he described as "relatively unproblematic," at least in comparison with the other two concepts (Whelan 2010: 3).

The 1993 *Vienna Declaration and Programme of Action* effectively called an end to the Cold War in human rights, announcing that the universality of human rights was "beyond question" and noting, "All human rights are … indivisible and interdependent and interrelated" (UN General Assembly 1993: 20). Removed from the historical context that gave them salience, the indivisibility and interdependence of human rights (interrelatedness has largely fallen by the wayside) has become a kind of catechism that "invokes the continued sanctity of the Universal Declaration and seeks to fulfill its promise as a 'common standard of achievement for all mankind'" (Whelan 2010: 208).[2] Like many a catechism or mantra, its deeper meaning has been quietly lost in its familiarity, so that in contemporary usage to call human rights indivisible and interdependent is simply a standard way of affirming that they are an integrated and holistic package and that states may not pick and choose which rights to honor and enforce.

When the *Vienna Declaration* proclaimed that the indivisibility, interdependence, and interrelatedness of rights should be treated as settled, it papered over lingering uncertainty about what interdependence, in particular, might actually mean. According to Scott (1989: 781), it could describe either a relationship of empirical necessity or of logical entailment among rights, such that the enjoyment of some rights is either functionally or conceptually predicated on the enjoyment of (some) others.[3] It is rarely specified which rights depend on which others, but the indivisibility and interdependence of rights has become such a ubiquitous trope that it seems safe to assume that, for many commentators who invoke, it, each right requires the enjoyment of all the others.

However widely accepted this stock understanding of interdependence might be, it has proven almost impossible to validate. To enjoy a right is to realize or "possess" the object or substance of that right; one enjoys the right not to be tortured when one is not, in fact, being tortured. Empirically, it is straightforwardly *not* a condition of the actual enjoyment of most rights that some other right(s) also actually be enjoyed. Purely as a matter of fact, one can enjoy the right against torture without enjoying a right to vote or a right to subsistence. Quantitative studies confirm this: Minkler and Sweeney (2011) found that there is only a weak correlation between security and subsistence. Interdependence is not a functional requirement of the enjoyment of rights.

It is equally difficult to show logically or conceptually that interdependence is somehow a necessary feature of rights. Most of the debate on this subject has focused on the work of Henry Shue (1996), who famously argued that a right cannot be considered *secure* unless other basic rights are also secure—that is, unless the right is adequately protected against standard threats.[4] Shue illustrated this idea using the right to physical security, which he considered uncontroversial.

> No one can fully enjoy any right that is supposedly protected by society if someone can credibly threaten him or her with murder, rape, beating, etc., when he or she tries to enjoy the alleged right. Such threats to physical security are among the most serious and—in much of the world—the most widespread hindrances to the enjoyment of any right. If any right is to be exercised except at great risk, physical security must be protected. In the absence of physical security people are unable to use any other rights that society may be said to be protecting without being liable to encounter many of the worst dangers they would encounter if society were not protecting the rights (Shue 1996: 21–22).[5]

Unless a society has made adequate arrangements to ensure that all (basic) rights are respected, the enjoyment of any right is precarious.

As influential as Shue's work has been, it is not a successful argument for the conceptual interdependence of rights (Pogge 2009). To show why, Ashford (2009) used Shue's own example of the right against torture and the right to subsistence. Shue had argued that, unless the right to subsistence is secure, people desperate for something to eat might agree to be tortured a little in exchange for food. (Although such examples may seem far-fetched, Ashford (2009: 97) observed that if one substitutes "child labor" for "torture," the idea of a rights-violating contract to secure subsistence becomes tragically plausible). Critics responded that strict enforcement of the no-torture rule and a ban on such "torture contracts" would be enough to adequately secure the right against torture even in the absence of subsistence rights (Ashford (2009: 94–96).

Ashford conceded that Shue failed to establish a logical entailment regarding the enjoyment of rights. It *is* conceptually possible to fully secure the right to freedom from torture without securing the right to subsistence, but the arguments establishing this conclusion miss what Ashford took to be Shue's larger point: If people lack subsistence, they can readily be coerced into giving up the objects of their other rights. In such cases, those other rights cannot be said to be secure (Ashford 2009: 99). She reminded us, in other words, that what matters is not whether interdependence really is a characteristic of human rights but whether people can enjoy their rights in a substantively meaningful way.

It is tempting to argue that Shue never intended to say anything about the conceptual interdependence of rights. His argument about securing rights was always focused on the mechanisms needed to ensure that people's enjoyment of their rights was not merely contingent but robust against standard and predictable threats. The security of rights is therefore a question to do with the social arrangements in place to guarantee their respect, protection, and fulfillment. Admittedly, Shue obscured this point by talking about basic rights as if "basicness" were a property or feature of rights themselves. (This way of framing the debate also suggests a hierarchy of rights, which unhelpfully implies that some "nonbasic" rights might be dispensable or of lower priority than others.) The crucial point is that securing rights is about putting in place the social arrangements necessary to protect against standard threats. Politically, the most important aspect of interdependence has little to do with what rights are or how they relate to one another conceptually, and everything to do with the practical conditions of their enjoyment. In this sense, interdependence can be understood as a political project.

Negative interdependence

If interdependence means anything, it means taking seriously that the insecurity of some rights makes other rights insecure. This "negative interdependence" is not a claim about the nature of rights but, rather, a practical lesson drawn from the practice of rights in everyday life.[6] Systemic disruptions like those caused by SARS-CoV-2 provide a lens through which the widespread shortcomings in human rights protections come into sharp focus. The erosion of rights set off by the COVID-19 pandemic and by governmental responses to it shows just how poorly many societies are doing when it comes to creating the social arrangements needed to secure rights. As it turns out, many people's rights are, at best, contingently enjoyed.

In the United States, the fragility of the right to healthcare is perhaps the most glaring and offensive example, but lack of food and income, housing insecurity, poor workplace conditions, weak protections for labor rights, and many other deprivations are rampant. Of course, this insecurity is not uniform: Negative interdependence does not affect everyone equally. Although well-meaning pundits have proclaimed that "the virus doesn't discriminate," the loud rejoinder has been that societies do: The misery wrought by this pandemic and the efforts to check it has spread and intensified along familiar vectors of discrimination and vulnerability defined by race, gender, ethnicity, ability, legal status, and other social positions. These social positions are strongly correlated with greater prepandemic vulnerability (e.g., well-known disparities in health outcomes, levels of wealth, and incarceration rates) and strongly predict pandemic-related deprivation (e.g., higher rates of infection and mortality, involuntary job loss, and higher risk of eviction and foreclosure). The lens of crisis also focuses our attention on how the arrangements in place (or missing) in a given society reflect—and, to a significant extent, constitute—familiar structures of privilege and injustice.

There are thus good epistemological and normative reasons to stop thinking of interdependence as a feature of rights (in addition to the fact that it is not). Epistemologically, negative interdependence highlights failures and fractures in the social arrangements in place to secure rights; normatively, it highlights how insecurity promotes and perpetuates injustice. When interdependence is taken for granted—either as a feature of rights or simply as a settled fact—there is *nothing to do* politically. The focus on insecurity helps to conceive of (negative) interdependence as a political project; it activates the idea critically and analytically, providing a framework for evaluating a society's commitment to everyone's equal enjoyment of rights and for identifying the kinds of policies and institutions needed to advance that commitment. The political commitment is crucial: In its absence, the insecurity of rights becomes merely a set of empirical regularities.

Because negative interdependence (insecurity) most severely affects people in disadvantaged social positions, a grounded, intersectional approach to insecurity is required.[7] In a wide-ranging research project, Bouchard and Meyer-Bisch (2016) demonstrated the advantages of such an approach for understanding and addressing rights violations caused or compounded by the interaction between multiple and interlocking forms of oppression. Their team studied how "intersectional human rights violations," in which multiple forms of discrimination are at work, triggered "chain reactions" or spirals of insecurity much like those revealed by the current crisis. Greater vulnerability led to increased violations, and those violations spread horizontally (to similarly situated others) and vertically (across generations; Bouchard and Meyer-Bisch 2016: 197–199). In the eight cases they examined, the severity of these chain reactions limited the capacity of victims to seek redress; the interdependent effects of multiple violations became a compounding factor in precipitating further violations; and, as the "contamination" spread, it encouraged outsiders in the belief that victims were responsible for their own plight. In a striking metaphor, the authors likened these insecurity spirals to a "bottomless pit" (Bouchard and Meyer-Bisch 2016: 199).

COVID-19, negative interdependence, and the insecurity of rights

> I am an essential worker. I have been working through the whole pandemic. … I have to choose between 3 bills at the beginning of the month to pay and I have no money. This $97.50 a month [of transit fares], I can't afford it. (Deanna Turner, Pittsburghers for Public Transit)[8]

The negative interdependence of human rights finds a kind of grounding in the lives of people experiencing domination, oppression, and exploitation; from their perspective, the many interrelated dimensions of insecurity become plainly visible (Scott 1989: 787–788). People like Deanna Turner might well feel like they are descending into a bottomless pit: They put their health and families at risk to do their jobs, but they still struggle to make ends meet.

Many activists have adopted versions of the slogan that, following the pandemic, we can't go back to normal—that "normal is the problem." That is because, for many people, "normal" means a society in which their rights are, at best, contingently realized, in which they live one crisis away—whether global or personal—from spirals of insecurity. Situations like Deanna Turner's are not caused by the pandemic; rather, the pandemic lays bare the precarity of those situations.

As Künnemann (1995: 323) put it, indivisibility and interdependence are part of the daily reality of struggles against oppression and for human rights. Historically, rights are achieved through such struggles, making them "first and foremost a tool in the hands of vulnerable individuals and groups against powerful mechanisms of oppression" (Künnemann 1995: 342). A crisis like the COVID-19 pandemic, therefore, has a lot to teach us about oppression and vulnerability, about negative interdependence, and also about the kind of politics through which it might be possible to mobilize against them.

Let me highlight one organization, Pittsburghers for Public Transit (PPT), that puts many of the ideas and arguments discussed here into action in its work. PPT "is a grassroots organization of transit riders, workers, and residents who defend and expand public transit"[9] (PPT 2020b). It has long advocated for public transit as a human right, working in collaboration with partner organizations in the Pittsburgh region to address the multiple sources of rights insecurity (PPT 2020c). The organization understands its broader aims and strategy intersectionally, recognizing, for instance, that struggles for racial justice are central to its work: "We are in the same fight: for a world where all people have the freedom to move, to be in public space without fear or threat."

(PPT 2020d). PPT has drawn attention to the use of local buses in ferrying state police to protests against racism, opposed the use of these public assets to transport arrested protestors, and highlighted how the abrupt cancellations of bus service during curfews strands essential workers and transit users, exposing them to militarized police violence perpetrated against protestors and bystanders (PPT 2020d).

Throughout the pandemic, PPT has amplified its advocacy for transit riders and operators, shining a light on how reductions in bus routes and frequencies threaten not only people's mobility but their health and their livelihoods. In one fascinating example of learning from the crisis, PPT is analyzing ridership data gathered during the state-mandated "lockdown" period (March–May 2020) to assess transit dependency, and advocate for the redistribution of transit service, and to help prevent bus overcrowding and rider "pass-ups" on high-demand routes. (Wiens 2020; a pass-up occurs when a bus or other transit vehicle skips a regular stop or station where passengers are waiting, usually due to overcrowding.)

I use PPT and transit rights as my example in part because they are important to me and to my community. Yet transit rights are also instructive in broader ways. There is no internationally recognized right to public transit, and it is nearly impossible to find transit mentioned in discussions of basic rights, rights security, interdependence, or really in any academic discussion of human rights. Yet the work of PPT shows—and the pandemic underscores—the essential role transit plays in securing some people's core rights, including health, free expression, affordable housing, access to food, and more. I stress "some people's" rights because affordable and comprehensive public transportation is clearly among the key social arrangements needed to secure the enjoyment of human rights, especially for those (mostly poorer) people who are most likely to depend on transit. For PPT, securing the right to public transportation is part of a broader political project of securing everyone's human rights.

Conclusion

When interdependence is taken for granted, treated as a feature of or fact about rights, it remains politically inert. Negative interdependence focuses our analytical and critical attention on the insecurity of rights. It can best be comprehended by foregrounding the lived experiences of vulnerable and oppressed people, using intersectional approaches to demonstrate how chain reactions of deprivation and violation create and sustain structures of injustice in our societies. Crises like the current pandemic bring negative interdependence clearly into focus, inviting a critical analysis of rights insecurity. Such an analysis reveals the gaps and deficiencies in our social arrangements and highlights that filling and correcting them is a political project, one that calls us to imagine and construct a solidaristic, democratic politics oriented toward the secure enjoyment of human rights for everyone.

Notes

1. "Since human rights and fundamental freedoms are indivisible, the full realization of civil and political rights without the enjoyment of economic, social and cultural rights is impossible. The achievement of lasting progress in the implementation of human rights is dependent upon sound and effective national and international policies of economic and social development" (International Conference on Human Rights 1968).
2. Whelan attributed this sanctity only to indivisibility; I have taken the liberty of applying his description to the entire locution.
3. Scott explored the possibility that, legally, interdependence might be understood as a kind of interpretive permeability among rights, a fascinating argument I cannot engage here (see Quane 2012).
4. Basic rights are just those necessary to the secure enjoyment of (all) other rights (Shue 1996).

5. It is impossible to provide absolute surety; attempts to do so would lead to myriad inefficiencies and absurdities. It is better to think probabilistically about minimizing the likelihood of violations (see Shue 1996; Pogge 1999, 2000).
6. I use the term "negative interdependence" to contrast this empirical focus on insecurity from claims that the actual enjoyment of rights is conditioned on the enjoyment of other rights.
7. For a discussion of a democratic methodologies for analyzing injustice, see Goodhart (2018: 139–162) and Ackerly (2018).
8. See Pittsburghers for Public Transit (PPT 2020a).
9. For transparency, I want to disclose that I am a member (financial supporter) of PPT and also of the steering committee for the Pittsburgh Human Rights City Alliance, in which PPT participates.

References

ABALAKA, Ojima. (2020) *Women Face Rising Risk of Violence During COVID-19: Leave No Woman Behind in Governments' Response.* [Online]. Available: https://www.hrw.org/news/2020/07/03/women-face-rising-risk-violence-during-covid-19 [3 September 2020].

ACKERLY, Brooke. (2018) *Just Responsibility: A Human Rights Theory of Global Justice* (New York, NY: Oxford University Press).

ASHFORD, Elizabeth. (2009) The alleged dichotomy between positive and negative rights and duties. In *Global Basic Rights*, Charles R. Beitz and Robert E. Goodin (eds.) (Oxford, UK: Oxford University Press).

BOUCHARD, Johanne, and MEYER-BISCH, Patrice. (2016) Intersectionality and interdependence of human rights: Same or different? *Equal Rights Review, Special Focus: Intersectionality*, 16, 186–203.

DESPARD, Mathieu, GRINSTEIN-WEISS, Michal, CHUN, Yung, and ROLL, Stephen. (2020) *COVID-19 Job and Income Loss Leading to More Hunger and Financial Hardship.* [Online]. Available: https://www.brookings.edu/blog/up-front/2020/07/13/covid-19-job-and-income-loss-leading-to-more-hunger-and-financial-hardship/ [13 July 2020].

DUNCAN, Ian. (2020) Reeling from the loss of gas tax revenue during pandemic, states are deferring billions of dollars of transportation projects. *The Washington Post*, 10 July.

DUNN, Caroline G., KENNEY, Erica, FLEISCHHACKER, Sheila E., and BLEICH, Sara N. (2020) Feeding low-income children during the COVID-19 pandemic. *New England Journal of Medicine*, 382(18), e40. doi:10.1056/NEJMp2005638

GOODHART, Michael. (2018) *Injustice: Political Theory for the Real World* (New York, NY: Oxford University Press).

GUPTA, Anubhav. (2020) *In Modi's India, Rights and Freedoms Erode Further Amid COVID-19.* [Online]. Available: https://www.worldpoliticsreview.com/articles/28863/in-modi-s-india-rights-and-freedoms-erode-further-amid-covid-19 [24 June 2020].

INTERNATIONAL CONFERENCE ON HUMAN RIGHTS. (1968) *Proclamation of Teheran: Final Act of the International Conference on Human Rights, Teheran*, April 22 to May 13, 1968. A/CONF. 32/41 at 3. New York, The United Nations.

JOHNSON, Marty. (2020) *States Tell Workers They'll Lose Unemployment Benefits if They Refuse to Return to Jobs.* [Online]. Available: https://thehill.com/homenews/state-watch/495050-states-telling-workers-theyll-lose-unemployment-benefits-if-they-refuse [30 July 2020].

KÜNNEMANN, Rolf. (1995) A coherent approach to human rights. *Human Rights Quarterly*, 17(2), 323–342.

MINKLER, Lanse, and SWEENEY, Shawna. (2011) On the indivisibility and interdependence of basic rights in developing countries. *Human Rights Quarterly*, 33(2), 351–396. doi:10.1353/hrq.2011.0017

O'DONOVAN, Caroline. (2020) *Amazon Fired an Employee Involved in Workplace Organizing in Minnesota, Sources Say.* [Online]. Available: https://www.buzzfeednews.com/article/carolineodonovan/amazon-fired-employee-involved-in-workplace-organizing-in [30 July 2020].

PITTSBURGHERS FOR PUBLIC TRANSIT (PPT). (2020a) *PPT members Call on Port Authority Board to Take Action for Transit Workers during COVID-19.* [Online]. Available: https://www.pittsburghforpublictransit.org/ppt-members-call-on-port-authority-board-to-take-action-for-transit-equity-during-covid-19/ [28 July 2020].

PITTSBURGHERS FOR PUBLIC TRANSIT (PPT). (2020b) *Who We Are.* [Online]. Available: https://www.pittsburghforpublictransit.org/about-us/ [9 September 2020].

PITTSBURGHERS FOR PUBLIC TRANSIT (PPT). (2020c) *Transit is a Human Right! Residents at Hilltop Parkview Manor Demand Restoration of the 59 Bus!* [Online]. Available: https://www.pittsburghforpublictransit.org/transit-is-a-human-right-residents-at-hilltop-parkview-manor-demand-restoration-of-the-59-bus/ [9 September 2020].

PITTSBURGHERS FOR PUBLIC TRANSIT (PPT). (2020d) *Black Lives Matter Must Be at the Heart of the Fight For Transit Justice.* [Online]. Available: https://www.pittsburghforpublictransit.org/black-lives-matter-must-be-at-the-heart-of-the-fight-for-transit-justice/ [9 September 2020].

POGGE, Thomas W. (1999) Human flourishing and universal justice. *Social Philosophy and Policy*, 16(1), 333–361. doi:10.1017/S0265052500002351

POGGE, Thomas W. (2000) The international significance of human rights. *Journal of Ethics*, 4(1), 45–69. doi:10.1023/A:1009852018252

POGGE, Thomas W. (2009) Shue on rights and duties. In *Global Basic Rights*, Charles R. Beitz and Robert E. Goodin (eds.) (Oxford, UK: Oxford University Press).

QUANE, Helen. (2012) A further dimension to the interdependence and indivisibility of human rights: Recent developments concerning the rights of indigenous peoples. *Harvard Human Rights Journal*, 25(1), 49–83.

ROSENBAUM, Lisa. (2020) The untold toll—The pandemic's effects on patients without COVID-19. *New England Journal of Medicine*, 382(24), 2368–2371. doi:10.1056/NEJMms2009984

SCHULZE, Elizabeth (2020) *As Unemployment Surges, Essential Workers Fear Calling Out Sick Could Cost Them Their Jobs.* [Online]. Available: https://www.cnbc.com/2020/05/08/unemployment-is-surging-and-essential-workers-fear-calling-out-sick.html [29 July 2020].

SCOTT, Craig. (1989) Interdependence and permeability of human rights norms: Towards a partial fusion of the International Covenants on Human Rights. *Osgoode Hall Law Journal*, 27(3), 769–878.

SHUE, Henry. (1996) *Basic Rights: Subsistence, Affluence, and U.S. Foreign Policy* (Princeton, NJ: Princeton University Press).

UN GENERAL ASSEMBLY. (1993) *Vienna Declaration and Programme of Action.* UN Doc. A/CONF.157/23 (New York, NY: United Nations).

UN OFFICE OF THE HIGH COMMISSIONER FOR HUMAN RIGHTS, COMMITTEE ON ECONOMIC, SOCIAL AND CULTURAL RIGHTS. (2000) *CESCR General Comment No. 14: The Right to the Highest Attainable Standard of Health.* UN Doc. Art. 12, E/C.12/2000/4 (New York, NY: United Nations).

WEINS, Laura Chu. (2020) "City budgets in tough times: Ensuring equity and justice," *Learning from COVID 19: Shaping a Health and Human Rights Agenda for our Region* (Webinar, 30 April 2020).

WHELAN, Daniel, J. (2010) *Indivisible Human Rights: A History* (Philadelphia, PA: University of Pennsylvania Press).

A forecasted failure: Intersectionality, COVID-19, and the perfect storm

Kimberly Theidon

ABSTRACT
This article is one chronicle of a pandemic foretold. The consequences of COVID-19 in the United States were not inevitable, and my goal is to trace the humanly and inhumanely authored trajectory this pandemic has taken. Who could be surprised that the burden of morbidity and mortality would follow the color/class/poverty/gender lines that riddle this society? I begin by considering history — specifically the 1918 flu epidemic — and what public health messages from that pandemic reveal about gender, health behavior, and messaging aimed at men who were resistant to barrier methods of flu prevention. I then consider the politics of disposability. How are certain communities made "unimaginable," such that their deaths provoke a presidential "it is what it is"? Disposability and the lack of national grieving invites us to consider the drastic interruption in rituals of mourning, and to investigate Donald Trump for crime against humanity.

In April 2020, I joined a group of colleagues for a podcast about COVID-19 and intersectionality (Facebook 2020). By viral reckoning, April 15 seems a long time ago; the pandemic was poised to spiral out of control in the United States, a biological disaster well on its way to becoming a man-made crisis of mismanaged proportions. I began by noting that many of us had heard COVID-19 was the "great equalizer," and that I hoped my comments would convince our viewers it was not. Just days before, Chicago Mayor Lori Lightfoot had said, "we are all experiencing this crisis together, but we are not all experiencing this crisis in the same way" (Matthews 2020). These were prescient words from the mayor of a city in which African-Americans account for 30 percent of the population yet comprise more than 70 percent of all COVID-19 deaths.

Native American leaders were also clearly aware of the danger that lay in their path. The Yankton Sioux Tribe of South Dakota issued a Declaration of Disaster (Ortiz 2020). Navajo Nation president Jonathan Nez lamented that, once again, the US government had ignored indigenous people. His nation alone had, at that time, more confirmed cases of COVID-19 than any states except for New Jersey and New York. In the previous two weeks, deaths in the Navajo Nation had increased a staggering 367 percent (Miller 2020). Histories of slavery, Jim Crow, and red lining converged with histories of settler colonialism, ethnic discrimination, and economic dispossession. These are components of the "underlying conditions" that shape disease occurrence, progression, and outcome. No, this virus was not the great equalizer.

Another term also appeared in the headlines, alerting the public to the "silent pandemic" of domestic and intimate partner violence (Reykjavik Global Forum, 2020). As citizens were warned to shelter in place—to stay home and stay safe—feminist scholars pushed back on the notion that "home" was a safe place to be for many women and, I might add, children. Trapped at home with an abuser whose proverbial fuse was further shortened by working from home, working at risk of infection, or perhaps being unemployed, domestic violence would predictably increase even if reporting was limited due to the closure of shelters or the restriction on mobility.

Writing now in the summer of 2020, equalizing rhetoric and concerns about a silent pandemic have ceded to the metaphor of a "perfect storm" to capture the convergence of structural inequalities. Yet, how could this storm have passed below forecasting radar? How could this tempest have caught anyone by surprise when it so clearly traced the fault lines that fracture the United States and have done so since the country's founding? To be clear: The consequences of COVID-19 were not inevitable, and viruses morph in unpredictable ways. I refer, however, not to the coronavirus *per se* but to the *humanly* and *inhumanely* authored trajectory this pandemic has taken in the United States. Who could be surprised that the burden of morbidity and mortality would follow the color/class/poverty/gender lines that riddle this society? Anyone with even a cursory grasp of the salient concept of intersectionality developed by Crenshaw (1991) could see the menacing clouds on the horizon.

My intent in this article is to unsettle any claim that the impact and consequences of COVID-19 in the United States are shocking; that language is self-serving. If we return to the inflammatory rhetoric that characterized Donald Trump's 2016 presidential campaign, the reader will grasp that behind the nationalist, white supremacist, swaggering masculine bravado lay the promise of where we stand now. There was a sector of the population who seized on those promises and voted for their realization. When Trump boasted about grabbing women's pussies because being rich entitled him to do so; when he implied that women (including his own daughter) are ranked on a scale whose best cuts of meat are labeled a great piece of ass; when he invoked herd immunity as a solution to the pandemic; when he suggested injecting bleach to kill the virus; when he withheld assistance to "blue states" unless the governors took the knee (no, not the #BLM knee, the other one)—encapsulated in those words and actions were the all the elements necessary to forecast how COVID-19 would devastate the United States. Some lives were deemed disposable; science was in the service of FAKE NEWS; there were "good people" on both sides in Charlottesville; and the death toll from COVID-19 in the United States is a tragedy for which the President stated he assumes no responsibility. Although we should not be shocked by how this has unfolded, we should not lose our capacity for indignation and protest.

In this article, I begin by considering history—specifically, the 1918 flu epidemic—and what public health messages from that pandemic reveal about gender, health behavior, and messaging aimed at men who were resistant to barrier methods of flu prevention. Time depth is important for what it can reveal about prior gendered responses to a viral pandemic, and for tracing out slower forms of dying that may elude the short-term data collection of COVID-19 mortalities. I suspect that although more men are dying from the direct medical effects of COVID-19 (Ducharme 2020), more women and girls will ultimately die from the socio-economic legacies and the spike in domestic and partner violence that are coterminous with and will outlive this pandemic. In sum, more men may be killed by COVID, but more women and girls will die (Paskin 2020; Alon, Doepke, Olmstead-Rumsey, Tertilt 2020).

I then consider the politics of disposability and the 57 percent of Republicans who state that the US death toll from COVID-19 is "acceptable" (CBS News 2020; Salvanto, DePinto, Backus, Khanna, and Cox 2020). How are certain communities made "unimaginable," such that their deaths provoke an indifferent shrug, or a presidential, "It is what it is."[1] Disposability and the lack of national grieving invites us to consider the drastic interruption in rituals of mourning, painfully illustrated by those refrigerated vans parked outside of New York City hospitals. Among the legacies of this pandemic will be delayed bereavement, intergenerational trauma, and the loss of many elders and their wisdom. I conclude this chronicle of a perfect storm foretold by considering the possibility of holding Donald Trump and his collaborators criminally negligent, on a scale that might warrant a judgment of crimes against humanity.

At the crossroads: Intersectionality and why it matters

In her influential article, "Mapping the Margins: Intersectionality, Identity Politics, and Violence Against Women of Color," feminist legal theorist Kimberlé Crenshaw coined the term *intersectionality* (1991). Her aim was to capture the "multilayered and routinized forms of domination that often converge" to create "burdens, largely the consequence of gender and class oppression" that are then compounded by discriminatory policies and practices (1991: 1245–1246). All people, of course, inhabit multiple identities, but for some the crossroads of these identities result in the multiplication of forms of symbolic, political, and representational inequalities. To grasp these inequalities requires that we explore how one's gender identity intersects with race, class, sexual orientation, religion, ethnicity, disability, and other salient axes of differentiation and stratification to exacerbate vulnerabilities or to enhance privileges. Intersectionality allows us to focus on those saturation points where the accumulation of disadvantage truncates people's lives and life chances.[2]

Importantly, the spectrum of gendered identities exceeds any binary reductionism. When teaching gender theory, I caution students that if they read a text and can replace the word "gender" with "women" without any significant shift in meaning, then something (and someone) is missing in the analysis. When gender defaults to women, men—white, heterosexual, middle-class, and able-bodied men—are left as the unquestioned, unmarked category of the human from which other genders somehow diverge. Lost in this default is the full spectrum of humanity that comprises the LGBTQ + communities, as well as the fluidity of gender identities across space and time.

We cannot understand how the COVID-19 pandemic has impacted people in the United States without applying an intersectional lens to the distribution of morbidity and mortality. Intersectionality allows us to grasp how certain individuals and communities were made structurally vulnerable to the virus's virulent impact. From this perspective, the "preexisting conditions" that should be measured and redressed go beyond Type 2 diabetes, chronic asthma, high-blood pressure, and other medical conditions. Preexisting conditions would include histories of racial and ethnic discrimination, economic dispossession, environmental exposures, urban segregation, and racism as a pathogen (Krieger 2005; Lock 2015). Just as racism can be toxic, so can certain performances of masculinity.

Unmasking toxic masculinity

One of many striking moments in the 2016 presidential campaign involved the size of Trump's hands and, metonymically, his penis. As he traded barbs with Marco Rubio—whom Trump nicknamed "little Marco"—Rubio took advantage of a rally to note that Trump "is taller than me, he's like 6'2", which is why I don't understand why his hands are the size of someone who is 5'2"," Rubio joked. "Have you seen his hands? And you know what they say about men with small hands … " As the crowd waited for the familiar other shoe to drop, Rubio paused for comedic effect and finished with a sly surprise: "You can't trust them" (Shapiro 2016). The crowd roared. Trump predictably took the bait. Standing in front of a sea of red MAGA baseballs caps, Trump raised his outstretched hands. "Look" he invited the crowd. "[Little Marco] referred to my hands—if they are small, something else must be small." Pause for a smirk. "I guarantee you there is no problem. I guarantee you."

These dueling hand barbs draw on familiar tropes of masculinity. As Connell (1995: 71) originally argued, "Masculinity, to the extent the term can be briefly defined, is simultaneously a place in gender relations, the practices through which men and women engage that place in gender, and the effects of these practices on bodily experience, personality and culture." Connell would subsequently expand those gender relations beyond the binary, but for the purpose of this essay the thread I wish to follow is that of masculinities (in the plural) as patterned gender behaviors that are relationally defined and performed. It is not only in large arenas and political rallies that forms of masculinity are performed, although both Rubio and Trump did swagger in their respective venues. Masculinities are performed in the realm of the everyday, the performance always addresses some real or imagined audience of other gendered beings, certain forms of masculinity may be compulsory, and in any given time and context a particular way of performing "maleness" may become privileged. During these Trumpian times, the performance has increasingly been described, at least in certain circles, as toxic.

The term *toxic masculinity* was coined during the mythopoetic men's movement of the 1980s and 1990s—think male-only wilderness retreats and banging the drum to a virile beat. The toxicity referred to by Robert Bly (1990) and others consisted of society denying young boys and men participation in the rites and rituals that would allow them to be in touch with a protective, warrior masculinity that allegedly constituted the "deep maleness" that feminism was eroding. From this perspective, men's aggression and violence were consequences of masculinity thwarted and frustrated—by women.

This is not how I use the term. Rather than referencing some long-lost masculine essence, I am concerned with the here, the now, and the angry. Michael Kimmel has suggested that part of the anger fueling white men is the result of "aggrieved entitlement" (2017). For a sector of white males in America, this is an emotion grounded in a sense of loss and disenfranchisement, such that aggrieved entitlement is "a fusion of that humiliating loss of manhood and the moral obligation and entitlement to get it back" (Kalish and Kimmel 2010: 454). As Kimmel defined it, "manhood" refers to the rights men have historically exercised over women, rights they feel slipping away from them in a changing society. Importantly, Kimmel argued that men "tend to feel their sense of aggrieved entitlement because of the past; they want to restore what they *once had*. Their entitlement is not aspirational; it is nostalgic" (Kimmel 2017: 63). So yes, they fervently hope to make America great *again*.

The "angry white males" that were the focus of Kimmel's research perform toxic masculinity. Scholar Colleen Clemens (2017) defined the term accessibly this way:

> Toxic masculinity is a narrow and repressive description of manhood, designating manhood as defined by violence, sex, status and aggression. It's the cultural ideal of manliness, where strength is everything while emotions are a weakness; where sex and brutality are yardsticks by which men are measured, while supposedly "feminine" traits—which can range from emotional vulnerability to simply not being hypersexual—are the means by which your status as "man" can be taken away.

I note that the status, rather than being a solid and permanent achievement, is one that can be lost or taken away: In short, for all of the bluster and bravado, it is a fragile masculinity.

It is a masculinity that may also take a toll on those socialized into its compulsory components. In 2019, the American Psychological Association issued guidelines for working with boys and men, noting the harmful effects of feeling obligated to enact "traditional masculinity," marked by stoicism, competitiveness, dominance, and aggression (Pappas 2019: 34). The authors of the report noted that men socialized this way are less likely to engage in healthy behaviors, a claim for which a robust body of research exists.[3] The APA also emphasized the psychological harm this form of masculinity may cause, and the reluctance men have to reach out for counseling and therapeutic assistance to address their distress.

These themes are powerfully addressed in the 2015 documentary, *The Mask You Live In*.[4] The film draws on lengthy interviews with boys and men, in which they discuss the challenges of maintaining a sense of self and self-worth when confronted by societal expectations of what constitutes a "real man." A recurrent theme is that of feeling as though one walks through this world wearing a mask that hides a more authentic self. The mask is thus obligatory yet oddly protective: A failure to perform the appropriate maleness could leave one open to the accusation of being a "sissy" or a "wuss."

Cue the pandemic irony. Being a tough guy means wearing the mask of masculinity: Being a tough guy means refusing to don a mask that might preserve one's life and the lives of others. History provides a cautionary tale of toxic masculinity turned lethal.

Lessons unlearned?

The 1918–1919 influenza pandemic was among the most severe pandemics in recent history. It is estimated that about 500 million people, or one-third of the world's population, became infected with the virus. The number of deaths was estimated to be at least 50 million worldwide, with about 675,000 deaths occurring in the United States (US Centers for Disease Control n.d.). Attempts to control the spread of the virus included social distancing, bans on public gatherings, and the promotion of personal hygiene campaigns focused on hand washing, handkerchiefs, and protective masks (Tomes 2010: 49). In the United States, influenza was first identified in military personnel in the spring of 1918. Control of the virus would thus require making sure men were on board, so to speak, with prevention and control measures. This proved to be a challenge for public health practitioners and medical professionals.

In addition to an insistence on personal freedoms, a key point of resistance to the personal hygiene measures was masculinity itself. Cautions against spitting and sneezing in public sounded, to "modern men and boys," less like the "gospel of germs" and more like the hygiene rules they associated with "mothers, schoolmarms, and Sunday school teachers" (Tomes 2010: 58). In an effort to counter this resistance, public health messaging focused on more "modern, manly form[s] of public health, steeped in discipline, patriotism, and personal responsibility" (Tomes 2010: 58). Sneezing into large, manly handkerchiefs (banish the lacy trim) was positioned as a civic duty. Advertisements for disposable paper tissues featured mothers instructing their sons on how to manage their "man-sized sneezes." And mask wearing was promoted as a sign of public spiritedness and manly discipline.

Flash forward to 2020. The president himself refused to wear a mask for months, and his mask-wearing heyday was brief indeed, ceding to his desire to project strength and downplay the risk of a pandemic he had denied and allowed to spin out of control. At one Trump rally in Arizona, men told reporters, "Wearing a mask is submission," and, "It's muzzling yourself, it looks weak, especially for me" (Canales 2020). What is it about men and barrier methods of disease prevention that chafes? In one lively article, Emily Willingham (2020) suggested that masks are "the condoms of the face," harking back to HIV/AIDS education and prevention efforts that attempted to convince men that wearing a condom was desirable. As someone who spent several years in the HIV/AIDS education field, I recall the men who insisted that thin layer of latex reduced stimulation and interfered with their sexual pleasure. Fair enough, but how could masks be seen in the same light? If condoms were tied to a reduction in sensation, how does that translate to rejecting face masks?

I suggest we consider a spectrum of masculine behaviors and the logic that undergirds them: an unsheathed penis; the right to bear arms, if doing so while white; unbridled white male privilege; and a nostalgia for unquestioned entitlement. The right to be "in-your-face," which Merriam-Webster defines as "characterized by or expressive of bold and often defiant aggressiveness," parallels the discourse of those who praised Trump for "telling it like it is," which equates to unvarnished misogyny and racism. Unmasking toxic masculinity reveals its defensive posture, indifference to the well-being and wishes of others, and its mooring in Kimmel's (2017) case study of angry white males.

And the women who love them? Amid that sea of red MAGA caps, amid the monochromatic panorama of white faces, there are women wearing American flag sweatshirts and cheering wildly. What do we make of this? I think of complicit femininities: the forms of femininity that cast their fate with those angry white men, shoring up their racial privilege by backgrounding their gendered identity. Natalie Moore (2020) has insisted that we can trace white women's support for Trump back to

> the white women who lined up behind Schlafly as defending their own status in this country. They were, in their own words, "protecting their way of life." White womanhood and femininity is revered and white women historically have benefited from white supremacy. They have been heralded as virtuous and lean in the arms of white men in our racial caste system. Whiteness is aspirational for women, too.

For those men who refuse to wear an "emasculating" protective face mask, there is likely a female partner who has accepted the sexual contract and whatever benefits it confers. Now to consider the costs, which extend beyond any individual woman, any country—beyond race, class, or ethnicity. I turn now to times of crises and the impact on domestic violence and gendered harm.

Domesticating violence and gendering harm

> Make the prevention and redress of violence against women a key part of nationl response plans for COVID-19. (UN Secretary General António Guterres, April 5, 2020)

One of the first articles I ever published was "Domesticando la Violencia: Alcohol y las Secuelas de la Guerra" (Thiedon 1999). I had been conducting research in postwar Peru and was struck by the level of alcohol consumption and domestic violence in the highland communities in which I lived. This was, after all, supposedly a postconflict setting, and yet the "postviolence violence" was resulting in horrible injuries to the girls and women who were overwhelmingly the targets. Dead bodies in the streets and streams had abated; the ongoing violence occurred in what should have been a place of refuge—the home. The violence was driven inward, and women were grappling with the impact of "domesticating violence."

Peruvian women were not alone. Research has indicated that natural disasters and crises are key factors associated with intimate partner violence (IPV). In one thoughtful overview of the literature, Stanley (2020: 3–5) noted several recurrent themes among the causal narratives: isolation, stress, economic anxiety and joblessness, alcohol consumption, and a lack of social service resources to address all of the above. COVID-19 has affected each of these stressors, with a predictable upsurge in cases of IPV and domestic violence. Globally, the numbers are staggering. According to the UN Fund for Population Activities ([UNFPA] 2020):

> [The] COVID-19 pandemic is also expected to increase levels of violence. In the immediate term, the largest contributor is likely to come from the effects of stay-at-home orders and movement restrictions, which could increase women's exposure to violent partners. Mounting household tensions and economic stresses could also play a role. There are already indications that violence incidence is indeed growing, including increases in calls to violence prevention hotlines and media reports of rising domestic abuse and homicide. Projections show that if violence increases by 20 per cent during periods of lockdown, there would be an additional 15 million cases of intimate partner violence in 2020 for an average lockdown duration of 3 months, 31 million cases for an average lockdown of 6 months, 45 million for an average lockdown of 9 months, and 61 million if the average lockdown period were to be as long as one year. (2020: 4)

Although the study focused primarily on low- and middle-income countries, COVID-19 defies any geographic partition. As Gupta and Stahl (2020) reported, in the United States more than one in three women has experienced rape, physical violence, and/or stalking by an intimate partner (defined as current or former spouses or partners) in her lifetime, and in recent years, the number of domestic violence cases (which includes violence by intimate partners and family members) has spiked, making up about 20 percent of all violent crimes in the United States in 2018.

This violence and the lack of resources to address the violence has potentially long-term legacies. The UNFPA study also noted that the pandemic lockdown means less or erratic access to contraceptive methods, interruptions in ob/gyn doctor and hospital visits, more unplanned (and perhaps unwanted) pregnancies, and giving birth under quarantine conditions. These are violations of sexual and reproductive rights, and the violations will fall heaviest on the girls and women who inhabit intersectional saturation points.

Disposability and final reflections

> I said to my people, slow the testing down please. (Donald Trump, June 20, 2020; quoted in Atkins 2020)

> herd im·mu·ni·ty
>
> noun
>
> noun: herd immunity; plural noun: herd immunities
>
> the resistance to the spread of a contagious disease within a population that results if a sufficiently high proportion of individuals are immune to the disease, especially through vaccination. (*Oxford Learner's Dictionaries*)

The idea behind herd immunity is that if enough people become immune to the virus at the center of the COVID-19 pandemic (either through mass vaccination or prior infection) the disease will slow its spread. Scientists are still working to answer the questions that would make this strategy feasible, questions that include how long immunity lasts and who is most vulnerable to infection. On the surface, herd immunity—when achieved via natural immunity or vaccination—sounds innocuous, even salutary. Otherwise healthy people become infected and recover; tests and contact tracing are efficiently provided; a vaccination is tested and made available; and the most vulnerable are, ostensibly, protected from the virus while the steps are sequenced. That has not happened in the United States.

In light of the current political context, herd immunity strikes me as a euphemism for a eugenics mindset (Klein 2020). When we consider the death toll in the United States, we see a painful overrepresentation of the elderly nursing home population and members of the African-American, Native American, and Latinx communities. Although data collection in the United States has been sketchy and incomplete—perhaps due to the lack of leadership at the federal level—these are the trends to date. These are populations that have been made structurally vulnerable due to history, to "essential worker" status in the service sector, and to the uneven levels of care afforded to those elderly who have been warehoused in substandard institutions.[5] There is also evidence that the Trump administration knowingly withheld assistance to "blue states" in which Democratic voters would bear the brunt of this political calculus (Steib 2020).

The Trump administration has committed crimes of commission ("I said to my people, slow the testing down please") and crimes of omission (denying that COVID-19 was reaching a pandemic level of infection), to cite two examples from a potential litany of criminally negligent behavior. I strongly advocate that Congress convene an independent investigative body with subpoenae powers to determine the breadth and depth of these crimes, which may be of such magnitude as to warrant the charge of crimes against humanity.

Epilogue

Two months ago my partner, Kathleen, was returning from her morning walk. Our next door neighbor, Claudette, was standing at the foot of her driveway, her big black Labrador playfully tugging on his leash.

"How are you?" Kathleen asked, sensing distress.

Our neighbor shook her head: "Terrible." She paused as tears filled her eyes.

"What's wrong?" my partner asked.

Claudette exhaled. "Everything. My mother just died after four months of not being able to hug her or see her any way other than with a thick pane of glass between us."

Pointing down the hill, she added that her mother had been in a nursing home in town and said, "The COVID virus went through it like wild fire. She got sick and died without my even being able to go to the hospital to see her, to be with her. And now we can't even have a proper funeral for her."

Notes

1. For more on "unimagined communities," see Nixon (2013).
2. For a powerful analysis of the accumulation of disadvantage, see Coates (2014).

3. For a synthesis of this research, see Galdas, Cheater, and Marshall (2005).
4. *The Mask You Live In* is a 2015 documentary film written, directed, and produced by Jennifer Siebel Newsom.
5. The data indicate that 40 percen of all COVID-19 deaths have occurred among the nursing home population (see *New York Times* 2020).

References

ALON, Titan, DOEPKE, Matthias, OLMSTEAD-RUMSEY, Jane, and TERTILT, Michéle. (2020) *The Impact of the Coronoavirus Pandemic on Gender Equality*. [Online]. Available: https://voxeu.org/article/impact-coronavirus-pandemic-gender-equality [2 September 2020].

ATKINS, Davis. (2020) *Trump Just Admitted to a Crime Against Humanity. No, He Wasn't Joking*. [Online]. Available: https://washingtonmonthly.com/2020/06/21/trump-admitted-to-a-crime-against-humanity-last-night-and-no-he-wasnt-joking/ [2 September 2020].

BLY, Robert. (1990) *Iron John: A Book About Men* (Boston, MA: Addison-Wesley).

CANALES, Katie. (2020) *These Surpisingly Relevant Vintage Ads Show How Officials Tried to Convince People to Wear Masks After they Refused During the 1918 Flu Pandemic*. [Online]. Available: https://www.businessinsider.com/people-vintage-mask-ads-spanish-flu-1918-pandemic-2020-5 [30 August 2020].

CBS NEWS. (2020) *CBS News Poll, 2020*. [Online]. Available: https://ropercenter.cornell.edu/ipoll/study/31117438 [30 August 2020].

CLEMENS, Colleen. (2017) *What We Mean When We Say 'Toxic Masculinity.'* [Online]. Available: https://www.tolerance.org/magazine/what-we-mean-when-we-say-toxic-masculinity [30 August 2020].

COATES, TaNehisi. (2014) The case for reparations. *The Atlantic*, June.

CONNELL, R. W. (1995) *Masculinities* (1st ed.) (Berkeley, CA: University of California Press).

CRENSHAW, Kimberlé. (1991) Mapping the margins: Intersectionality, identity politics, and violence against women of color. *Stanford Law Review*, 43(6), 1241–1299. doi:10.2307/1229039

FACEBOOK. (2020) *COVID-19 and Intersectionality: A Discussion Among Fletcher Faculty and Students*. [Online]. Available: https://www.facebook.com/watch/live/?v=228573798372945&ref=watch_permalink [15 April 2020].

DUCHARME, Jamie. (2020) *Why is COVID-19 Striking Men Harder than Women?* [Online]. Available: https://time.com/5829202/covid-19-gender-differences/ [2 September 2020].

GALDAS, Paul, CHEATER, Francine, and MARSHALL, Paul. (2005) Men and health-seeking behaviour: A literature review. *Journal of Advanced Nursing*, 49(6), 616–623.

GUPTA, Alisha Haridasani, and STAHL, Aviva. (2020) *For Abused Women, a Pandemic Lockdown Holds Dangers of its Own*. [Online]. Available: https://www.nytimes.com/2020/03/24/us/coronavirus-lockdown-domestic-violence.html?searchResultPosition=6 [2 September 2020].

GUTERRES, António. (2020) *Make the Prevention and Redress of Violence Against Women a Key Part of National Response Plans for COVID-19*. [Online]. Available: https://www.un.org/en/un-coronavirus-communications-team/make-prevention-and-redress-violence-against-women-key-part [30 August 2020].

KALISH, Rachel, and KIMMEL, Michael. (2010) Suicide by mass murder: Masculinity, aggrieved entitlement, and rampage school shootings. *Health Sociology Review*, 9(4), 451–464. doi:10.5172/hesr.2010.19.4.451

KIMMEL, Michael. (2017) *Angry White Men: American Masculinity at the End of an Era* (London, UK: Hachette).

KLEIN, Charlotte. (2020) *Trump's New Favorite COVID Advisor Thinks 'Herd Immunity' is a Good Idea*. [Online]. Accessible: https://www.vanityfair.com/news/2020/08/trump-new-favorite-covid-adviser-scott-atlas-thinks-herd-immunity-is-a-good-idea [30 August 2020].

KRIEGER, Nancy. (2005) Embodiment: A conceptual glossary for epidemiology. *Journal of Epidemiology and Community Health*, 59, 350–355. doi:10.1136/jech.2004.024562

LOCK, Margaret. (2015) Comprehending the body in the era of the epigenome. *Current Anthropology*, 56(2), 151–177. doi:10.1086/680350

MATTHEWS, David. (2020) *Chicago Mayor Lori Lightfoot: 'Breathtaking' that African-Americans, Latnix Community Dying at Higher Rates*. [Online]. Available: https://www.nydailynews.com/coronavirus/ny-coronavirus-20200407-bzj3npnydjclrey4gt5ootjc5u-story.html [30 August 2020].

MERRIAM-WEBSTER. (2020) *In Your Face*. [Online]. Available: https://www.merriam-webster.com/dictionary/in-your-face [30 August 2020].

MILLER, Hayley. (2020) *Navajo Nation President: US Government Ignoring Native Americans Amid Coronavirus.* [Online]. Available via: https://www.huffpost.com/entry/navajo-nation-coronavirus_n_5e838c96c5b6871702a59ee8 [30 August 2020].

MOORE, Natalie. (2020) *Why did 57% of White Women Vote for Trump? The Story of Phyllis Schlafley Tells Why.* [Online]. Available: https://chicago.suntimes.com/columnists/2020/5/21/21266599/phyllis-schlafly-feminism-equal-rights-amendment-mrs-america-era-culture-wars [30 August 2020].

NEW YORK TIMES. (2020) *More than 40% of U.S. Coronavirus Deaths are Linked to Nursing Homes.* [Online]. Available: https://www.nytimes.com/interactive/2020/us/coronavirus-nursing-homes.html [30 August 2020].

NIXON, Rob. (2013) *Slow Violence and the Environmentalism of the Poor* (Cambridge, MA: Harvard University Press).

ORTIZ, Erik. (2020) *Native American Tribes Brace for Coronavirus: 'It's Going to Be a Test.'* [Online]. Available: https://www.nbcnews.com/news/us-news/native-american-tribes-brace-coronavirus-it-s-going-be-test-n1156961 [30 August 2020].

OXFORD LEARNER'S DICTIONARIES. (2020) *Herd Immunity.* [Online]. Available: https://www.oxfordlearners-dictionaries.com/us/definition/english/herd-immunity [30 August 2020].

PAPPAS, Stephanie. (2019). *APA Issues First-Ever Guidelines for Practice with Men and Boys.* [Online]. Available: https://www.apa.org/monitor/2019/01/ce-corner [30 August 2020].

PASKIN, Janet. (2020) *Women are Bearing the Brunt of Coronavirus Disruption.* [Online]. Available: https://www.bloomberg.com/news/articles/2020-03-11/coronavirus-will-make-gender-inequality-worse [2 September 2020].

REYKJAVIK GLOBAL FORUM. (2020) *The Silent Pandemic: Gender-Based Violence and the Cost of Inaction.* [Online]. Available: https://reykjavikforum.global/the-silent-pandemic-gender-based-violence-and-the-cost-of-inaction/[30 August 2020].

SALVANTO, Anthony, DEPINTO, Jennifer, BACKUS, Fred, KHANNA, Kabir, and COX, Elena. (2020) *Republicans See US as Better Off Now than 4 Years Ago Ahead of Convention: Battleground Tracker Poll.* [Online]. Available: https://www.cbsnews.com/news/republicans-economy-coronavirus-opinion-poll-cbs-news-battleground-tracker/ [30 August 2020].

SHAPIRO, Emily. (2016) *The History Behind the Donald Trump 'Small Hands' Insult.* [Online]. Available: https://abcnews.go.com/Politics/history-donald-trump-small-hands-insult/story?id=37395515 [30 August 2020].

STANLEY, Maclen. (2020) *Why the Increase in Domestic Violence During COVID-19?* [Online]. Available: https://www.psychologytoday.com/us/blog/making-sense-chaos/202005/why-the-increase-in-domestic-violence-during-covid-19 [29 August 2020].

STEIB, Matthew. (2020) *Trump's Disregard for Blue States is at the Heart of his Shoddy COVID Response.* [Online]. Available: https://nymag.com/intelligencer/2020/07/trumps-war-on-blue-states-is-worse-than-previously-thought.html [2 September 2020].

THEIDON, Kimberly. (1999) Domesticando la violencia: Alcohol y las secuelas de la guerra. *Ideele: Revista del Instituto de Defensa Legal*, 120(July): 56–63.

TOMES, Nancy. (2010) 'Destroyer and teacher': Managing the masses during the 1918–1919 influenza pandemic. *Public Health Reports*, 125(Suppl 3): 48–62. doi:10.1177/00333549101250S308

UN FUND FOR POPULATION ACTIVITES. (2020) *Impact of COVID-19 on Family Planning and Ending Gender-Based Violence, Female Genital Mutilation and Child Marriage.* [Online]. Accessible: https://www.unfpa.org/sites/default/files/resource-pdf/COVID-19_impact_brief_for_UNFPA_24_April_2020_1.pdf [2 September 2020].

US CENTERS FOR DISEASE CONTROL. (n.d.) *1918 Pandemic (H1N1 Virus).* [Online]. Accessible: https://www.cdc.gov/flu/pandemic-resources/1918-pandemic-h1n1.html [30 August 2020].

WILLINGHAM, Emily. (2020) *The Condoms of the Face: Why Some Men Refuse to Wear Masks.* [Online]. Available: https://www.scientificamerican.com/article/the-condoms-of-the-face-why-some-men-refuse-to-wear-masks/ [30 August 2020].

Solidarity in times of crisis

Kathryn Libal and Prakash Kashwan

ABSTRACT
The 2019 COVID-19 pandemic has amplified inequalities and human rights challenges; in some states, COVID-19 policies have been introduced that further curtail human rights. Although some limits may be justified in the time of a public health emergency, other rights are vital to secure precisely because of pandemic conditions. Following a discussion of the concept of political solidarity, we examine how COVID-19 has underscored democratic "deficits" and human rights failures within the United States and India. Emergency "stay-at-home" orders and social distancing measures make political dissent challenging, yet this extreme moment has created opportunities for solidarity, initially in restrained ways via the internet or local forms of collective support and protest, and later through mass mobilizations to end racial injustice (in the United States). Our assessment of the challenges and promises of solidarist action in two of the largest democracies offers reasons for guarded optimism.

Introduction

The 2019 COVID-19 pandemic has amplified existing inequalities and related human rights challenges globally and within many societies. In powerful and increasingly authoritarian states – such as the United States, India, Brazil, and South Africa – where democracy and the rule of law are weakened or under assault, a range of COVID-19 policies has tended to curtail human rights. Although some limits on rights may be justified in the time of a public health emergency, others are vital to secure precisely because of the pandemic conditions; these include, for example, freedom of expression, rights to information, due process, right to seek asylum, and access to health care and social security. As Kathryn Sikkink (2020) has underscored, "A quarantine is a legitimate state policy in times of health emergencies, but the state must also attend to the rights of individuals caught in the quarantine to adequate health care, food, and shelter."

Less clear are the limits on rights to mobilize through public protest, such as in the United States in the aftermath of the killing of George Floyd (Sykes 2020) or the residents of the state of Kashmir in India, protesting against the "perennial lockdown" imposed on August 5, 2019, after the government of India scrapped Kashmir's autonomous status (BBC News 2020). UN human rights experts and bodies recognize these risks, and have been critical of the US government's severe policing tactics in the wake of "a national uprising against systemic racism in law enforcement," noting that the government "has reenacted the very injustices that have driven people into the streets in the first place" (United Nations 2020).

A deeper meditation on the challenges of protecting political and civil liberties during an emergency such as the COVID-19 pandemic is important because authoritarian leaders and governments may use the emergency – a form of "national trauma" – to justify weakening rights

(Nay 2020: e238). And as the international human rights system faces serious challenges from increasingly illiberal regimes at state and regional levels (Neuman 2020), we must think more intensively about how solidarity matters in human rights work (Mander 2019; Satterthwaite 2020). Brysk (2013: 169) asked how human rights activists and defenders, embedded within social movements for human rights, can "sustain solidarity." She pointed to the need to recognize our interconnectedness: "Human rights as an ethos of social responsibility promotes a worldview of moral interdependence, in which we are invested in each others' well-being" (2013: 168).

Solidarity has become a keyword during COVID-19, initially in a call to people at local, national, and global levels to work together through maintaining social distancing practices to slow the spread of the SAR CoV-2 virus. In Europe and the United States, solidarity has been invoked in television advertisements, on social media, and in public displays of support through bell-ringing to foster a sense of social commitment for sacrifice of personal freedoms and to show support for healthcare and other workers critical for daily survival (e.g., agricultural workers, janitors, manufacturing, and grocery store workers). Solidarity has also been demonstrated through voluntarism to help those too vulnerable to shop for food or supplies or to provide informal support to those who may face eviction or food insecurity. Yet global pandemics or planetary climate crises also require international solidarity and global action.

The European Network of National Human Rights Institutions (ENNHRI; 2020) recognized the need for solidarity at many levels early in the pandemic: "Respect for human rights during the COVID-19 pandemic calls for solidarity at all levels. Within states, measures to combat the pandemic should be motivated by the conviction of all people to contribute to preventing the virus' spread, while states must stand by those most at risk." Although to date the European Union has made substantial strides to arrest the rapid spread of the virus, in two other democracies – the United States and India – solidarity actions from below have been significant, but often undermined by the state. Moreover, these governments have been largely ineffectual at the national level in stemming the spread and addressing the consequences of the pandemic. As others have commented before us, these weaknesses are a result of at least a four-decade-long neoliberal onslaught on social and environmental protections and the institutions of the state in general (Alston 2017; Fouskas and Gokay 2020).

This article focuses on how COVID-19 has presented challenges to human rights as well as a potential catalyst for transformative change in two large democracies – the United States and India. Both states illustrate how the recent history of neoliberalism, politics of illiberalism, and ongoing structural inequalities have generated new obstacles to human rights. We outline the situation in which US and Indian civil society have faced daunting barriers to solidarity activism. These cases are also instructive because of their shared histories of the dominance of neoliberal ideology, although it is relatively more recent in the Indian case. But the Indian exemplar is also instructive because India has often been cited as an exceptional case of a successful democracy despite very high levels of poverty. The pandemic and its aftermath offer an opportunity to investigate the depth and responsiveness of India's democratic institutions *vis-à-vis* myriad civil society initiatives and social movements of the poor and marginalized. Growing public awareness in the United States of the long-term effects of "structural adjustment" – often framed as "downsizing big government" – has also led to increased action by civil society and social movements to challenge poverty and inequality, particularly as they relate to racial justice (Schrecker and Bambra 2015).

The Trump administration in the United States as well as the Modi government in India have greatly enhanced their efforts to roll back environmental and labor regulations, while continuing to clamp down aggressively on all forms of dissent. Moreover, Indian government agencies have continued to label Rohingya refugees who fled Myanmar and took refuge in India as "illegal migrants," which makes them ineligible for whatever meager aid government agencies have offered in the wake of the pandemic (Bose 2020). The pandemic has thrown into stark focus both the democratic "deficits" within the United States and India and the failure to realize human rights. Adding to these challenges are the imperatives of quarantine, stay-at-home orders, and social distancing measures being implemented unevenly across both nations.

Yet this extreme moment has created opportunities within these same societies, initially in relatively restrained ways through the internet or local forms of solidarity-making and protest. However, as the pandemic continued to develop in summer 2020, initial acts of protest flourished into profound acts of public dissent in support of the Black Lives Matter movement both in the United States and globally. For reasons we will discuss below, India has seen few overt protests during the pandemic, even as the Indian government has continued to target social activists and dissenting academics.

Solidarity and human rights

The proposal that a particular set of rights can be understood as "solidarity rights" – or a third generation of rights requiring cooperation and responsibilities transcending nation-state boundaries – has been debated in international human rights law for some time (Alston 1982; Scholz 2014). Whereas some scholars have pointed to the challenges of rights proliferation or establishing rights that have little opportunity for remedy, Alston (1982: 318) asserted that "solidarity is an essential ingredient in the promotion and realization of all human rights." Although the debate over whether or not solidarity itself is a human right has garnered some attention since the 1980s, recently human rights practitioners have begun to invoke solidarity in both national and transnational contexts as critical to human rights campaigning.

As a concept, solidarity has a long history, stemming from the emergence of the social welfare state in the nineteenth century (Bayertz 1999; Ewald 2020), labor rights mobilizations of the nineteenth and twentieth centuries (Dibben 2004; Anner 2011), and postcolonial struggles that often exceeded imperial or national borders (Mahler 2018). The Polish Solidarity Movement of the 1970s–1980s embodied an understanding of solidarity mobilizations to transform states and played an important role in the transformation of the so-called Soviet bloc (Barker 2001). More recently, the term has gained currency in light of mass displacement and forced migration of refugees, asylum seekers, and migrants to Europe, where "solidarity" became a clarion call for support by EU citizens, regardless of nationality, for refugees (Ataç, Rygiel, and Stierl 2016). Calls for global solidarity have also been evoked, at least symbolically, by environmental justice activists in the face of climate change (Routledge and Cumbers 2013).

Normative definitions of human solidarity often focus on social cohesion or "a feeling of sympathy shared by subjects within and between groups, impelling supportive action and pursuing social inclusion" (Wilde 2013: 1). Scholz (2008) developed a taxonomy of solidarity distinguishing between three forms: social solidarity, civic solidarity, and political solidarity. Scholz recognized that there is often overlap between these three types of action and belonging. She associated social solidarity with group cohesiveness – a "community relation that also entails some binding obligations" (Scholz 2008: 21). Civic solidarity refers to relations between citizens and between citizens and the state, including "the obligations of the state, society, or community, of which the individual is a contributing part, to protect individuals against vulnerabilities" (Scholz 2008: 31). State obligation for provision of social welfare is deeply rooted in most of Europe, but less fully recognized in the United States, likely because of wider acceptance within Europe of democratic socialism as well as trade unionism (Bayertz 1999; Ewald 2020). Civic solidarity in European contexts implies commitments to social rights, including social security, access to healthcare, and workers' rights. Civic solidarity in other contexts is often devolved to local or provincial/state levels and is often visible in efforts for mutual aid.

Political solidarity, in contrast to social and civic, requires more radical forms of action and participation in the collective. "Instead of basing solidarity on varying notions of dependence and group control, the political conception of solidarity highlights individual conscience, commitment, group responsibility, and collective action" (Scholz 2008: 33). Political solidarity is "a unity of individuals each responding to a particular situation of injustice, oppression, social vulnerability, or tyranny (Scholz 2008: 51). When an individual or group is "threatened with severe harm, violence, or death because of an injustice" some are led to joining collective political movements in the name of solidarity (Scholz 2008: 51–52). Brysk (2013) observed that political solidarity cannot be taken for granted. It must be constructed and fostered through socialization and proximity of individuals who may not share the same community or social ties. She noted, "We manifest care in individual actions, social attitudes, transformations of communities, and political campaigns for human rights" (2013: 163). She linked solidarity to an "implicit notion of human rights," but both the foundations of and threats to solidarity emerge from the broader processes in politics and economy.

For example, neoliberalism has undermined the efficacy of the social democratic or other kinds of protections available for the poor within the Global North and the efforts related to international development and global environment (Deeming and Smyth 2015). The debilitating effects of neoliberal policy on welfare protections were evident even before the pandemic dealt another blow. Philip Alston, the former UN Special Rapporteur on extreme poverty and human rights, has criticized the global community for its "self-congratulatory message of impending victory over poverty" (2020). Alston has argued that the World Bank's international poverty line of $1.90 (2011 Purchasing Power Parity [PPP]) per day is "deeply flawed and yields a deceptively positive picture," even though "it doesn't even cover the cost of food or housing in many countries." Moreover, Alston (2020) argued that this "misplaced triumphalism" has blocked the "very reforms that could have prevented the worst impacts of the pandemic." The theoretically flawed and morally impoverished philosophy of trickle-down economics promoted by multilateral and regional institutions is arguably one of the most significant barriers against the protections of fundamental human rights.

COVID-19 exposed inequalities and fractures in the United States and India

The pandemic has underscored how deeply we are interconnected "as human beings and societies, including the sheer depth of our mutual vulnerability," said Abioma Okafor, UN Independent Expert on Human Rights and International Solidarity (Okafor 2020). This mutual vulnerability also is a source for activation of power from below, or what Piven (2014) has called "interdependent power." Chenoweth (2020: 82) noted that responses to the pandemic have provided "publics a view of the stark contrast between populists and autocrats on the one hand and liberal or social democrats on the other."

These contrasts have been cast into relief in the United States and India. The pandemic has revealed the precarious status of the United States as a "global leader," even as it further exposes its domestic human rights failures on numerous fronts (UN Special Rapporteur on Extreme Poverty and Human Rights, 2018). The Indian Prime Minister's "highly-personalised, muscular leadership style" was evident in the "draconian lockdown," which he declared with "no warning, no planning and no transparency into the policy deliberations or scientific advice behind it" (Kazmin 2020). It caused immense "human suffering," yet, India failed to "even slightly bend" the coronavirus curve (Kazmin 2020).

As community transmission of COVID-19 became more evident and intense in the US Northeast in early 2020, residents of New York City and other urban and suburban locales demonstrated solidarity as a matter of civic engagement: They organized to make masks and protective clothing for "essential workers"; set up informal places to give out hot meals or share food; raised funds for local food banks; and, following the lead of local officials, by and large observed social distancing measures. Yet, as the spread of the pandemic continued – even as case numbers were increasing in other parts of the country – these forms of civic solidarity became less visible, at least in mainstream media. Two months into the public emergency, some states began to reduce social distancing measures and hoped that allowing residents to return to businesses (restaurants, bars, salons, and other services) would help reboot local economies and get people off unemployment rolls and back to work. In late April 2020, small-scale protests erupted calling for an end to social distancing practice, framing wearing masks and distancing as an infringement on constitutional rights. President Trump endorsed these views, at times even making incendiary comments about distancing measures potentially limiting the 2nd Amendment of the Constitution, which outlines the right to bear firearms (DeBrabander 2020).

As the pandemic grew, it became increasingly evident that racial minorities were disproportionately affected (Hathaway 2020). The resentment against the injustices of COVID may have played a role in rekindling protests against racial injustices that had been ongoing for the past year. On May 25, 2020, when a video of George Floyd's murder by a police officer in Minneapolis, Minnesota, spread rapidly across the internet, public protest erupted throughout the country (Buchanan, Bui, and Patel 2020; Chenoweth 2020). The Black Lives Matter movement harnessed and spurred nationwide protests that quickly took on a global scale; activists took to social media and the streets to call for defunding and remaking how policing takes place in communities across the country, as well as a range of other structural changes to address a legacy of structural racism and white supremacy (Black Lives Matter n.d.).

The wave of protests that spread across the country in the midst of the pandemic has been unprecedented in the United States in recent decades. Chenoweth (2020: 81) wrote,

> [M]any protests continue – either in outright defiance of social-distancing measures or in spite of them. But this makes such actions all the more striking – and compelling. The fact that people are willing to risk their health to resist injustice raises awareness of the gravity and urgency of their claims.

These demands for justice explicitly invoke human rights in some cases, but more often they appeal for people to engage in public dissent, to vote, and to challenge all US social institutions to do transformative antiracist, work to dismantle white supremacy without explicitly naming human rights. Yard signs proclaiming "Black Lives Matter" have cropped up in communities around the country, and episodic protests have continued to erupt in unexpected locales, including largely white, rural communities in different parts of the country.

As the protest movement gained momentum in June and July 2020, its targets exceeded questions of policing to address dismantling visible symbolic markers of racial oppression. Activists demanded removing monuments and replacing building, street, or community names and other symbols of slavery, segregation, and racial inequality. The Black Lives Matter movement has been able to spur changes in local legislation on policing and have induced businesses and other nonprofits across the country to express support for the movement's aim to tackle structural racism. In this movement, "collective action in political solidarity" is creating a broader group or societal consciousness of systemic oppression (Scholz 2008: 134).

The signs of cultural transformation are evident, even in the face of counterprotests and mobilization by white supremacist groups. As Chenoweth (2020: 82) noted, gross negligence in handling the pandemic "could also sharpen public awareness of the urgency of political change, reminding voters that mismanaged crises affect everyone living in the country." Yet, it remains to be seen if the current momentum will be sustained in the context of November presidential and congressional elections. Even outside the electoral process, how might a broad set of civil society organizations and actors work in solidarity to press for universal health care, housing rights, and labor rights, along with other civil and political rights that have yet to be fully realized?

The prepandemic context in India was rife with nationwide movements to protest the discriminatory provisions of the Citizenship Amendment Act (CAA). These historic protests were triggered after the Delhi police mounted a violent attack on the students of Delhi's Jamia Milia Islamia University who were protesting the CAA. The most inspiring of these movements was the women-led peaceful protest and round-the-clock sit-in at Delhi's Shaheen Bagh. Over time, the women of Shaheen Bagh became the symbol of the CAA protest, motivating hundreds of other large protests throughout the country. These women also became the prime targets of anti-Muslim hatred launched by the leaders of India's ruling Bhartiya Janata Party (BJP) in the run up to and following the elections to the Delhi legislative council in February 2020 (Anwar 2020). These systematically orchestrated hate campaigns, which started while President Trump was on a state visit to India in February 2020, eventually culminated in targeted and apparently preplanned attacks against Muslim businesses, mosques, and homes in Delhi, killing 53 and injuring more than 200 hundred, most of them Muslims (The Wire Staff 2020). These mobs were apparently working with police complicity and setting mosques, shops, and homes on fire (Mohanty 2020).

Despite the still festering wounds, Delhi's streets have witnessed hundreds of volunteers and civil society groups working with meager resources and at great risk to personal safety to fight hunger and destitution caused by one of the most authoritarian lockdowns anywhere in the world. Prime Minister Modi appeared on national television late in the evening of March 24, 2020, to announce that the entire country was to shut down at midnight. Around 140 million vulnerable migrant workers saw their earnings collapse with a stroke of the proverbial pen (Kazmin 2020). Thousands were left with no choice but to walk back to their homes, some delivering babies while others lost their lives on the way. All they had for support were distraught volunteers, who rose to the occasion. One of these efforts was led by *Karwan e Mohabbat* (the Caravan of Radical Love), whose volunteers had rescued scores of residents from neighborhoods facing violent threats from lynch mobs during the Delhi riots of February 2020 (Mohanty 2020). *Karwan e Mohabbat* started off as a journey "of atonement, solidarity, healing, conscience and justice with people who had been targets of hate attacks across our wounded land" (Salvi 2018). As of this writing, the founder of the campaign and the writer of those words, Harsh Mander, also a veteran human rights defender, faces imminent arrest. Delhi police have charged Mander with crimes of rioting for a speech in which he called for love and nonviolence in the face of unprecedented police violence against the students of Jamia Millia Islamia University in Delhi (Apoorvanand 2020). Mander's *Karwan e Mohabbat* and many inspiring citizen groups and volunteer networks have stepped up to help the poor and migrant workers left without work in the wake of the pandemic.

Neither the onset of pandemic nor the valiant efforts launched by civil society seems to matter to India's ruling regime, which has been ruthless in its clamp down on dissent. More than a dozen human rights defenders, academics, public interest lawyers, and anticaste activists, including a pregnant doctoral scholar, have been arrested and kept in jails that saw COVID-19 infections. The apparent insensitivity of a government trying to capitalize on a crisis to dismantle environmental laws, suppress dissent, and arrest human rights defenders has been noted in various commentaries (Mohanty 2020). Yet, speaking at the UN Economic and Social Council (ECOSOC), Prime Minister Narendra Modi claimed, "In India, we have tried to make the fight against the pandemic a people's movement" (*New Indian Express* 2020). This is a rather cynical attempt to exploit the language of movements to obfuscate the Indian government's botched lockdown that did little to stem the rising tide of COVID-19 positive cases, and its miserably poor response that *The Economist* assessed as one of the stingiest. Modi's claims illustrate a form of parasitical solidarity, which as Scholz (2008) suggested, is often deployed as a "rhetorical tool rather than a moral relation." India's civil society has sought not just to lay bare the hollowness of the Prime Minister's rhetoric but to articulate a much better vision of a society in solidarity (Mander 2019). The following lines penned and recited powerfully by student activist Amir Aziz reflect these sentiments best:

> You write jokes in court;
>
> We will write 'justice' on the walls.
>
> You write 'injustice' on the earth;
>
> We will write 'revolution' in the sky ... (Prasad 2020)

Challenges to and opportunities for solidarity-making in this emergency era

Candice Delmas (2020: 129) characterized solidarity as "meaningful cooperation and collective action to advance shared goals and values." How civil society – including organizations and individuals acting collectively to achieve justice – builds on traditional approaches to resist oppression and hones new techniques to expand and sustain movements is a critical concern. "Historically, human rights progress has occurred as a result of struggle, and has often been spearheaded by oppressed groups. Where it has occurred, human rights progress has not been at all inevitable, but rather contingent on continued commitment and effort" (Sikkink 2018: 172).

Established international human rights organizations, such Amnesty International, have recognized the need for new alliances and approaches to human rights mobilization that supplement international legal approaches (Lettinga and van Troost 2014). These approaches must acknowledge the scale of human rights harms that exist, but also must highlight pragmatic solutions and approaches to create positive change. Human rights actors have begun to shift frames toward constructive, positive, hope-based goals in the wake of rising illiberalism and right-wing authoritarianism (Rodríguez-Garavito and Gomez 2018). A tract published in a practitioner/civil society forum, OpenGlobalRights, titled, "A Guide to Hope-Based Communications" underscores this turn; the movement must "show how human rights is a practical application of universal shared values like compassion, solidarity and dignity, rather than defining rights by the absence of their violations (a world without torture,' 'protection from harm')" (OpenGlobalRights n.d.). This hope-based messaging, grounded in notions of solidarity and constructive action, is vital, but it must also be tempered with the realities of ongoing structural oppression pervasive even in large democracies like the United States and India.

Both the United States and India have a strong network of groups working on the protection of rights of vulnerable and marginalized groups. Yet they also have fared poorly so far in efforts to slow or even mitigate the spread of COVID-19. Some evidence from European countries, India, and the United States suggests that authoritarians are losing some ground amid this crisis (Ulmer and Miglani 2020). Chenoweth (2020: 70) posited that COVID-19 may have actually helped to address some of the structural weaknesses of social movements in the United States in recent years, by "driving movements to turn their focus back to relationship-building, grassroots organizing, strategy, and developing narratives that resonate with a captive audience." Chenoweth may well have been channeling the spirit of large-scale social mobilizations that India witnessed in the winter of 2019, even prior to the pandemic.

Yet, in the face of a political leadership intent on exploiting the pandemic toward repressive means, India's human rights defenders, social activists, dissenters, and journalists have faced unprecedented challenges (Rezaian 2020). Instead of rethinking his administration's approach to social protections and development, Prime Minister Modi presided over a grand ceremony to lay the cornerstones of a major Hindu temple on the site where Hindu extremists armed with pick-axes tore down a sixteenth-century mosque in December 1992, sparking riots that killed thousands of Muslims (Frayer and Pathak 2020). As if to restate its significance to the Hindu nationalist base, the temple ceremony coincided with the first anniversary of India's revocation of special rights in Kashmir.

Indeed, hope and anxiety have pervaded progressive politics in the United States as well, particularly as the November 2020 elections near. In the wake of the COVID-19 disaster and obvious failures to enlist institutions and the broader public in many parts of the country to take measures of social distancing seriously, the economy is teetering on substantial recession and unemployment is at record highs. These harsh economic and social realities may lead to a backlash against the Republican president, Senate, and Republican-led state governments in many parts of the country. The COVID pandemic has revealed the need to both strengthen social institutions and foster a collective understanding of interdependence; that such a sensibility is growing is evidenced by the increasing public support for the Black Lives Matter movement and visible demands for universal healthcare and labor protections.

COVID-19 has led to some extraordinary acts of political solidarity in the United States and India, often in the face of severe repression or other harms. From the vantage point of the midst of the pandemic, we can see the potential for transforming societal structures through political engagement, including social media campaigning and other forms of public acts of dissent. The Indian case, in particular, offers a somber reminder of the work that remains to be done to make political repression morally reprehensible and unacceptable to the general public. Both the pre-pandemic movement against the anti-Muslim Citizenship Amendment Act (CAA) in India and the Black Lives Matter mobilization in the United States kindle hopes of a stronger solidarist world. Yet, as we have signaled in this article, solidarist currents must be fostered across social groups and must be constructed, to use Brysk's (2013) term, to be meaningful and transformative. The COVID-19 pandemic has created an opportunity for addressing longstanding and deeply entrenched forms of social exclusion and inequalities. A successful pursuit of these goals will take those engaged in progressive social movements, working alongside "traditional" human rights organizations, to catalyze action at domestic and international levels. These forms of grassroots, interorganizational, and transnational solidarities will be central to protecting and strengthening human rights in a postpandemic world.

References

APOORVANAND. (2020). With Harsh Mander named in Delhi riots chargesheet, Indian democracy has slipped into a dark hole. *Scroll In*, 20 June. [Online]. Available: https://scroll.in/article/965111/with-harsh-mander-named-in-delhi-riots-chargesheet-indian-democracy-has-slipped-into-a-dark-hole [15 August 2020].

ALSTON, Philip. (1982) A third generation of solidarity rights: Progressive development or obfuscation of international human rights law? *Netherlands International Law Review*, 29(03), 307–322. doi:10.1017/S0165070X00012882

ALSTON, Philip. (2017) The populist challenge to human rights. *Journal of Human Rights Practice*, 9(1), 1–15. doi: 10.1093/jhuman/hux007

ALSTON, Philip. (2020) *Philip Alston Condemns Failed Global Poverty Eradication Efforts*. [Online]. Available: https://chrgj.org/2020/07/05/philip-alston-condemns-failed-global-poverty-eradication-efforts/ [14 August 2020].

ANNER, Mark S. (2011) *Solidarity Transformed: Labor Responses to Globalization and Crisis in Latin America*. (Cornell, NY: Cornell University Press).

ANWAR, Tarique. (2020) We'll return after Corona pandemic ends, say Shaheen Bagh protesters after forceful eviction. *Newsclick*, 24 March. [Online]. Available: https://www.newsclick.in/well-return-after-corona-pandemic-ends-say-shaheen-bagh-protesters-after-forceful-eviction [15 August 2020].

ATAÇ, İlker, RYGIEL, Kim, and STIERL, Maurice. (2016) Introduction. The contentious politics of refugee and migrant protest and solidarity movements: Remaking citizenship from the margins. *Citizenship Studies*, 20(5), 527–544. doi:10.1080/13621025.2016.1182681

BARKER, Colin. (2001) Fear, laughter, and collective power: The making of solidarity at the Lenin Shipyard in Gdansk. Poland, August 1980. In *Passionate Politics: Emotions and Social Movements*, Jeff Goodwin, James P. Jasper, and Francesca Polletta (eds.) (Chicago, IL: University of Chicago Press).

BAYERTZ, Kurt. (1999) Four Uses of 'Solidarity.' In *Solidarity*, Kurt Bayertz (ed.) (Boston, MA: Kluwer Academic).

BBC NEWS. (2020) *Article 370: Curfew in Kashmir as Protesters Plan 'Black Day.'* [Online]. Available: https://www.bbc.com/news/world-asia-india-53646322 [15 August 2020].

BLACK LIVES MATTER. (n.d). *What Matters* (Episodes 1–6) [Online]. Available: https://blacklivesmatter.com/whatmatters/ [13 August 2020].

BOSE, Tapan Kumar. (2020) COVID-19: Rohingya refugees in India are battling islamophobia and starvation. *The Wire*, 1 May. [Online]. Available: https://thewire.in/rights/india-rohingya-refugees-starvation-covid-19 [15 August 2020].

BRYSK, Allison. (2013) 'Why we care': Constructing solidarity. In *Human Rights at the Crossroads*, Mark Goodale (ed.) (New York, NY: Oxford University Press).

BUCHANAN, Larry, BUI, Quotrong, and PATEL, Jugal K. (2020) Black Lives Matter may be the largest movement in U.S. history. *The New York Times*, 3 July. [Online]. Available: https://www.nytimes.com/interactive/2020/07/03/us/george-floyd-protests-crowd-size.html [13 August 2020].

CHENOWETH, Erica. (2020) The future of nonviolent resistance. *Journal of Democracy*, 31(3), 69–84. doi:10.1353/jod.2020.0046

DEBRABANDER, Firman. (2020) The great irony of America's armed anti-lock down protesters. *The Atlantic*, 13 May. [Online]. Available: https://www.theatlantic.com/ideas/archive/2020/05/guns-protesters/611560/ [8 August 2020].

DELMAS, Candace. (2020) *A Duty to Resist: When Civil Disobedience Should Be Uncivil* (New York, NY: Oxford University Press).

DEEMING, Christopher, and SMYTH, Paul. (2015) Social investment after neoliberalism: Policy paradigms and political platforms. *Journal of Social Policy*, 44(2), 297–318. doi:10.1017/S0047279414000828

DIBBEN, Pauline. (2004) Social movement unionism. In *Trade Unions and Democracy: Strategies and Perspectives*, Mark Harcourt and Geoffrey Wood (eds.) (Manchester, UK: Manchester University Press).

EUROPEAN NETWORK OF NATIONAL HUMAN RIGHTS INSTITUTIONS. (2020). *Now Is the Time for Solidarity on Human Rights: The Need for Human Rights in COVID-19 Responses in Europe*. [Online]. Available: http://ennhri.org/statement-on-covid-19/ [13 August 2020].

EWALD, François. (2020/1986) *The Birth of Solidarity: The History of the French Welfare State* (Durham, NC: Duke University Press).

FOUSKAS, Vassilis K., and GOKAY, Bulent. (2020) COVID-19 and the bankruptcy of neoliberalism in the context of the global shift. *Open Democracy*, 5 May. [Online]. Available: https://www.opendemocracy.net/en/can-europe-make-it/covid-19-and-bankruptcy-neoliberalism-context-global-shift/ [13 August 2020].

FRAYER, Lauren, and PATHAK, Sushmita. (2020) At site of razed mosque, India's Modi lays foundation for controversial Hindu temple. *NPR*, 5 August. [Online]. Available: https://www.npr.org/2020/08/05/899247507/at-site-of-razed-mosque-indias-modi-lays-foundation-for-controversial-hindu-temp [13 August 2020].

HATHAWAY, Bill. (2020) *New Analysis Quantifies Risk of COVID-19 to Racial, Ethnic Minorities*. [Online]. Available: https://news.yale.edu/2020/05/19/new-analysis-quantifies-risk-covid-19-racial-ethnic-minorities [15 August 2020].

KAZMIN, Amy. (2020) Modi stumbles: India's deepening coronavirus crisis. *Financial Times*, 26 July. [Online]. Available: https://www.ft.com/content/53d946cf-d4c2-4cc4-9411-1d5bb3566e83 [August 15, 2020].

LETTINGA, Doutje, and VAN TROOST, Lars (eds). (2014) *Debating the Endtimes of Human Rights: Activism and Institutions in a Neo-Westphalian World*. [Online]. Available: https://www.amnesty.nl/content/uploads/2016/12/debating_the_endtimes_of_human_rights.pdf [9 August 2020].

MAHLER, Anne Garland. (2018) *From the Tricontinental to the Global South: Race, Radicalism, and Transnational Solidarity* (Durham, NC: Duke University Press).

MANDER, Harsh. (2019) Employing the politics of solidarity against the rise of populism. *Open Global Rights*, 10 October. [Online]. Available: https://www.openglobalrights.org/employing-politics-of-solidarity-against-the-rise-of-populism/ [13 August 2020].

MOHANTY, Sobhi. (2020) From communal violence to lockdown hunger: Emergency responses by civil society networks in Delhi. *India. Interface: A Journal for and about Social Movements*, 12(1), 47–52.

NAY, Olivier. (2020) Can a virus undermine human rights? *The Lancet: Public Health*, 5(5), e238–e239. doi:10.1016/S2468-2667(20)30092-X

NEUMAN, Gerald L. (2020) Populist threats to the international human rights system. In *Human Rights in a Time of Populism: Challenges and Responses*, Gerald L. Neuman (ed.) (Cambridge, UK: Cambridge University Press).

NEW INDIAN EXPRESS. (2020) *India Made Fight against COVID-19 a People's Movement: PM Modi at Virtual UN Ecosoc Session*. [Online]. Available: https://www.newindianexpress.com/nation/2020/jul/17/india-made-fight-against-covid-19-a-peoples-movement-pm-modi-at-virtual-un-ecosoc-session-2171183.html [15 August 2020].

OKAFOR, Obiora C. (2020) Solidarity key to post COVID-19 response. *Open Global Rights*, 28 April. [Online]. Available: https://www.openglobalrights.org/solidarity-key-to-post-covid-19-response/ [13 August 2020].

OPENGLOBALRIGHTS. (n.d). *A Guide to Hope-Based Communications*. [Online]. https://www.openglobalrights.org/hope-guide/ [13 August 2020].

PIVEN, Frances Fox. (2014) Interdependent power: Strategizing for the Occupy movement. *Political Sociology*, 62(2), 223–231.

PRASAD, Vijay. (2020) *You Write Injustice on the Earth, We Will Write Revolution in the Skies.* [Online]. Available: https://mronline.org/2020/02/21/you-write-injustice-on-the-earth-we-will-write-revolution-in-the-skies/#lightbox/1/ [13 August 2020].

REZAIAN, Jason. (2020) In India, the pandemic is cover for Modi's war on journalists. *The Washington Post*, 1 June. [Online]. Available: https://www.washingtonpost.com/opinions/2020/06/01/india-pandemic-is-cover-modis-war-journalists/ [15 August 2020].

RODRÍGUEZ-GARAVITO, César, and GOMEZ, Krizna (eds.) (2018) *Rising to the Populist Challenge: A New Playbook for Human Rights Actors.* [Online]. Available https://www.dejusticia.org/wp-content/uploads/2018/04/Rising-to-the-populist-challenge_1.pdf [15 August 2020].

ROUTLEDGE, Paul, and CUMBERS, Andrew. (2013) *Global Justice Networks* (Manchester, UK: Manchester University Press).

SALVI, Puja. (2018) *Book Review: Reconciliation.* [Online]. Available: https://www.dnaindia.com/just-before-monday/review-book-review-reconciliation-2669675 [15 August 2020].

SATTERTHWAITE, Meg. (2020) In a world of radical inequality, solidarity is a cornerstone of justice. *Open Global Rights*, 13 February. [Online]. Available: https://www.openglobalrights.org/in-a-world-of-radical-inequality-solidarity-is-a-cornerstone-of-justice/ [13 August 2020].

SCHOLZ, Sally J. (2008) *Political Solidarity* (Philadelphia, PA: University of Pennsylvania Press).

SCHOLZ, Sally J. (2014) Solidarity as a human right. *Archiv Des Völkerrechts*, 52(1), 49–67. doi:10.1628/000389214X14056754359509

SCHRECKER, Ted, and BAMBRA, Clare. (2015) *How Politics Makes Us Sick: Neoliberal Epidemics* (New York, NY: Springer).

SIKKINK, Kathryn. (2018) *A Cautionary Note about the Frame of Peril and Crisis in Human Rights Activism.* [Online]. https://www.dejusticia.org/wp-content/uploads/2018/04/Rising-to-the-populist-challenge_1.pdf [13 August 2020].

SIKKINK, Kathryn. (2020) Solidarity key to post-COVID19 response. *Open Global Rights*, 28 April. [Online]. Available: https://www.openglobalrights.org/solidarity-key-to-post-covid-19-response/?lang=English [13 August 2020].

SYKES, Emerson. (2020) *How to Protest in a Pandemic.* [Online]. Available: https://www.aclu.org/news/free-speech/how-to-protest-in-a-pandemic/ [10 August 2020].

THE WIRE STAFF. (2020). *Delhi Riots Death Toll at 53, Here are the Names of the Victims.* [Online]. Available: https://thewire.in/communalism/delhi-riots-identities-deceased-confirmed [15 August 2020].

ULMER, Alexandra, and MIGLANI, Sanjeev. (2020) India's Coronavirus lockdown hits poor, tests Modi's support. *Reuters*, 3 April. [Online]. Available: https://www.reuters.com/article/us-health-coronavirus-india-modi/indias-coronavirus-lockdown-hits-poor-tests-modis-support-idUSKBN21L0ZH [13 August 2020].

UNITED NATIONS. (2020). *Urgent Debate of the Human Rights Council on 'the Current Racially Inspired Human Rights Violations, Systemic Racism, Police Brutality and the Violence against Peaceful Protest': Statement from the UN Special Rapporteur on Contemporary Forms of Racism, Racial Discrimination, Xenophobia and Related Intolerance, and The Working Group of Experts on People of African Descent. Joined by the Special Rapporteur on the Rights of Freedom of Assembly and Association, and the Coordination Committee of the UN Human Rights Special Procedures.* [Online]. Available: https://www.ohchr.org/EN/NewsEvents/Pages/DisplayNews.aspx?NewsID=25969&LangID=E [14 August 2020].

UN SPECIAL RAPPORTEUR ON EXTREME POVERTY AND HUMAN RIGHTS. (2018) *Report of the Special Rapporteur on Extreme Poverty and Human Rights on His Mission to the United States of America*, a/HRC/38/33/Add.1 (Geneva, Switzerland: United Nations).

WILDE, Lawrence. (2013) *Global Solidarity* (Edinburgh, Scotland: Edinburgh University Press).

Re-examining health

Global health and human rights in the time of COVID-19: Response, restrictions, and legitimacy

Lisa Forman and Jillian Clare Kohler

ABSTRACT
Policy responses to the COVID-19 pandemic have impacted a range of human rights, with the pandemic being used to justify police violence, authoritarian power grabs, and corruption. Health systems in high- and low-income countries have struggled to provide adequate COVID-19 testing, tracing, and treatment, with non-COVID-19 healthcare-restricted, vulnerable populations at high risk of infection and negative health and social impacts, and lockdowns exacerbating poverty, domestic violence, and mental health problems. If underresourced health systems are overwhelmed by COVID-19, and individuals are forced to bear testing and treatment costs, there is a stronger likelihood of health system failures, for higher mortality from a range of causes, and for people to be pushed further into poverty and insecurity. COVID-19 thus underscores the urgent need for clearer rules about legitimate restrictions of the right to health in responding to the pandemic, and for safeguarding global health policy initiatives in its aftermath. This article focuses on key right-to-health challenges, including realization of universal health coverage, and potential challenges in access to future COVID-19 therapies and vaccines. We conclude with reflections on what the pandemic may mean for the evolution of human rights, and the right to health in particular.

Introduction

Since the World Health Organization (WHO) proclaimed COVID-19 a pandemic in March 2020, almost all countries globally have introduced extraordinary and unprecedented legal and policy measures to combat the spread of SARS-CoV-2, the virus that causes COVID-19, including quarantines, emergency orders, extensive lockdowns, and travel restrictions. The impact on a range of human rights has been significant, with the pandemic being used to justify police violence, authoritarian power grabs, and corruption. Yet as a health crisis, this pandemic directly invokes the right to health in international human rights law and its specific protections regarding healthcare and the social determinants of health. Health systems in high-income countries have struggled to provide adequate COVID-19 testing, tracing, and treatment (Cousins 2020; Alonso-Zaldivar 2020), with non-COVID-19 healthcare-restricted (*RTL News* 2020), vulnerable populations at high risk of infection and negative health and social impacts, and lockdowns exacerbating poverty, domestic violence, and mental health problems (Human Rights Watch–India 2020; WHO 2020d; Forani 2020). Similar impacts are starting to be seen in low- and middle-income countries (LMIC) where COVID-19 infection rates are rising and will place significant pressures on clinical and public health systems already grappling with the challenge of realizing universal health coverage (UHC) under the Sustainable Development Goals (SGDs). These challenges are likely to intensify as we draw closer to an effective vaccine, making equitable domestic and global access to effective COVID-19 treatment and care a fundamental human rights challenge.

The right to health is an important framework for advancing more equitable COVID-19-related law and policy, both prescribing appropriate care and policy and delimiting restrictions of this right in service of public health. In this article, we first outline the relevance of right to health standards for related COVID-19 policy. We then focus on two key right to health challenges: COVID-19-related impacts on realization of the right to health and UHC, and potential challenges in access to future COVID-19 therapies and vaccines. We conclude with reflections on what the pandemic may mean for the evolution of human rights, and the right to health in particular.

Right to health standards and COVID-19

The extraordinary impact of COVID-19 on human rights underscores that all human rights are indivisible and interrelated (United Nations, 1993), and that health and human rights are inextricably intertwined (Mann, Gruskin, Grodin, and Annas 1999). These interconnections are evident in how race, income, age, and disability are proving to be key determinants of both COVID-19-related morbidity and mortality (Public Health Ontario 2020) and of the disproportionate enforcement of COVID-19 policies on such groups (Human Rights Watch–India 2020; allAfrica 2020; Morales and Joseph 2020; Alindogan 2020). This recognition underscores the recognition of the WHO (2020a), the United Nations (UN Office of the High Commission for Human Rights 2020), and the Council of Europe for Human Rights (2020), among others, that a human rights approach is crucial to an effective public health response to COVID-19.

The standards of the right to health hold particular importance for effective pandemic care and responses. The most authoritative form of this right is found in the *International Covenant on Economic, Social and Cultural Rights* (ICESCR), a treaty ratified by a majority of states globally (UN Office of the High Commission for Human Rights n.d.). Article 12 of the ICESCR recognizes "the right of everyone to the enjoyment of the highest attainable standard of physical and mental health," and elaborates steps to be taken to fully achieve this right include to prevent, treat, and control epidemics and other diseases and to assure medical services for all in the event of sickness (ICESCR 1976). These duties have obvious significance for state responses to COVID-19. Indeed, the UN Committee on Economic, Social and Cultural Rights (the Committee) specifically elaborated these duties in relation to infectious disease outbreaks to include creating systems of "urgent medical care in cases of … epidemics and similar health hazards," and requiring states to use "technologies, epidemiological surveillance and data collection, immunization programmes and other strategies of infectious disease control" (UN Committee on Economic, Social, and Cultural Rights 2000: para. 16). Similarly relevant to COVID-19 is the general right to health duty to ensure access to available, accessible, acceptable, and good-quality health facilities, goods, and services, and to provide the underlying determinants of health such as safe and potable water, sanitation, food, housing, health-related information and education, and gender equality (paras. 11–12). Although state duties under the ICESCR are generally limited to taking steps to progressively realize rights to the maximum of available resources (ICESCR 1976), states also hold core obligations to ensure the satisfaction of, "at the very least, minimum essential levels" of treaty rights. These core obligations include nondiscriminatory access to health facilities, goods, and services; essential drugs, as defined by the WHO; and adopting and implementing a national public health strategy and plan of action addressing the health concerns of the whole population, with particular attention to vulnerable or marginalized groups (UN Committee on Economic, Social and Cultural Rights 2000: para. 43).

In April 2020, the Committee issued a statement applying these duties to the emerging pandemic, emphasizing that in "responding to the pandemic, the inherent dignity of all people must be respected and protected, and minimum core obligations imposed by the Covenant should be prioritized" (UN Committee on Economic, Social and Cultural Rights 2020: para. 12). In other words, efforts to realize universal, nondiscriminatory, and affordable access to COVID-19-related healthcare and social determinants of health should be prioritized in government responses. This interpretation is reinforced in the statement that emphasizes that states must "adopt appropriate regulatory measures to ensure that health-care resources in both the public and the private sectors are mobilized and shared among the whole population to ensure a comprehensive, coordinated health-care response to the crisis" (UN Committee on Economic, Social and Cultural Rights 2020: para. 21). Moreover, states must "devote their maximum available resources for the full realization of all economic, social and cultural rights, including the right to health … [and] mobilize the necessary resources to combat COVID-19 in the most equitable manner, in order to avoid imposing a further economic burden on these marginalized groups" (para. 14).

These duties suggest, at a minimum, that states must provide free or affordable essential COVID-19-related healthcare (including COVID-19 testing, tracing, and treatment), protect healthcare workers from infections through adequate and effective protective personal equipment (PPE), and work to advance toward an effective treatment and/or vaccine. The right to health also suggests mitigating the negative impacts of COVID-19 infections on vulnerable populations (such as women, children, the elderly, people with disabilities, and prisoners), and mitigating the impact of broader policy responses on food, water, housing and sanitation (Forman, Ooms, and Brolan 2015; Forman, Beiersmann, Brolan, McKee, Hammonds, and Ooms 2016).

Key right to health challenges

We foresee two major emerging challenges in the broader impacts on realization of the right to health, and around equitable access to an eventual vaccine.

COVID-19-related impacts on the right to health

The pandemic has ushered in virtually unprecedented legal and policy measures to control its spread, which have considerably restricted rights to free movement, privacy, and economic activity. Yet many such measures are not of limited duration, proportionate, necessary, or nondiscriminatory, as required by the *Siracusa Principles.*[1] Indeed, some governments have used the pandemic as a pretext to grab power, use excessive force, and harass vulnerable populations, with these impacts often disproportionately experienced by poor, racialized, and marginalized people. For example, in South Africa and Kenya, people were killed when police used live ammunition to disperse crowds and exerted disproportionate force to enforce lockdowns (Human Rights Watch–India 2020; allAfrica 2020). In the United States, a reported 80 percent of social distancing summonses in New York City were issued to people of color (Morales and Joseph 2020). And in the Philippines, more than 100,000 people have been cited and 50,000 arrested under lockdown enforcement (Alindogan 2020).

These are troubling trends, as emergency laws once introduced can become fixtures, and there has been a global trend away from democracy and rights for more than a decade (Freedom House 2019). Yet there is considerably less focus in the media and human rights scholarship on the extent to which the right to health can be restricted in service of public health or emergencies. In addition, there is a paradox in restricting access to healthcare in service of a public health imperative like COVID-19 when state duties to provide healthcare arguably become more rather than less important. Evidence from the Ebola epidemic in West Africa underscores that measures like quarantine can weaken health systems and restrict rights to essential healthcare (e.g., basic maternal services; Shannon, Horace-Kwemi, Najjemba, Owiti, Edwards, Shringarpure, Bhat, and Kateh 2017), shelter, food, and water (Meier, Evans, and Phelan 2020). Evidence of similar impacts during COVID-19 is emerging from Uganda (Center for Health, Human Rights, and Development 2020), Kenya (Odhiambo 2020), and Nigeria (Adepoju 2020).

Yet extant human rights standards do not directly or adequately address such restrictions of the right to health. For one thing, the *Siracusa Principles* were drafted to address the civil and political rights contained in the International Covenant on Civil and Political Rights (ICCPR) rather than those in the ICESCR, and these treaties have different limitations provisions. Nor were these principles specifically drafted to address a health crisis, albeit that public health is a recognized ground on which to limit certain ICCPR rights. Yet the *Principles* say little about public health, other than indicating that its invocation must be restricted to serious threats to individual or population health, and be specifically aimed at preventing disease or injury or providing care for the sick and injured (UN Commission on Human Rights 1984). The Committee has not provided sufficient guidance in its interpretation of the right to health as to how public health restrictions should apply to the right to health and to health needs falling within core obligations, or of the varying standards of scrutiny that should attach to such restrictions (UN Committee on Economic, Social and Cultural Rights 2000: paras. 28–29). This absence belies the extent to which COVID-19 lockdowns take into account restrictions on the right to health, including core obligations such as nondiscrimination. These impacts are likely to be amplified if the pandemic generates austerity cutbacks like those adopted in high- and low-income countries alike after the 2008 financial crisis.[2]

There seems considerable cause to be concerned about how the pandemic will impact the roll-out of UHC and its right to health synergistic ambition of ensuring “financial risk protection, access to quality essential health-care services, and access to safe, effective, quality, and affordable essential medicines and vaccines for all” (UN General Assembly 2015). UHC is an important policy focus for governments to strengthen their health systems and for people globally to realize their rights to access affordable good quality healthcare.[3] Yet UHC had, in important respects, already been going in the wrong direction before the pandemic, with insufficient domestic and international health financing (World Bank 2019) and catastrophic health expenditures continuously growing since 2000 (WHO 2019). If underresourced health systems are being overwhelmed by COVID-19 and individuals are forced to bear testing and treatment costs, there is a stronger likelihood of health system failures, for higher mortality from a range of causes, and for people to be pushed further into poverty and insecurity. COVID-19 thus underscores the urgent need for clearer rules about legitimate restrictions of the right to health in responding to the pandemic, and for safeguarding global health policy initiatives in its aftermath. The United States’ recent proclamation that it will withdraw from the WHO only adds fuel to the global health and human rights crisis the pandemic may usher in.

Access to vaccines

One of the most important right-to-health questions unleashed by COVID-19 is how to ensure equitable access of the global population to forthcoming COVID-19 treatments and vaccines, which will invoke core state obligations to provide access to essential medicines. Here, we need to consider fundamental right-to-health questions related to affordability, resource allocations, and accountability. The COVID-19 crisis underscores the importance of ensuring everyone’s right to access affordable needed therapies and vaccines, and of bypassing the usual pricing barriers that new medicines face when entering the market. As we have seen in past pandemics (such as with HIV/AIDS) and in treatments for diseases from cancer to diabetes, public need for essential therapies can raise significant policy dilemmas regarding public health, equity, and human rights, on the one hand, and corporate pricing, intellectual property rights, and trade agreements, on the others (Forman and Kohler 2012). Equally important, we need to identify and mitigate against barriers to equitable access. Here, we will focus on these possible barriers: corruption, nationalism and attendant trade restrictions, and pricing.

Corruption

Corruption is defined by Transparency International (2020) as, "the abuse of entrusted power for private gain." Corruption in the health sector results in lives lost and public monies wasted, and creates barriers to healthcare services and products for the most vulnerable and marginalized members of a population. Human rights bodies and scholars recognize corruption as an "enormous obstacle to the realization of all human rights" (UN Human Rights Council 2015), and to the right to health in particular, because of how it undercuts the availability of resources upon which realization of the right to health depends.[4] Recent health crises have illuminated how corruption can emerge in the health system and undercut critical responses to emergencies, as was the case with Ebola virus disease (EVD) in Sierra Leone and other countries in West Africa. The EVD crisis demanded quick and nimble responses from the international community that was in many ways learning how to respond to EVD. Sierra Leone, as one example, was the beneficiary of a significant amount of international aid that was provided to UN agencies, NGOs, and other entities to help the government combat the EVD. Yet the Audit Service of Sierra Leone detailed in a 2014 report that there was a lack of documentation for the payment of US$3.3 million from the government of Sierra Leone's Ebola accounts, and that US$2.5 million in disbursements had incomplete documentation. The report also included many examples of apparent fraud and corruption in the procurement of supplies and Ebola response worker payments.

In the midst of this COVID-19 pandemic, as we experienced with the EVD, the health systems vulnerabilities to corruption are clear. Examples of corruption have been found globally in drug and medical equipment procurement and price gouging of essential supplies, such as hand sanitizer and 3M masks (Radio Canada International 2020). The European Medicines Agency (EMA) and the WHO have both issued public warnings about the increase in the circulation of falsified medicines (EMA 2020). The risk of falsified medicines is not only for those products that may potentially treat COVID-19 but also for other drugs and products, particularly when shortages exist (UN Office on Drugs and Crime 2020). Newton and Bond (2020) explained that the circulation of substandard and falsified products is heightened when shortages are taking place and quality assurance standards are lax. They advanced the importance of information-sharing among countries to ensure that global demand and supplies are being met and noted that countries need to ensure sufficient regulatory controls. They also pointed out that this will be even more critical once valid COVID-19 treatments are available.

Governments and health institutions are also under pressure to purchase and import quickly needed medical equipment and supplies for COVID-19 through emergency procurement processes. The Organisation for Economic Co-operation and Development (OECD) has reported a number of bribery cases in the health industry and the risk of the purchase of inferior or falsified goods (OECD 2020). Furthermore, when there is weak or nonexistent recordkeeping when emergency procurement processes are invoked, anticorruption mechanisms—such as audits, inspections, or investigations—are limited in terms of what they can investigate.

There is also worrisome political pressure on regulatory agencies to allow the entry of unproven treatments into the market. A case in point is the use of hydroxychloroquine, which was granted an emergency use authorization (EUA) for off-label use in the United States despite limited observational and clinical trials efficacy data, risking harm to both patients and public confidence in the pandemic response. This is particularly dangerous when an EUA is mistaken by the public as FDA approval, as was the case during a media briefing by President Trump, Vice President Pence, and members of the Coronavirus Task Force (Goodman and Borio 2020).

Vaccine nationalism and trade restrictions as a barrier

The second barrier to equitable access is vaccine nationalism (and attendant trade restrictions) or a "my nation first" approach to the production and distribution of vaccines or other pharmaceutical treatment related to COVID-19. Such approaches undercut the promise of economic, social, and cultural rights like health because they undermine states' willingness to engage in international cooperation and assistance to achieve their realization (ICESCR 1976).

There are bountiful examples of how national interests are superseding a globally coordinated response. For example, Sanofi's CEO expressed that the United States "has the right to the largest pre-order," given the company had signed an agreement with the US Biomedical Advanced Research and Development Authority (BARDA; Weintraub, Bitton, and Rosenberg 2020). In another example, the Serum Institute India, the world's largest producer of vaccine doses, issued a statement that the majority of its products "would have to go to our countrymen before it goes abroad" (Weintraub et al. 2020). Finally, US Operation Warp Speed is an America-first vaccine policy that rejects international cooperation in an effort to advance research and development of a vaccine for people in the United States (Cohen 2020).

Vaccine nationalism, albeit, is not a new phenomenon. During the H1N1 outbreak, high-income countries secured large advance orders for the vaccine for their own populations. The vaccine was thus distributed commensurate with a country's purchasing power rather than its public health needs (Human Rights Watch–India 2020; allAfrica 2020; Morales and Joseph 2020; Alindogan 2020).

In April 2020, the World Economic Forum reported that 59 World Trade Organization members did not report their restrictions on exports, breaking trade regulations. As many as 80 countries/custom territories banned or limited exports of medical supplies critical for the COVID-19 pandemic, including face masks, personal protective gear (PPE), and gloves (Shalal 2020). Global health systems depend largely on imports for essential medical supplies. For example, China is a major global supplier of PPE, India of generic medicines, and Malaysia of gloves (Tripathi 2020). In April 2020, Canada had to deal with a critical PPE shortage, given that trade restrictions from as many as 68 countries curbed exports of PPE and, what is more, with supply shortages, prices rose significantly (Reynolds 2020). Export restrictions that countries implement to secure domestic stockpiles can create not only supply shortages but also opportunities for corruption to thrive. Shortages of critical supplies can result in price gouging and may incentivize the production and entry into the marketplace of products that may be falsified and substandard in quality, if appropriate oversight is not in place.

Pricing as a barrier

Pre-COVID-19, fair pricing of medicines was a major global policy concern. Today, its import remains. The 2020 WHO Fair Pricing Milestones identified financial sensitivity in health systems and incentivising pharmaceuticals' research and development as two key policy areas requiring further study (WHO 2020e). Pricing of therapies and vaccines for the treatment and prevention of COVID-19 will remain a key public health concern as treatments and vaccines for COVID-19 become available. Already, Médecins Sans Frontières (MSF) is advocating for governments to ensure that the pharmaceutical industry prices any future COVID-19 vaccines at cost. GAVI, the Vaccine Alliance, is seeking to implement a global mechanism that will aim to negotiate fair prices of vaccines with manufacturers in an effort to recognize the nature of a vaccine as a global public good (MSF 2020). On March 31, 2020, the Medicines Patent Pool broadened its voluntary licensing mechanism mandate to include, at least in the short term, all possible health technologies that may help with the global COVID-19 response (Medicines Patent Pool 2020).

In the United States, congressional leaders are advancing a pathbreaking policy on COVID-19 drug pricing that is rejecting any manufacturer exclusivity for vaccine, drug, or therapeutic products; rejecting any pricing of a COVID-19 therapy or vaccine at an unreasonable price; and demanding transparency of the true costs involved in a product's research and development, manufacturing, and regulatory approval (Schakowsky 2020). As the pharmaceutical industry seeks to repurpose existing drugs for the treatment of COVID-19, fair pricing will again be absolutely critical to ensuring global equity and access to products. Gilead has pledged to donate Remdesivir to the United States government until its current supply chain is exhausted, but has not specified its pricing plan (Lui 2020). Johnson & Johnson, on the other hand, has committed to supply eventual COVID-19 vaccines on a no-profit basis at an estimated cost of $10 per dose (McConaghie 2020). Of course, time will tell if this pledge is honored.

Positively as many as 165 countries to date have expressed interest in the newly created COVAX Facility, which aims to ensure the "fair and equitable access to COVID-19 vaccines worldwide" (WHO 2020c). Yet if access to a COVID vaccine becomes constrained by price, nationalist hoarding, or misallocated resources, it is likely that, as with antiretrovirals, human rights strategies such as litigation and mobilization may prove critical interventions in the fight for affordable and accessible medicines and vaccines.

Conclusion

Human rights continue to offer standards, principles, and rules that could center equity and vulnerable populations in COVID-19-related law, policy, and practice, and offer key protections to challenge inequities in these domains. At the same time, the sheer scale of the pandemic will test the capacity of the current standards and rules of the international human rights law system to withstand the pressures of a global pandemic of this nature. We may need to rethink the parameters of necessity and proportionality when it comes to legitimate restrictions of rights in service of public health. We may also need to reinforce the until-now relatively understated rules and standards within international human rights law that promote global solidarity in the context of crises like COVID-19, particularly when it comes to global access to a future vaccine. Human rights may offer tools to address COVID-19, but the pandemic is already underscoring that these are tools that need updating and revision if they are to effectively address the emerging right-to-health and global health challenges of our age.

Notes

1. The *Siracusa Principles* are a set of criteria created by human rights experts to guide policymakers in what constitutes legitimate restrictions of human rights.
2. For a related discussion, see Nolan (2014: 2–3), Cummins (2013: i), and Kyrili and Martin (2010: 38).
3. For a related discussion, see WHO (2012, 2013: 5); Norheim (2015: 712); and Ooms, Abdul Latif, Waris, Hammonds, Friedman, Brolan, and Forman (2014: 1-7).
4. For a related discussion, see Durojayé and Mirugi-Mukundi (2012: 3–6) and Toebes (2009: 102–134).

References

ADEPOJU, Paul. (2020) Tuberculosis and HIV responses threatened by COVID-19. *The Lancet*, 7(3), 319–320.

ALINDOGAN, Jamela. (2020) *HRW: COVID-19 Lockdown Violators in Philippines Abused.* [Online]. Available: https://www.aljazeera.com/news/2020/04/hrw-covid-19-lockdown-violators-philippines-abused-200429080703660.html [13 August 2020].

ALLAFRICA. (2020) *Uganda: Police Shoot Two on Bodaboda for Defying Museveni COVID-19 order.* [Online]. Available: https://allafrica.com/stories/202003300087.html [14 August 2020].

ALONSO-ZALDIVAR, Rocardo. (2020) *U.S. Faces 'Truly Daunting' Challenges on Needed COVID Tests.* [Online]. Available: https://www.ctvnews.ca/health/coronavirus/u-s-faces-truly-daunting-challenges-on-needed-covid-tests-1.4929649 [13 August 2020].

AUDIT SERVICE OF SIERRA LEONE. (2014) *Report on the Audit of the Management of Ebola Funds.* [Online]. Available: https://reliefweb.int/report/sierra-leone/audit-service-sierra-leone-report-audit-management-ebola-funds-may-october-2014 [13 August 2020].

CENTER FOR HEALTH, HUMAN RIGHTS, AND DEVELOPMENT. (2020) *Sexual Reproductive Health and COVID-19 in Uganda: Avoiding the Pitfalls of Unintended Consequences for Maternal, Newborn, Child, Adolescent, and Nutrition Health in the National Response.* [Online]. Available: https://www.jasprogramme.ug/publication/sexual-reproductive-health-and-covid-19-in-uganda-avoiding-the-pitfalls-of-unintended-consequences [13 August 2020].

COHEN, Jon. (2020) *Unveiling 'Warp Speed,' the White House's America-First Push for a Coronavirus Vaccine.* [Online]. Available: https://www.sciencemag.org/news/2020/05/unveiling-warp-speed-white-house-s-america-first-push-coronavirus-vaccine [14 August 2020].

COUNCIL OF EUROPE FOR HUMAN RIGHTS. (2020) *Learning from the Pandemic to Better Fulfill the Right to Health.* [Online]. Available: https://www.coe.int/en/web/commissioner/-/learning-from-the-pandemic-to-better-fulfil-the-right-to-health [13 August 2020].

COUSINS, Ben. (2020) *Lack of Resources Led to Limited COVID-19 Testing, but New Options Are on the Way.* [Online]. Available: https://www.ctvnews.ca/health/coronavirus/lack-of-resources-led-to-limited-covid-19-testing-but-new-options-are-on-the-way-1.4891161 [13 August 2020].

CUMMINS, Isabel Ortiz Matthew. (2013) *The Age of Austerity: A Review of Public Expenditures and Adjustment Measures in 181 Countries. Isabel Initiative for Policy Dialogue and the South Centre Working Paper* (Geneva, Switzerland: The South Centre).

DUROJAYÉ, Ebenezer, and MIRUGI-MUKUNDI, Gladys. (2012) The implications of corruption for the enjoyment of the right to health in Africa. *ESR Review*, 13(3), 3–6.

EUROPEAN MEDICINES AGENCY (EMA). (2020) *COVID-19: Beware of Falsified Medicines from Unregistered Websites.* [Online]. Available: https://www.ema.europa.eu/en/news/covid-19-beware-falsified-medicines-unregistered-websites [13 August 2020].

FORANI, Jonathan. (2020) *Half of Canadians Report Worsening Mental Health, Experts Say Woes Just Beginning.* [Online]. Available: https://www.ctvnews.ca/health/coronavirus/half-of-canadians-report-worsening-mental-health-experts-say-woes-just-beginning-1.4913642 [13 August 2020].

FORMAN, Lisa, BEIERSMANN, Claudia, BROLAN, Claire E., MCKEE, Martin, HAMMONDS, Rachel, and OOMS, Gorik. (2016) What do core obligations under the right to health bring to universal health coverage? *Health and Human Rights Journal*, 18(2), 23–34.

FORMAN, Lisa, and KOHLER, Jillian Clare. (2012) *Access to Medicines as a Human Right: Implications for Pharmaceutical Industry Responsibility* (Toronto, ON: University of Toronto Press).

FORMAN, Lisa, OOMS, Gorik, and BROLAN, Claire E. (2015) Rights language in the Sustainable Development Agenda: Has right to health discourse and norms shaped health goals? *International Journal of Health Policy and Management*, 4(12), 799–804. doi:10.15171/ijhpm.2015.171

FREEDOM HOUSE. (2019) *Freedom in the World: 2019 Democracy in Retreat.* [Online]. Available: https://freedomhouse.org/report/freedom-world/freedom-world-2019/democracy-in-retreat [13 August 2020].

GOODMAN, Jesse L., and BORIO, Luciana. (2020) Finding effective treatments for COVID-19: Scientific integrity and public confidence in a time of crisis. *Journal of the American Medical Association*, 323(19), 1899–1900. doi: 10.1001/jama.2020.6434

HUMAN RIGHTS WATCH–INDIA. (2020) *COVID-19 Lockdown Puts Poor at Risk.* [Online]. Available: https://www.hrw.org/news/2020/03/27/india-covid-19-lockdown-puts-poor-risk [13 August 2020].

INTERNATIONAL COVENANT ON ECONOMIC, SOCIAL, AND CULTURAL RIGHTS (ICESCR). (1976) *G.A. Res. 2200A (XXI), 21 U.N. GAOR Supp. (No. 16) at 49,* U.N. Doc. A/6316 (1966), *993* U.N.T.S. 3, entered into force 3 January 1976, article 12.1, and 12.2.d and c (New York, NY: United Nations).

KYRILI, Katerina, and MARTIN, Matthew. (2010) *The Impact of the Global Economic Crisis on the Budgets of Low-Income Countries.* [Online]. Available: https://www.oxfam.de/system/files/the_impact_of_the_economic_crisis_on_the_budget_of_low-income_countries.pdf [13 August 2020].

LUI, Angus. (2020) *Fair Price for Gilead's COVID-19 Med Remdesivir? $4,460, Cost Watchdog Says.* [Online]. Available: https://www.fiercepharma.com/marketing/gilead-s-covid-19-therapy-remdesivir-worth-4-460-per-course-says-pricing-watchdog [13 August 2020].

MANN, Jonathan, GRUSKIN, Sofia, GRODIN, Michael A., and ANNAS George J. (1999) *Health and Human Rights: A Reader* (New York, NY: Routledge).

MCCONAGHIE, Andrew. (2020) *COVID-19 Vaccine Could Cost as Little as $10 a Dose, Says Janssen.* [Online]. Available: https://scrip.pharmaintelligence.informa.com/SC141970/COVID19-Vaccine-Could-Cost-As-Little-As-10-A-Dose-Says-Janssen?mod=article_inline. [13 August 2020].

MÉDECINS SANS FRONTIÈRES (MSF). (2020) *MSF: Any Future COVID-19 Vaccines Must Be Sold at Cost and Accessible to All.* [Online]. Available: https://msfaccess.org/msf-any-future-covid-19-vaccines-must-be-sold-cost-and-accessible-all [13 August 2020].

MEDICINES PATENT POOL. (2020) *COVID-19.* [Online]. Available: https://medicinespatentpool.org/what-we-do/our-work/covid-19/ [13 August 2020].

MEIER, Benjamin Mason, EVANS, Dabney P., and PHELAN, Alexandra. (2020) Rights-based approaches to preventing, detecting, and responding to infectious disease outbreaks. In *Infectious Diseases in the New Millennium: Legal and Ethical Challenges,* Mark Eccleston-Turner and Iain Brassington (eds.) (Cham, Switzerland: Springer).

MORALES, Mark, and JOSEPH, Elizabeth. (2020) *Blacks and Latinos are Overwhelmingly Ticketed by NYPD for Social Distancing Violations.* [Online]. Available: https://www.cnn.com/2020/05/08/us/social-distancing-stats-nyc/index.html [13 August 2020].

NEWTON, Paul N., and BOND, Katherine C. (2020) COVID-19 and risks to the supply and quality of tests, drugs, and vaccines. *The Lancet Global Health,* 8(6), e754–e755. doi:10.1016/S2214-109X(20)30136-4

NOLAN, Aoife. (2014) *Economic and Social Rights After the Global Financial Crisis* (Cambridge, UK: Cambridge University Press).

NORHEIM, Ole Frithjof. (2015) Ethical perspective: Five unacceptable trade-offs on the path to universal health coverage. *International Journal of Health Policy Management,* 4(11), 711–714. doi:10.15171/ijhpm.2015.184

ODHIAMBO, Agnes. (2020) *Tackling Kenya's Domestic Violence Amid Covid-19 Crisis.* [Online]. Available: https://www.hrw.org/news/2020/04/08/tackling-kenyas-domestic-violence-amid-covid-19-crisis [13 August 2020].

OOMS, Gorik, ABDUL LATIF, Laila, WARIS, Attiya, HAMMONDS, Rachel, FRIEDMAN, Eric E., BROLAN, Claire E., and FORMAN, Lisa. (2014) Is 'universal health coverage' the practical expression of the right to health? *BMC International Health and Human Rights,* 14(3), 1–7. doi:10.1186/1472-698X-14-3

ORGANISATION FOR ECONOMIC CO-OPERATION AND DEVELOPMENT (OECD). (2020) *Policy Measures to Avoid Corruption and Bribery in the COVID-19 Response and Recovery.* [Onine]. Available: https://read.oecd-ilibrary.org/view/?ref=133_133216-hn3bqtlvkw&title=Policy-measures-to-avoid-corruption-and-bribery-in-the-COVID-19-response-and-recovery [13 August 2020].

PUBLIC HEALTH ONTARIO. (2020) *Synopsis: COVID-19—What We Know so far About … Social Determinants of Health.* [Online]. Available: https://www.publichealthontario.ca/-/media/documents/ncov/covid-wwksf/2020/05/what-we-know-social-determinants-health.pdf?la=en [13 August 2020].

RADIO CANADA INTERNATIONAL. (2020) *COVID-19: Company Charged for Price Gouging During Pandemic.* [Online]. Available: https://www.rcinet.ca/en/2020/05/12/covid-19-company-charged-for-price-gouging-during-pandemic/ [27 July 2020].

REYNOLDS, Christopher. (2020). *Coronavirus: Canada Looks to Secure PPE, but 68 Countries have Restricted Exports.* [Online.] Available: https://globalnews.ca/news/6769162/canada-medical-supplies-coronavirus/ [14 August 2020].

RTL NEWS. (2020) *Judge Rorbids Abortion Pill by Mail Despite Corona Crisis.* [Online]. Available: https://www.rtlnieuws.nl/nieuws/nederland/artikel/5088361/corona-maatregelen-quarantaine-abortus-pil-post-rechter [13 August 2020].

SCHAKOWSKY, Jan. (2020) *Congressional Progressive Leaders Announce Principles on COVID-19 Drug Pricing for Next Coronavirus.* [Online]. Available: https://schakowsky.house.gov/media/press-releases/congressional-progressive-leaders-announce-principles-covid-19-drug-pricing [13 August 2020].

SHALAL, Andrea. (2020) *80 Countries Are Hoarding Medical Supplies—Here's Why It Damages the Global Response to COVID-19.* [Online]. Available: https://www.weforum.org/agenda/2020/04/wto-report-80-countries-limiting-exports-medical-supplies [14 August 2020].

SHANNON, Fulton Q., HORACE-KEWMI, Elizabeth, NAJJEMBA, Robinah, OWITI, Philip, EDWARDS, Jeffrey, SHRINGAPURE, Kalpita, BHAT, P., and KATEH, Frances. (2017) Effects of the 2014 Ebola outbreak on antenatal care and delivery outcomes in Liberia: A nationwide analysis. *International Union Against Tuberculosis and Lung Disease*, 7(1), S88–S93.

TOEBES, Brigit. (2009) Human rights and health sector corruption. In *Global Health and Human Rights: Legal and Philosophical Perspectives*, John Harrington and Maria Stuttaford (eds.) (Oxford, UK: Routledge).

TRANSPARENCY INTERNATIONAL. (2020) *What is Corruption?* [Online]. Available: https://www.transparency.org/en/what-is-corruption [13 August 2020].

TRIPATHI, Salil. (2020) *The World Needs to Change How It Trades Drugs*. [Online]. Available: https://foreignpolicy.com/2020/04/21/trading-drugs-during-coronavirus-pandemic/ [13 August 2020].

UNITED NATIONS. (1993) *Vienna Declaration and Programme of Action*, adopted by the World Conference on Human Rights, 25 June (Geneva, Switzerland: United Nations).

UN COMMISSION ON HUMAN RIGHTS. (1984) *The Siracusa Principles on the Limitation and Derogation Provisions in the International Covenant on Civil and Political Rights*. UN Doc. E/CN.4/1985/4. [Online]. Available: https://www.refworld.org/docid/4672bc122.html [22 July 2020].

UN COMMITTEE ON ECONOMIC, SOCIAL, AND CULTURAL RIGHTS. (2000) *General Comment No. 14 (2000): The Right to the Highest Attainable Standard of Health*. UN Doc. E/C.12/2000/4, 11 (See General Comment 14) (Geneva, Switzerland: United Nations).

UN COMMITTEE ON ECONOMIC, SOCIAL AND CULTURAL RIGHTS. (2020) *Statement on the Coronavirus Disease (COVID-19) Pandemic and Economic, Social and Cultural rights*. UN Doc. E/C.12/2020/1 (See Para. 12) (Geneva, Switzerland: United Nations).

UN GENERAL ASSEMBLY. (2015) *Transforming Our World: The 2030 Agenda for Sustainable Development*. [Online]. Available: http://unctad.org/meetings/en/SessionalDocuments/ares70d1_en.pdf [13 August 2020].

UN HUMAN RIGHTS COUNCIL. (2015) *Final Report of the Human Rights Council Advisory Committee on the Issue of the Negative Impact of Corruption on the Enjoyment of Human Rights, Assembly UNG, ed.* UN Doc. A/HRC/28/73 (Geneva, Switzerland: United Nations).

UN OFFICE OF THE HIGH COMMISSION FOR HUMAN RIGHTS. (n.d.) *170 Countries Have Ratified the ICESCR*. [Online]. Available: https://indicators.ohchr.org [13 August 2020].

UN OFFICE OF THE HIGH COMMISSION FOR HUMAN RIGHTS. (2020) *UN Human Rights Treaty Bodies Call for Human Rights Approach in Fighting COVID-19*. [Online]. Available: https://www.ohchr.org/EN/NewsEvents/Pages/DisplayNews.aspx?NewsID=25742 [13 August 2020].

UN OFFICE ON DRUGS AND CRIME. (2020) *COVID-19-Related Trafficking of Medical Products as a Threat to Public Health, 2020*. [Online]. Available: https://www.unodc.org/documents/data-and-analysis/covid/COVID-19_research_brief_trafficking_medical_products.pdf [13 August 2020].

WEINTRAUB, Rebecca, BITTON, Asaf, and ROSENBERG, Mark L. (2020) *The Danger of Vaccine Nationalism*. [Online]. Available: https://hbr.org/2020/05/the-danger-of-vaccine-nationalism [13 August 2020].

WORLD BANK. (2019) *High-Performance Health Financing for Universal Health Coverage: Driving Sustainable, Inclusive Growth in the 21st Century*. [Online]. Available: http://documents.worldbank.org/curated/en/641451561043585615/pdf/Driving-Sustainable-Inclusive-Growth-in-the-21st-Century.pdf [13 August 2020].

WORLD HEALTH ORGANIZATION (WHO). (2020a) *Addressing Human Rights as Key to the COVID-19 Response*. [Online]. Available: https://www.who.int/publications-detail/addressing-human-rights-as-key-to-the-covid-19-response [13 August 2020].

WORLD HEALTH ORGANIZATION (WHO). (2020b) *Medical Product Alert N°3/2020*. [Online]. Available: https://www.who.int/news-room/detail/31-03-2020-medical-product-alert-n-3-2020 [13 August 2020].

WORLD HEALTH ORGANIZATION (WHO). (2020c) *More than 150 Countries Engaged in COVID-19 Vaccine Global Access Facility*. [Online]. Available: https://www.who.int/news-room/detail/15-07-2020-more-than-150-countries-engaged-in-covid-19-vaccine-global-access-facility [21 July 2020].

WORLD HEALTH ORGANIZATION (WHO). (2020d) *COVID-19: Responding Quickly to the Wave of Domestic Violence*. [Online]. Available: https://unric.org/nl/covid-19-snel-reageren-op-de-golf-van-huiselijk-geweld-who-europa/ [13 August 2020].

WORLD HEALTH ORGANIZATION (WHO). (2020e) *WHO Fair Pricing Forum, 2020–21: Milestones*. Available: https://www.who.int/medicines/access/fair_pricing/2020FairPricingWorkplan.pdf?ua=1 [13 August 2020].

WORLD HEALTH ORGANIZATION (WHO). (2019) *Primary Health Care on the Road to Universal Health Coverage: 2019 Global Monitoring Report*. [Online]. Available: https://www.who.int/docs/default-source/documents/2019-uhc-report.pdf [13 August 2020].

WORLD HEALTH ORGANIZATION (WHO). (2013) *The World Health Report 2013: Research for Universal Health Coverage*. [Online]. Available: https://www.who.int/whr/2013/report/en/ [13 August 2020].

WORLD HEALTH ORGANIZATION (WHO). (2012) *Positioning Health in the Post-2015 Development Agenda*. [Online]. Available: https://www.who.int/topics/millennium_development_goals/post2015/WHOdiscussionpaper_October2012.pdf?ua=1 [13 August 2020].

Human rights obligations of drug companies

Michael Santoro and Robert Shanklin

ABSTRACT
This article addresses the human rights obligations of pharmaceutical companies regarding access to vaccines and other drugs developed to prevent and treat COVID-19, and more broadly regarding access to essential medicines. We examine two United Nations guidelines–the Guiding Principles on Business and Human Rights and the Human Rights Guidelines for Pharmaceutical Companies in relation to Access to Medicines–which assert that pharmaceutical companies have human rights responsibilities to make essential medicines available to patients in the global South, and that member-states are responsible for enforcing these obligations. We develop a moral theory that justifies such human rights duties based on the idea of a "social contract" that more broadly underpins the idea of corporate social responsibility. We conclude by offering practical advice enabling pharmaceutical companies to balance their human rights duties to the global South with their responsibilities to shareholders and the need to sustainably incentivize drug discovery.

COVID-19 and HIV/AIDS: Renewed human rights concerns for the global South

The COVID-19 global pandemic has raised anew human rights concerns that last erupted on the world stage during the HIV/AIDS crisis roughly three decades ago. Once again there are uncertainties and worries about access to and the affordability of life-saving medications for poor patients, particularly in the Global South. Back then, the private sector developed a number of significant antiretroviral therapies treatments to treat HIV/AIDS patients. To this day, there is no vaccine to protect against HIV/AIDS, owing to the rapid and nimble mutation of the virus. Thus, treatment with antiretrovirals rather than vaccination has become the medical standard of care.

Relying on recently enacted World Trade Organization patent protections, the pharmaceutical industry set off a global human rights firestorm by pricing those drugs out of reach for citizens in the Global South, where the virus impacted most tragically. At one point the industry was so tone deaf that it took the unusual step of suing Nelson Mandela in a South African court to assert patent rights. It took almost a decade of global protests, litigation, public shaming, and competition from mostly India-based low-cost generic manufacturers to finally bring the pharmaceutical industry to a reasonable compromise position in which profits and the need for financial incentives to spur innovation were appropriately balanced against the human rights and medical needs of poor patients in the Global South (Joseph 2003; Leisinger 2005; Santoro 2006).

Pharmaceutical companies are once again engaged in a race for a cure for a global scourge. Once again, a collision between profits and human rights appears inevitable. Because the SARS-CoV-2 virus does not mutate in the manner of HIV/AIDS, the development of a vaccine is theoretically achievable. Normally vaccines take from two to five years to develop and bring to market, but in the summer of 2020, just months after the virus caused nation after nation to enter into prolonged economic and social lockdowns, there were hundreds of candidates for potential vaccines. Small, previously obscure companies like Moderna and large, well-established ones like AstraZeneca (working closely with Oxford University) as well as Pfizer and Johnson & Johnson, all with substantial government backing from the United States and/or the United Kingdom, are racing at "warp speed" to conduct clinical trials, with large numbers of volunteers to test for efficacy, safety, and side effects. There is no guarantee that any of these vaccine candidates will prove to be safe and effective or that they will confer immunity for any extended period. However, in the summer of 2020 hopes ran high that a vaccine with limited effectiveness would be available at the beginning of 2021. At the same time, doctors and drug companies are testing various treatments to ameliorate the effects of the SARS-CoV-2 virus and reduce the probability of death for those contracting the disease.

The access and pricing issues arising in the case of HIV/AIDS and COVID-19 medications are illustrative of a fundamental economic and moral dilemma. Medical progress and innovation often ineluctably result in healthcare inequality. There is a tension between scientific progress and universal access to medicines.[1] The economic incentives and patent protection that spur private industry investment and invention are the same forces that restrict supply, raise prices, and put the drugs out of reach for many patients, particularly in the Global South. This tension becomes more dramatic in the case of global pandemics. The pandemic aspect creates panic and fear. The global part means large differences in affordability of medicines between rich and poor counties.

There is some reason to hope that history will not repeat itself in the case of drugs developed to treat the SARS-CoV-2 virus and immunize patients from the disease. Public funding and university laboratories are important contributors to the research being conducted, and governments worldwide are unlikely to tolerate the kind of insensitive pricing that occurred at the outset of the global HIV/AIDS crisis. French President Emmanuel Macron has called COVID-19 drugs a "public good for the world, and not subject to the laws of the market." German Chancellor Angela Merkel has also spoken of "a global public good, to produce this vaccine and to distribute it in all parts of the world." South African President Cyril Ramaphosa, chairman of the African Union, warned that the continent, because of its poor standards of healthcare, was "extremely vulnerable to the ravages of this virus and is in need of support" (Nebehay and Shields 2020). Even some pharmaceutical executives have acknowledged that maximizing profit is not appropriate in the current public health crisis (Ip 2020).

Despite these positive signs that there will not be a repeat of the humanitarian scandal pitting profits over people in the case of HIV/AIDS, there are plenty of reasons for human rights advocates to remain skeptical and vigilant. When vaccines and treatments are eventually developed, the question of pricing and access to these drugs in the Global South is bound to become a matter of urgent concern.

A cautionary tale again can be found from the past. At the peak of the HIV crisis in 2010, over a million adults and children died of HIV-related causes, and still today the World Health Organization (WHO) estimates that with better access to antiretroviral treatments, hundreds of thousands of deaths, primarily in Africa, could be prevented (World Health Organization 2020b). As of 2019, countries in sub-Saharan Africa have some of the highest annual infection rates in the world, with up to 23 percent of the population living with HIV/AIDS (Roser and Ritchie, 2019).

Of particular concern is the rise of what has been called "vaccine nationalism," whereby rich countries like the United States, in return for funding the basic research, attempt to siphon off and control the supply of vaccines for their own citizens, and thereby choke off supply to the Global South. The conditions of poor infrastructure, population displacement, poor sanitation and drinking water, and overcrowding in the Global South, combined with a lack of access to testing and resources for effective contact-tracing, all provide a lethal cocktail for a humanitarian catastrophe that largely remains out of sight and out of mind in rich nations (Lapidor 2020). Moreover, because the testing capacities in the Global South are so wanting, it is impossible to calculate the true prevalence of the SARS-CoV-2 virus.

This article addresses the human rights obligations of the pharmaceutical industry with regard to vaccines and treatments developed to prevent and treat COVID-19. Although our analysis is motivated by the current pandemic, the questions we address and the conclusions we express are meant to apply more broadly to the issue of global access to essential medicines. In particular, we address the following questions: Do pharmaceutical corporations have human rights responsibilities to make medicines available to disadvantaged populations, especially in the Global South, or do they have something more binding, such as an obligation?[2] If so, on what grounds?

We begin by examining two sets of guidelines promulgated by the United Nations—the *Guiding Principles on Business and Human Rights* (2011) and the *Human Rights Guidelines for Pharmaceutical Companies in Relation to Access to Medicines* (2008). These guidelines, taken together, support the idea that pharmaceutical companies have a responsibility to help make essential medicines available to patients in the Global South. Moreover, they support the view that it is the human rights obligation of member states to enforce this moral obligation during the COVID-19 pandemic. We then develop a model of the moral basis of corporate responsibility (including human rights responsibilities) that is based on the idea of a "social contract." Our purpose in doing so is to demonstrate that the human rights responsibilities outlined in the UN documents are, in fact, moral obligations.

We conclude our analysis by offering some practical advice for pharmaceutical companies manufacturing COVID-19 essential medicines that will enable them to balance their human rights responsibilities to the Global South with their fiduciary responsibilities to shareholders. In the process, we try to arrive at an appropriate balance to resolve the underlying tension between the need to economically incentivize drug discovery and the human rights claims of citizens in the Global South.

The UN Guiding Principles on Business and Human Rights and the UN Human Rights Guidelines for Pharmaceutical Companies in Relation to Access to Medicines

The UN *Guiding Principles on Business and Human Rights* (widely known informally as the Ruggie Principles, after Special Representative John Ruggie) were unanimously adopted by the UN Human Rights Council in 2011. They provide that businesses and member states each have particular responsibilities and obligations with respect to human rights. According to the "protect, respect, remedy" framework, member states are obligated to protect against human rights violations by third parties, including businesses, within their jurisdictions (United Nations 2011: Principle 1). This obligation includes an obligation to remedy violations and abuses: "States must take appropriate steps to ensure, through judicial, administrative, legislative or other appropriate means, that when such abuses occur within their territory and/or jurisdiction those affected have access to effective remedy" (United Nations 2011: Principle 25). Importantly, these obligations are strict, not mere responsibilities but duties that states bear by virtue of being members of the United Nations. In addition, the *International Covenant on Economic, Social and Cultural Rights* (ICESCR; United Nations 1966) and the *CESCR General Comment No. 14: The Right to the Highest Attainable Standard of Health* (2000) explicitly lay out legal responsibilities and obligations relating globally to the right to health for states that are party to the Covenant, including "the obligation to … adopt appropriate legislative, administrative, budgetary, judicial, promotional, and other measures towards the full realization of the right to health" (United Nations 2000: para. 33).

Furthermore, according to the Ruggie Principles, businesses bear responsibilities to "respect" human rights: "this means that they should avoid infringing on the human rights of others and should address adverse human rights impacts with which they are involved" (United Nations 2011: Principle 11). Responsibilities, being hortatory, are less strict than obligations, but importantly, this responsibility requires that businesses "seek to prevent or mitigate adverse human rights impacts that are directly linked to their operations … even if they have not contributed to those impacts" (United Nations 2011: Principle 13 b). The commentary indicates that business responsibility for impacts includes both actions and omissions. A straightforward application of the Ruggie principles, therefore, tells us that failing to take steps to make COVID-19 medications available to underprivileged populations, including in the Global South, would constitute such an omission by drug companies and thereby violate the Ruggie Principles.

One threshold issue is how to assign responsibility for the human right to healthcare. Not all states guarantee a legal right to health. In the United States, for example, the provision of and payment for healthcare is mostly conducted through the private sector and tied to employment benefits. Despite the lack of universal access to healthcare in the United States, however, the idea of human right to health is well established. Article 25 of the Universal Declaration of Human Rights, for example, provides that everyone has a right to medical care (UN General Assembly 1948). This is elaborated in the ICESCR (United Nations 1966) and the *CESCR General Comment No. 14* (United Nations 2000).

The substance of what the human right to medical care entails was addressed in the *Human Rights Guidelines for Pharmaceutical Companies in Relation to Access to Medicines* (the Hunt Guidelines) submitted to the United Nations General Assembly in 2008, by the Special Rapporteur on the Right to the Highest Attainable Standard of Health, Paul Hunt. The Hunt Guidelines set forth specific responsibilities of pharmaceutical companies, as developers and sellers of medicines, in regard to access to medicines (Hunt and Khosla, 2010). Although the Hunt Guidelines predate the later Ruggie Principles on business and human rights, taken in sum with the human right to health, they unequivocally establish that pharmaceutical companies bear human rights responsibilities, together with member states, to promote access to medications, in particular to what have been termed essential medicines (Moon 2003). Essential medicines, as defined by the WHO, are the medicines that "satisfy the priority health care needs of the population" (World Health Organization, 2020a). The WHO goes on to declare that "essential medicines are intended to be available within the context of functioning health systems at all times in adequate amounts, in the appropriate dosage forms, with assured quality, and at a price the individual and the community can afford" (World Health Organization, 2020) It is no great leap to conclude that if and when a COVID-19 vaccine or standard of therapeutic care is developed, it will be classified as an "essential medicine" (EM) by the WHO.

Several of the Hunt Guidelines are understandably more specific than the Ruggie Principles in declaring that pharmaceutical companies bear responsibilities to make EMs such as vaccines and other medicines relating to COVID-19 accessible to underprivileged populations, especially in the Global South. Guideline 5 states of any pharmaceutical company that, "its strategies, policies, programmes, projects and activities … should give particular attention to the needs of disadvantaged individuals, communities and populations such as children, the elderly and those living in poverty" (United Nations 2008).

Hunt Guidelines 26 through 28 indicate that pharmaceutical companies should respect the rights of countries to use provisions of the WTO's Agreement on Trade-Related Aspects of Intellectual Property Rights (TRIPS), which allows countries flexibility in recognizing patent ownership in discharging their human rights obligations, in particular those regarding the right to health (World Trade Organization 1994). This includes both respecting and not interfering with states' rights to protect public health and increase access to medicines pursuant to the WHO's Doha Declaration on the TRIPS Agreement and Public Health. That declaration clarifies the measures states may take in promoting access to medicines, especially EMs, to control diseases of public importance, such as HIV, tuberculosis, and malaria, and, undoubtedly, COVID-19 (World Health Organization 2001).

Our argument thus far may be summarized as follows: According to the Ruggie Principles, member states have obligations to protect and remedy human rights violations and abuses. Companies have responsibilities to respect human rights law, and not to interfere with states' fulfillment of their obligations. These rights include the right to health, which, according to the Hunt Guidelines, includes responsibilities to respect states' fulfillment of their obligations. This entails that companies, especially innovative ones that develop EMs relating to diseases of global importance such as COVID-19, are responsible for helping states fulfill their obligations. Fulfilling this responsibility requires companies not to impede states in fulfilling their obligations, for instance, by pricing vaccines out of reach for poor communities. Precisely how drug companies can be expected to help provide EMs to the Global South is a subject we will take up in the final section of this article.

The Ruggie Principles and the Hunt Guidelines, by virtue of their promulgation by the United Nations, have enormous prestige and influence. They might even be said to possess a certain moral authority by virtue of their reflecting, in some measure, an imperfect consensus of the "global community" about the human rights responsibilities and obligations of business. However, they are, in the manner of the Universal *Declaration* of Human Rights (emphasis added), merely pronouncements without independent moral authority or justification. Although the ICESCR is more binding, not all UN member states are party to it—including, notably, the United States.[3] In the following section, we make a moral argument for certain human rights responsibilities and obligations of business as contemplated by the Ruggie Principles and the Hunt Guidelines.

A social contract corporate social responsibility argument for drug company human rights obligations

Executives of private companies manage assets owned by shareholders and thus legally owe a fiduciary duty to competently manage those assets and return a profit for shareholders.[4] The idea that corporations have moral responsibilities other than maximizing profits and should act in a socially responsible manner has become an increasingly accepted notion in recent years.[5] However, it is worth reflecting on the philosophical foundations that underpin this idea. The moral argument for corporate social responsibility can be constructed from a number of philosophical premises. One useful approach is based on the idea of a "social contract."[6] Broadly speaking, the idea of a corporate social contract is based on the political social contract in the writings of John Locke, Jean-Jacques Rousseau, and Thomas Hobbes (D'Agostino, Gaus, and Thrasher 2019). The social contract is meant to describe the relationship of trust existing between corporations and society. The very existence of a corporation as a legal "person" is made possible by society. Society also enacts and enforces the legal norms and institutions that protect private property and the accumulation of capital and profits. In return for what society makes possible for them, corporations are accountable to society. They have a "contractual" moral duty to operate in a manner that benefits society—that is, in a socially responsible manner. Global businesses, including innovative pharmaceutical firms, are incorporated and enjoy legal personhood within the jurisdictions and territories of "home" member states. They also operate abroad in multiple jurisdictions or "host" states, where they might manufacture and, more commonly, sell their products. Multinational businesses thus enjoy various rights and privileges in both home and host countries. In return, they have a duty to act in a socially responsible manner in *both* the home and host countries in which they enjoy legal existence and operate.

A corporation's moral responsibility for human rights is a particular instance of its duty to act in a socially responsible manner. The moral nature and international character of human rights might be described as follows:

> Human rights are rights of such importance that they impose correlative duties on actors beyond a nation's borders. To call something a "human right" is to say that it imposes duties upon others across national borders to honor that right. Human rights are moral rights. Human rights exist regardless of whether a particular national government in actuality protects those rights. (Santoro 2009: 15).

Of course, the existence of human rights that impose moral duties with international reach begs a number of crucial questions: Who owes what human rights duties? What duties does business owe with respect to human rights, as opposed to duties owed by other entities such as governments and nongovernmental organizations? As described above, the Ruggie Principles and Hunt Guidelines offer a basis for answering these questions.[7] However, a crucial question remains: How, as a practical matter, can drug companies meet the obligations outlined in these frameworks? To this subject we now turn.

Implementing the human rights obligations of drug companies regarding essential medicines

Before we discuss the specific ways that drug companies can fulfill their human rights obligations with respect to COVID-19 vaccines and therapies, we must give due consideration to their fiduciary responsibilities to shareholders and the current incentive structures for innovation. The argument is sometimes made that corporate social responsibility is a win-win situation, by which is implied that "doing good" or behaving in a socially responsible way will result in "doing well" or making profits. This notion of whether ethics "pays" has been discussed, debated, and empirically studied for decades with no clear-cut answer emerging.[8] Although drug companies that help make COVID-19 drugs more affordable in the Global South might enjoy some reputational benefits, the number of people affected by COVID-19, when taken together with the costs of developing and producing vaccines, make it likely that providing such help will result in lower profitability.

Although the COVID-19 crisis, particularly because of its disproportionate impact on communities of color, has helped to undermine public support for how healthcare is paid for and delivered,[9] given current corporate governance frameworks and business incentive structures, the human rights responsibilities of drug companies cannot amount to the equivalent of a blank check.[10] To be sustainable, the corporate social responsibility to provide drugs at free or reduced prices must be reconciled with the fiduciary duties owed to shareholders to recoup research and development expenses and generate profits.[11] A crucial question remains: How much profit is enough to maximize access and incentivize innovation? Although no precise answer is possible, the principle for deciding this question is clear. It is a matter of balance and proportionality—that is, drug companies must to do their "fair share" in providing access, consistent with their obligations to shareholders and their economic sustainability. As we note below, a crucial corollary of this principle is that others—including, governments, nongovernmental organizations, philanthropy and foundations, as well as intergovernmental organizations—share the duty to assure access to healthcare.[12]

A second limitation on what might reasonably be expected from drug companies is imposed by the need to sustainably incentivize innovation. Much as it might surprise and upset some in the human rights advocacy community to hear, it would present a poor prospect for incentivizing cures for the future global pandemics that are sure to come, if companies were to reap meager rewards for successfully combatting the current pandemic. Again, how much reward is necessary to incentivize innovation is a matter of balance and proportionality. The human rights duty of a drug company to do its fair share in providing access to drugs must be weighed against the need to maintain its sustainability as an innovating organization that society will rely on to fashion cures and treatments for future diseases.

With these practical constraints in mind, there are a number of ways in which a socially responsible drug company can fulfill the human rights duties outlined in the Ruggie Principles and the Hunt Guidelines. We highlight three in particular: donations (particularly when working with multi-stakeholder initiatives), differential pricing, and relaxation of patent rights.

Donations through multi-stakeholder initiatives

The most direct method for drug companies to practice corporate responsibility in the era of COVID-19 is through philanthropic donations. After initial missteps in the HIV/AIDS era, a number of companies donated substantial resources to the Global South. Pfizer, for example, made free donations of its antifungal medicine Diflucan® (fluconazole) for the treatment of opportunistic infections associated with HIV infection (Diflucan Partnership Program 2012). Such donations are more impactful when they are conducted through multi-stakeholder initiatives. A good example is Merck's participation in the Masa (New Dawn) program of the African Comprehensive HIV/AIDS Partnership (ACHAP). ACHAP is a public–private partnership among the Republic of Botswana, the Bill and Melinda Gates Foundation, and the Merck Foundation. Thanks in part to ACHAP, Botswana became the first African nation to implement widespread distribution of antiretroviral drugs through its public health system.[13] Similar multi-stakeholder initiatives have already been formed to address the COVID-19 pandemic. The Gavi Foundation—a multi-stakeholder vaccine alliance including, among others, the Bill and Melinda Gates Foundation, UNICEF, the WHO, the London-based money transfer company TransferWise, and the World Bank—has set a goal to provide 2 billion doses of a vaccine by the end of 2021, an effort they estimate will require $18.1 billion in funding (Gavi 2020).

Differential pricing

In lieu of donating drugs at no cost, drug companies can still profitably sell drugs through differential or discounted pricing, whereby countries in the Global North and wealthy individuals therein pay more, sometimes substantially more, for a medicine than do underprivileged individuals in either the Global North or South. Here again the HIV/AIDS era provides an example of how such a policy can work. Thanks in part to competition from generic Indian manufacturers, antiretroviral medications that sold for $10,000 to $15,000 per patient per year in Global North countries were selling for $350 per patient per year in the Global South. That relative success was not a one-off; other successful examples of differential, discounted pricing include tuberculosis drugs as well as ring-vaccinations methods used to stop polio (Hassoun 2020).

Relaxation of patent rights

A third proven and practical way to increase access to EMs is by relaxing enforcement of patent rights.[14] This can be implemented in various ways, including voluntary licensing and shortening the duration of a patent (Wolitz 2019). By relinquishing patent rights for sales in underprivileged jurisdictions, innovative drug companies would, in effect, speed up the rate at which less expensive generic medicines become available. Patent sharing among innovative firms is another way that patent policy can contribute to the speedy development of new drugs. The UN-sponsored Medicines Patent Pool, for example, is designed to speed up drug development and at the same time reduce costs and increase access in the Global South (Hassoun and Khosla 2020).

Conclusion: Drug companies have a moral obligation to do their 'fair share' to assure access to essential medicines developed to prevent and treat COVID-19

Looking back on the historical corporate social responsibility of the pharmaceutical industry, UN Special Rapporteur Paul Hunt assessed the record as a checkered one. He observed that, although the pharmaceutical sector often helps to deliver the right to health—for example, through donations, differential pricing, and patent relaxation—companies do not always live up to their human rights responsibilities (Hunt and Khosla 2010).

In this article we have tried to clarify what human rights obligations drug companies have, their basis in international law, in UN guidelines, and in morality, as well as some specific steps that can be taken in the case of COVID-19 treatments and other EMs. We do not presume to be able to draw the line on precisely how far innovator companies must go in discharging their responsibilities and obligations. As our discussion of the importance of incentivizing innovation, fiduciary duties to shareholders, and economic sustainability should suggest, we are not covertly arguing anything as simple as putting human rights before profits, on the grounds that under those conditions, human rights and human betterment may not be served at all. We are cognizant that there will be ongoing debate about precisely how those lines should be drawn.

The approach we have adopted is that companies must do their fair share. This approach frames the issue more in terms of taking reasonable steps that nonetheless meaningfully address the relevant human rights at stake, in this case the right to health (Santoro 2009). An important point to emphasize is that by limiting the human rights obligations of drug companies to their fair share, we do not in any respect intend to dilute the human rights of citizens in the Global South to EMs. Duties with respect to human rights are owed not only by businesses but also by other actors. The portion of the obligation not taken up by drug companies is owed by others who also owe their fair share—governments, NGOs, private philanthropy and foundations, and intergovernmental organizations (Santoro 2010).

We have argued that drug companies have a moral obligation to promote access to EMs that is grounded in international standards such as the Ruggie Principles, the Hunt Guidelines, and the IESCR, as well principles of corporate social responsibility derived from the social contract business has with the international community. Moreover, drug companies have available to them a number of viable options to discharge that obligation in the COVID-19 pandemic by doing their fair share, while still retaining sufficient financial incentives to spur the innovation, development, and production of yet-to-be-discovered essential medicines when, inevitably, the international community confronts the next global pandemic, perhaps one that will be even more devastating than COVID-19.

Notes

1. A number of human rights scholars have criticized the "neo-liberalization" of health, and have questioned the inevitability of the trade-off between scientific progress and health access (Chapman 2016; Yamin and Farmer 2017; Yamin 2020). Moreover, the late economist Uwe Reinhard demonstrated that the high cost of healthcare in the United States, in large part driven by its private insurance system, does not result in optimal health outcomes as compared with the healthcare systems of other developed economies (Reinhardt, Cheng, Krugman, and Frist 2019).
2. Concepts such as responsibility and obligation are thought to have different strengths, such that an obligation is more binding (i.e., must be fulfilled) whereas a responsibility is less binding (i.e., ought to be fulfilled, or should be fulfilled). These concepts fall into different categories—legal obligations and responsibilities, moral obligations and responsibilities, and so on (Björnsson and Shanklin 2014). It is not always clear how those categories relate to one another. For example, Dr. Martin Luther King Jr. argued that a moral obligation to disobey a law can outweigh the legal obligation to obey, when a law is unjust (King 1963). Moreover, different categories of responsibility and obligation can interact in complex ways, as they relate to business, human rights, and international law (Rodríguez-Garavito 2017).

3. Some have argued that, for member states that are not parties to the ICESCR, constitutional litigation in national courts represents a promising avenue for establishing the right to healthcare (Gruskin and Dickens 2006; Gauri and Brinks 2008; Hunt 2016).
4. The extreme version of this responsibility was infamously enunciated by Milton Friedman who believed that the "sole responsibility of business is to increase its profits" (Friedman 1970).
5. It should be noted that some philosophers question the fundamental premise that corporations can be thought of as persons that have moral obligations in the same way that individuals do (French 1979).
6. In the business ethics literature, the seminal work applying social contract theory to the human rights responsibilities of multinational corporations is Thomas Donaldson's (1989). For other approaches, see Wettstein (2009) and Hsieh (2015).
7. Although the Ruggie Principles and the Hunt Guidelines offer answers to these questions, they have no moral authority beyond their promulgation by the United Nations on behalf of the "global community." We do not scoff at the persuasive power of these principles and guidelines. We merely wish to note that, just as the existence of corporate human rights duties required philosophical justification for moral persuasiveness, so too does the assignment of particular duties to any particular actors, including businesses. For one attempt to delineate and morally justify the extent and limits of corporate responsibility for human rights, see Santoro (2010).
8. For a thoughtful and sophisticated take on how to think about the question of whether ethics "pays," see Paine (2003: chap. 2).
9. Further fueling discontent with existing healthcare models in the United States is the fact that the high cost of healthcare—in large part driven by its private, employer-based health insurance system—does not achieve optimal health outcomes as compared with the healthcare systems of other developed economies (Reinhardt, Cheng, Krugman, and Frist 2019).
10. This is not to say that some business activities that violate human rights should not be undertaken regardless of their impact on profits. Rather, we refer to a very specific kind of business and human rights *positive duty to contribute to* healthcare.
11. Pogge, Rimmer, and Rubinstein (2010) suggested alternative ways to incentivize innovation in private industry (see also Gruskin and Dickens 2006; Chapman 2016; Hunt 2016).
12. For a discussion of the economics underlying the grants of patents for drugs and its effect on pricing, see Parker-Lue, Santoro, and Koski (2015).
13. Information about ACHAP can be found at http://www.achap.org/ and http://www.gatesfoundation.org/Globalhealth/ [July 22, 2020].
14. Alternatives to the patent system include a health incentive fund (HIF), whereby international bodies, states, or both offer financial incentives for the development of EMs, to compensate for lost profits under TRIPS. Financial awards would be given to firms for developing medicines relating to any particular global or local need, and studies have indicated substantial support for such programs, and that they would indeed be feasible (Pogge and Hollis 2008; Pogge 2016; Obi 2017; McMullan, Ajay, Srinivas, Bhalla, Prabhakaran, and Banjaree 2018).

References

BJÖRNSSON, Gunnar, and SHANKLIN, Robert. (2014) Must,' 'ought,' and the structure of standards. *Lecture Notes in Computer Science: Deontic Logic & Normative Systems*, 8554, 33–48.

CHAPMAN, Audrey R. (2016) *Global Health, Human Rights, and the Challenge of Neoliberal Policies* (Cambridge, UK: Cambridge University Press).

D'AGOSTINO, Fred, GAUS, Gerald, and THRASHER, John. (2019) *Contemporary Approaches to the Social Contract.* [Online]. Available: https://plato.stanford.edu/archives/fall2019/entries/contractarianism-contemporary/ [20 July 2020].

DIFLUCAN PARTNERSHIP PROGRAM. (2012) *Diflucan Partnership Program Factsheet.* [Online]. Available: https://pfe-pfizercom-d8-prod.s3.amazonaws.com/philanthropy/Diflucan_Partnership_factsheet.pdf [30 July 2020].

DONALDSON, Thomas. (1989) *The Ethics of International Business* (New York, NY: Oxford University Press).

FRENCH, Peter. (1979) The corporation as a moral person. *American Philosophical Quarterly*, 16(3), 207–215.

FRIEDMAN, Milton. (1970) The social responsibility of business is to increase profits. *The New York Times*, 13 September [Online]. Available: https://www.nytimes.com/1970/09/13/archives/a-friedman-doctrine-the-social-responsibility-of-business-is-to.html [5 November 2020].

GAURI, Varun, and BRINKS, Daniel (eds.). (2008) *Courting Social Justice: Judicial Enforcement of Social and Economic Rights in the Developing World* (Cambridge, UK: Cambridge University Press).

GAVI, THE VACCINE ALLIANCE. (2020) *New Private Sector Commitments to Fund Access to Future COVID-19 Vaccines Announced at International Pledging Summit.* [Online]. Available: https://www.gavi.org/news/media-room/new-private-sector-commitments-fund-access-future-covid-19-vaccines-announced [25 August 2020].

GRUSKIN, Sofia, and DICKENS, Bernard. (2006) Human rights and ethics in public health. *American Journal of Public Health*, 96(11), 1903–1905. doi:10.2105/AJPH.2006.099606

HASSOUN, Nicole. (2020) *Ending the Pandemic Will Take Global Access to Treatment and Vaccines—Which Means Putting Ethics Before Profits.* [Online]. Available: https://theconversation.com/ending-the-pandemic-will-take-global-access-to-covid-19-treatment-and-vaccines-which-means-putting-ethics-before-profits-141763 [20 July 2020].

HSIEH, Nien-hê. (2015) Should business have human rights obligations? *Journal of Human Rights*, 14(2), 218–236. doi:10.1080/14754835.2015.1007223

HUNT, Paul. (2016) Interpreting the international right to health in a human rights-based approach to health. *Health and Human Rights Journal*, 18(2), 109–130.

HUNT, Paul, and KHOSLA, Rajat. (2010) Are drug companies living up to their human rights responsibilities? The perspective of the former United Nations Special Rapporteur (2002–2008). *PLoS Medicine*, 7(9), e1000330. doi:10.1371/journal.pmed.1000330

IP, Greg. (2020) Vaccine race puts profits aside, for now. *The Wall Street Journal*, A2, 22 July.

JOSEPH, Sarah. (2003) Pharmaceutical corporations and access to drugs: The 'fourth wave' of corporate human rights scrutiny. *Human Rights Quarterly*, 25(2) 425--452. doi:10.1353/hrq.2003.0018

KING, Martin Luther. Jr. (1963) A letter from Birmingham Jail. *Ebony*, 23–32. (August).

LAPIDOR, Eden. (2020) *Out of the Spotlight: COVID-19 and the Global South.* [Online]. Available: https://www.justsecurity.org/71570/out-of-the-spotlight-covid-19-and-the-global-south/ [22 July 2020].

LEISINGER, Klaus M. (2005) The corporate social responsibility of the pharmaceutical industry: Idealism without illusion and realism without resignation. *Business Ethics Quarterly*, 15(4), 577–594. doi:10.5840/beq200515440

MCMULLAN, Patrick, AJAY, Vamadevan S, SRINIVAS, Ravi, BHALLA, Sandeep, PRABHAKARAN, Dorairaj, and BANERJEE, Amitava. (2018) Improving access to medicines via the Health Impact Fund in India: A stakeholder analysis. *Global Health Action*, 11(1), 1434935–1434920. doi:10.1080/16549716.2018.1434935

MOON, Suerie. (2003) *Respecting the Right to Access to Medicines: Implications of the UN Guiding Principles on Business and Human Rights for the Pharmaceutical Industry.* [Online]. Available: https://www.hhrjournal.org/2013/10/respecting-the-right-to-access-to-medicines-implications-of-the-un-guiding-principles-on-business-and-human-rights-for-the-pharmaceutical-industry/ [22 July 2020].

NEBEHAY, Stephanie, and SHIELDS, Michael. (2020) *World Leaders Launch Plan to Speed COVID-19 Drugs, Vaccine: US Stays Away.* [Online]. Available: https://www.usnews.com/news/world/articles/2020-04-24/world-leaders-due-to-launch-covid-19-drugs-vaccine-plan-who [21 July 2020].

OBI, Evaristus. (2017) *Post-Trial Access to Drugs in Developing Nations: Global Health Justice* (New York, NY: Springer Publishing).

PAINE, Lynn Sharp. (2003) *Power Shift: Why Companies Must Merge Social and Financial Imperatives to Achieve Superior Performance* (New York, NY: McGraw Hill).

PARKER-LUE, Sara, SANTORO, Michael A, and KOSKI, Greg. (2015) The ethics and economics of pharmaceutical pricing. *Annual Review of Pharmacology and Toxicology*, 55, 191–206. doi:10.1146/annurev-pharmtox-010814-124649

POGGE, Thomas. (2016) *Incentives for Global Health, Yale University.* [Online]. Available: http://www.unsgaccessmeds.org/inbox/2016/2/23/contributionincentives-for-global-healthyale-university [25 August 2020].

POGGE, Thomas, and HOLLIS, Aidan. (2008) *The Health Impact Fund.* [Online]. Available: https://healthimpactfund.org/pdf/High-level-panel-draft-016-02-22-formatted.docx.pdf [26 August, 2020].

POGGE, Thomas, RIMMER, and RUBENSTEIN, Kim (eds.). (2010) *Incentives for Global Public Health: Patent Law and Access to Essential Medicines* (Cambridge, UK: Cambridge University Press).

REINHARDT, Uwe, TSUNG-MEI, Cheng, KRUGMAN, Paul, and FRIST, William H. (2019) *Priced Out: The Economic and Ethical Costs of American Health Care* (Princeton, NJ: Princeton University Press).

RITCHIE, Hannah, ORTIZ-OSPINA, Esteban, BELTEKIAN, Diana, MATHIEU, Edouard, HASELL, Joe, MACDONALD, Bobbie, GIATTINO, Charlie, and ROSER, Max. (2020) *Coronavirus Pandemic (COVID-19)—Statistics and Research.* [Online]. Available: https://ourworldindata.org/coronavirus [25 August 2020].

RODRÍGUEZ-GARAVITO, César (ed.). (2017) *Business and Human Rights: Beyond the End of the Beginning* (New York, NY: Cambridge University Press).

ROSER, Max, and RITCHIE, Hannah. (2019) *HIV/AIDS.* [Online]. Available: https://ourworldindata.org/hiv-aids [31 July 2020].

SANTORO, Michael A. (2006) Human rights and human needs: Diverse moral principles justifying third world access to affordable HIV/AIDS drugs. *North Carolina Journal of International Law and Commercial Regulation*, 31(4), 923–942.

SANTORO, Michael A. (2009) *China 2020: How Western Business Can—and Should—Influence Social and Political Change in the Coming Decade* (Ithaca, NY: Cornell University Press).

SANTORO, Michael A. (2010) Post-Westphalia and its discontents: Business, globalization and human rights in political and moral perspective. *Business Ethics Quarterly*, 20(2), 285–297. doi:10.5840/beq201020221

UNITED NATIONS. (1966) *International Covenant on Economic, Social, and Cultural Rights.* [Online]. Available: https://www.ohchr.org/en/professionalinterest/pages/cescr.aspx [25 August 2020].

UNITED NATIONS. (2000) *CESCR General Comment No. 14: The Right to the Highest Attainable Standard of Health (Art. 12).* [Online] Available: https://www.refworld.org/pdfid/4538838d0.pdf [25 August 2020].

UNITED NATIONS. (2008) *Human rights guidelines for pharmaceutical companies in relation to access to medicines.* [Online]. Available: http://www.ohchr.org/Documents/Issues/Health/GuidelinesForPharmaceuticalCompanies.doc [21 July 2020].

UNITED NATIONS. (2011) *Guiding Principles on Business and Human Rights* (see Principles 1, 11, 13(b), 25). [Online]. Available: https://www.ohchr.org/Documents/Publications/GuidingPrinciplesBusinessHR_EN.pdf [21 July 2020].

WETTSTEIN, Florian. (2009) *Multinational Corporations and Global Justice: Human Rights Obligations of a Quasi-Governmental Institution* (Stanford, CA: Stanford University Press).

WORLD HEALTH ORGANIZATION. (2020a) *Essential Medicines and Health Products.* [Online]. Available: https://www.who.int/medicines/services/essmedicines_def/en/ [24 July 2020].

WORLD HEALTH ORGANIZATION. (2020b) *Number of Deaths Due to HIV/AIDS.* [Online]. Available: https://www.who.int/gho/hiv/epidemic_status/deaths_text/en/ [24 May 2020].

WORLD HEALTH ORGANIZATION. (2001) *The DOHA Declaration on the TRIPS Agreement and Public Health.* WT/MIN(01)/DEC/W/2 [Online]. Available: https://www.who.int/medicines/areas/policy/doha_declaration/en/ [21 May 2020].

WOLITZ, Rebecca. (2019) A corporate duty to rescue: Biopharmaceutical companies and access to medications. *Indiana Law Journal*, 94(3), 1164–1221.

WORLD TRADE ORGANIZATION. (1994) TRIPS: Agreement on Trade-Related Aspects of Intellectual Property Rights, Marrakesh Agreement Establishing the World. *Trade Organization, Annex 1C,* 1869 U.N.T.S. 299, 33 I.L.M. 1197. (Geneva, Switzerland: World Trade Organization).

YAMIN, Alicia Ely. (2020) *When Misfortune Becomes Injustice: Evolving Human Rights Struggles for Health and Social Equality* (Stanford, CA: Stanford University Press).

YAMIN, Alicia Ely, and FARMER, Paul. (2017) *Power, Suffering, and the Struggle for Dignity: Human Rights Frameworks for Health and Why They Matter* (Philadelphia, PA: University of Pennsylvania Press).

What COVID-19 revealed about health, human rights, and the WHO

Wendy H. Wong and Eileen A. Wong

ABSTRACT

As of July 2020, COVID-19 has caused over 600,000 deaths, with 17 million confirmed cases, and counting. The World Health Organization (WHO), the global governance organization charged with providing health for all, declared a pandemic of on March 11, signaling the beginning of the global response to the disease. Despite a commitment to human rights and health, the WHO and others have been virtually silent on how rights and pandemic management go together, and have largely relied on techniques that date back to the 1918 flu epidemic. COVID-19 has made painfully obvious the tension between the protection of public health and the protection of human rights. The "rights-based approach" to health espoused by the WHO needs to be reexamined in light of how public health and human rights may, in times of crisis, work at cross-purposes. We show this through an analysis of the WHO's COVID-19-related publications.

As a doctor I would say let's put tanks in the streets and let's do a police state. … But the Western world has different realities (Guido Marinoni, president of the Bergamo Doctor Association, in response to Italy's policies in the COVID-19 crisis (as quoted in the *New York Times*, April 24, 2020; Horowitz and Bubola 2020).

Health is a state of complete physical, mental, and social well-being and not merely the absence of disease or infirmity. The enjoyment of the highest attainable standard of health is one of the fundamental rights of every human being without distinction of race, religion, political belief, economic, or social condition. (WHO Constitution, October 2006 version; World Health Organization 2006)

Introduction

In the months since news of a novel coronavirus respiratory infection emerged from Wuhan, China, in December 2019, the disease has spread globally. As of July 2020, COVID-19 has caused more than 600,000 deaths, with 17 million confirmed cases, and it is rapidly rising with uncontrolled spread in the United States and beyond. The devastating disease caused by the novel coronavirus SARS-CoV-2 was officially named COVID-19 by the World Health Organization (WHO) on February 11, 2020, and declared a pandemic on March 11, 2020. We are left searching for answers often by remembering the 1918 flu, which killed an estimated 50 million worldwide in a series of three waves (Taubenberger and Morens 2006). But that was a world without global human rights, low levels of "global governance," and vaccines, much less modern antiviral treatments. It was also a remarkably different world in terms of social, political, and economic features: Disadvantaged groups had few resources at their disposal, the internet did not exist, colonies defined much of the world, and global supply chains were not "just in time."

Disappointingly, the gulf between 1918 and 2020 has led to similar pandemic-management policies. Despite a commitment to human rights and health, the WHO and others have been virtually silent on how rights and pandemic management go together. Governments have largely followed the same pandemic protocols, such as isolation and quarantine, school closures, and public gathering bans, based on public health authorities' advice. Physicians and public health officials have an elevated role in public discourse, governance, and decision making in ways we have not seen on such a global scale in some time. The focus is on health as disease management through blanket policies, rather than the conception of health as a fundamental human right that encompasses other aspects of well-being. Consequently, the focus has been on individual treatments and behaviors—how individuals can pitch in, how we can make prosocial choices about social distancing, mask wearing, and other activities. More importantly for this article, the focus on individual-level action has also led to governments' creation of systemic injustices, or the exacerbation of existing injustices, now left gaping by a lightning-speed disease. In some cases, government-mandated individual-level action infringes on fundamental human rights.

In this article, we take the view that continuing to use indiscriminate interventions from 1918 is the wrong strategy because we no longer inhabit that world. In 2020, we live in a world post-United Nations, where the gamut of international human rights are strongly accepted by the great majority of states and there exist many global institutions designed to mitigate harms to human rights. It is widely accepted that the right to health cannot be realized without the protection and/or realization of other rights (Gruskin, Mills, and Tarantola 2007). The WHO has explicitly adopted a rights-based approach to health (World Health Organization 2017a). In its own words, a rights-based approach to health includes, "accountability, equality and nondiscrimination, participation, and universal[ity], indivisibil[ity], and interdependen[ce]" (World Health Organization 2017a). A human rights-based public health approach to pandemics is absolutely necessary and perhaps urgently needed as never before.

Even in noncrisis times, fulfilling the expansive 1946 constitutional mandate of "the highest attainable standard of health as a fundamental right of every human being" is remarkably ambitious for an intergovernmental organization (IGO). COVID-19's devastating global run has shown that population-level well-being, or individual-level well-being, is insufficient to mitigate the effects of the disease.

"We're all in this together," a common slogan throughout the pandemic (Arthur 2020), might feel good, with its emphasis on what we all can do (and bear), but it also emphasizes the need to insert human rights in protecting global health. There is inherently a tension between the protection of public health and the protection of human rights, because public health is motivated by population health, whereas human rights are motivated by ensuring that remedies are provided to individuals and groups who are not living a life of basic human dignity. This tension means that "the population" must be understood as many subpopulations, each with its own (dis)advantages that make it more or less likely to realize a high standard of health.

"Neutral" policies, like a declaration of the right to the highest attainable standard of health, might be ethical, but they are not necessarily rights-oriented. Not only can they occlude the disproportionate struggles for some groups to attain any suitable standard of health, they also promote the idea that blanket approaches that emphasize sameness are appropriate for a pandemic that has exacerbated old inequities and brought on new ones. Rights emphasize to what we are all entitled, and focus on the *recipients* of policy rather than the *providers* of policy. Rights require that we understand that the right to health is held by both individuals and communities; that protecting the group may require trade-offs on individual rights; and the very rights that are traded off—such as freedom of assembly and expression—help build the conditions to protect the right to health. Although human rights can help in formulating health policy that accounts for gaps in power and access (Forman 2017), this gap has been perniciously difficult to fill with regard to COVID-19.

To illustrate the conundrum of protecting human rights and public health, we put together a timeline of recent WHO actions in response to COVID-19 crisis, including technical guidance to countries, scientific reports, and organizational responses. As the leader in global health-setting standards and policy options and in providing technical support across its 194 member states, the WHO shapes the public health response globally, especially for many countries with lower technical capacity. By assembling these actions, we illustrate the challenge for public health organizations to actualize their "rights-based" approaches in a real-time, rapidly changing emergency with many unknowns. Whereas adopting a rights-based approach in less fraught times may have seemed in line with an evolving norm emphasizing the importance of human rights, in pandemic times, the contradictions inherent in such an approach have come to the fore. In so doing, we actively connect three fields that are too often disconnected: human rights, global politics, and public health. The purpose of this article is to draw together some of the frustrations this pandemic has caused, and to offer insight into where the tensions lie. Resolving these tensions should be foremost in public health and human rights law practitioners' minds going forward.

First, we explain critical differences between a human rights and a public health perspective. Second, we make the claim that linking human rights and public health creates problematic tensions that come to the fore in crises. Although the contrast may not be as extreme as the epigraph above, the frustration expressed is not surprising from a public health perspective, but it is perturbing from a human rights perspective. Third, we demonstrate the tensions in documents released by the WHO in its efforts to address the COVID-19 pandemic while remaining true to its previous legally, ethically, and economically comprehensive guidance, finding that it provides insufficient rights guidance during the urgency of a pandemic. We conclude with an emphasis on the importance of the cross-pollination of human rights, global politics, and public health perspectives while understanding the limitations and contradictions inherent in such an approach.

Of health and human rights

The view from human rights and global politics

The recognition of human rights as universal, inalienable, and indivisible (since the 1993 Vienna Declaration and Program of Action) is also linked to tension among the long and ever-growing list of human rights. One person's exercise of rights can threaten another person's enjoyment of those rights, especially in situations of life or death. This is particularly poignant when individual and group rights conflict, or when individual sacrifice is viewed as part of the greater good. Global politics have long focused on conflict as an area of tradeoff. Violent events with global consequences, such as the September 11, 2001, terrorist attacks, increase real or perceived threats, which in turn can have the effect of increasing peoples' acceptance of human rights violations. Bussmann and Schneider (2015), moreover, found a weakening in the effectiveness of international humanitarian law over time.

Pandemics have been an area of less focus in global politics and human rights. Although theories of international relations have been used to explain certain outcomes—such as the lack of a united response to COVID-19 (Farrell and Newman 2019; Busby forthcoming), or how the securitization of health leads to domestic policies such as drug stockpiling (Elbe, Roemer-Mahler, and Long 2014), or the role of health in diplomacy (Fazal forthcoming)—threats to health are undertheorized in relation to public goods. Pandemics call into sharp relief how individual rights can and must be curbed for the sake of collective well-being (Colgrove and Bayer 2005; Bayer

2007), especially as the human right to health is both an individually held and a collectively shared right (Toebes 2015).

The duality of the right to health makes it a challenge to enforce when a disease like COVID-19 demands individual-level restrictions for the benefit of the community. Although derogations from certain human rights are permitted under instruments such as the International Covenant on Civil and Political Rights (ICCPR) and are built into the documents themselves (Toebes 2015), such restrictions are not unlimited. States must follow the Siracusa Principles in determining when and how to suspend derogable rights: The suspensions of rights should be temporary in nature and should follow the principle of reciprocity (Silva and Smith 2015) in order to ensure that access to *other* essential rights (such as access to food, water, and housing) is not denied as a result of such restrictions (Rubenstein and DeCamp 2020). The Siracusa Principles also make it clear that the nonderogable rights in the ICCPR must remain as such (Davies 2017). It is the burden of the state to justify such measures (Silva and Smith 2015).

Nevertheless, critics have argued that even such restraint results in disproportionate burdens on certain populations, such as disabled people (Gulati, Dunne, and Kelly 2020) and other marginalized populations, exacerbating injustices (Forman 2020). COVID-19 has brought into sharp relief the disproportionate burdens borne by front-line workers in low-paying service jobs, who bear high risk in interacting with the public during periods in which movement is restricted and have their rights curbed because of their roles in sustaining communities. These frontline worker (such as health and food industry workers) as well as migrants are particularly at risk (Rubenstein and DeCamp 2020).

More generally, individuals are more tolerant of restrictions on rights when there is increased health anxiety. Restrictions run the gamut, from limitations on freedom of movement and assembly to property losses (Gadarian and Albertson 2014) as well as more onerous policy choices, such as quarantine (Worsnop 2017). Because health and security are intertwined, it is important to think about protection in the context of security, including human security, although this conceptualization has its limits (Wenham and Farias 2019).

The view from public health

Public health has become a more prominent feature of public discourse since the rise of scientific knowledge in the nineteenth century, and the corresponding rise in public interest in and demand for a decrease in preventable diseases (Institute of Medicine 1988). At its core, public health "aims to provide maximum benefit for the largest number of people" (Krug, Dahlberg, Mercy, Zwi, and Lozano 2002), but it requires a balance of individual rights and common good. Ethics have been an integral part of healthcare, a codified set of principles to guide the actions and relationships of healthcare workers, researchers, and organizations, ever-evolving based on scientific or societal changes (Gruskin and Dickens 2006). Ethical health questions may address the protection of human rights, but they do not encompass all aspects of human rights (World Health Organization 2015). Public health ethics is distinct from bioethics because of the focus on the population and the involvement of governments in public health actions (Faden, Bernstein, and Shebaya 2020). The focus on populations in public health requires outcomes and goals to be aggregated, masking the individuals and subgroups who make up populations, leading to critical ethical questions as these strategies for the collective health may infringe upon individual rights—for example, the ethics of public health surveillance, restrictions on freedom of movement, and the equitable allocation of resources (Faden et al. 2020).

The WHO "is bound by internationally accepted principles of human rights, which provide an important—and nonnegotiable—ethical framework for work and research in health and healthcare," publishing series of documents for ethical consideration during the implementation of public health and creating the Global Health Ethics Unit in 2002 (World Health Organization 2015).

Most of the issues within public health ethics concern either justice and equity of public health actions or the legitimacy of the state to implement public health measures (Faden et al. 2020). More recently, the interconnectedness of human rights and ethics within public health have been exemplified through the HIV/AIDS epidemic, with traditional public health methods conflicting with individual human rights in policies such as compulsory testing, travel restrictions, and isolation or quarantine (Gruskin et al. 2007; Meier, Evans, Kavanagh, Keralis, and Armas-Cardona 2018). Principles protecting human rights like the Siracusa Principles have been evoked in previous disease outbreaks, most notably in the compulsory treatment and involuntary confinement of patients with drug-resistant tuberculosis (World Health Organization 2007a; Boggio, Zignol, Jaramillo, Nunn, Pinet, and Raviglione 2008; Amon, Girard, and Keshavjee 2009; Todrys, Howe, and Amon 2013).

Although ethics and human rights are integrally linked, ethics are about guidelines governing individual or group behavior. They are not, as human rights are, entitlements held by individuals or groups. This is a significant difference, and one that the COVID-19 crisis has demonstrated remains one of the core hurdles to overcome. It is one thing to judge recommendations, such as social distancing, as ethical. They are, after all, ethical in the sense that they are not asking people to hurt themselves or others. But they affect individuals in varied circumstances quite differently, as has been well-documented for populations such as the homeless (Danielson 2020) and households with domestic abuse (Mahdawi 2020).

The instability of rights-based health and international organization

Articulating a human rights-sensitive approach to health was seen as a major win in the context of development (London 2008). Although the operationalization of rights-based approaches has been harder to nail down (Gruskin et al. 2007), using a rights-based approach to make assessments and design programs certainly leads to more awareness of the variance in underlying factors that must be accounted for in different political and social contexts. This approach is hardly new, but implementing human rights within health work has proven challenging.

Most programs that rely on rights-based approaches focus on making *recipients* more active participants in the healthcare they receive by focusing on participation and inclusion, nondiscrimination and equality, and accountability (Broberg and Sano 2017), rather than emphasizing the ethics of *providers*. These concerns are at the tip of the human rights iceberg, as such concerns rarely bring up rights such as the freedom of expression and right to assembly, both of which have arisen as political wedges in the COVID-19 crisis. Given the fundamental differences in how public health and human rights proponents think about the effects and purposes of their actions, the nominal integration of human rights into health systems demonstrates the rights–health challenge (Backman, Hunt, Khosla, Jaramillo-Strouss, Fikre, Rumble, Pevalin, Páez, Pineda, Frisancho, Tarco, Motlagh, Farcasanu, and Vladescu 2008; Gruskin, Ahmed, Bogecho, Ferguson, Hanefeld, Maccarthy, Raad, and Steiner 2012).

Rights-based approaches to health will remain inherently unstable for a number of reasons. First, political factors—such as the regime type, legal system, level of development, and region (e.g., Simmons 2009; Ooms, Keygnaert, and Hammonds 2019)—affect how human rights are implemented at the national and subnational levels, so there should be no reason to expect the right to health and rights-based approaches to health not to experience the same limitations. Human rights can provide tools for public health advocates to push states to fulfill their health obligations (London and Schneider 2012), just as they provide means for domestic actors to force states to fulfill their obligations through courts (Smith-Cannoy 2012; Helfer and Voeten 2013), including right to health (Saiz 2004; Yamin 2017; Rodríguez-Garavito 2017).

Health is also dependent on a whole gamut of other rights (i.e., "development"), the fulfillment of which, through approaches like the Sustainable Development Goals and the Millennium

Development Goals before them, clearly illustrate the challenge of reaching development benchmarks (Perehudoff and Forman 2019). There is also clear evidence that protecting health rights is often dependent on protecting basic civil and political rights so that reporting is accurate (Davies 2017) and inequities are known and recognized; the Black Lives Matter-driven social mobilization in the wake of George Floyd's murder has made these linkages explicit (Abdul-Jabbar 2020). Countries with more resources and less inequality deal better with the effects of epidemics (Guillen forthcoming).

Second, the implementation of health as a right depends on the actor in question (Broberg and Sano 2017). Actors will have different interests and obligations in fulfilling rights-based approaches to health. Another important set of actors are IGOs, which provide institutional supports for many global governance aspects. The WHO has been at the forefront of the coronavirus pandemic, following a pattern of inserting itself into the global governance of infectious disease more generally (Davies 2008).

To be clear, we are *not* critiquing the performance of this organization during the COVID-19 pandemic as adequate or inadequate, a focus of extensive debate since early spring 2020 (e.g., Sohrabi, Alsafi, O'Neill, Khan, Kerwan, Al-Jabir, Iosifidis, and Agha 2020). Rather, we explore theoretically and empirically why COVID-19 brings into sharp relief the struggle with balancing human rights and health, whether this is framed as a "rights-based approach to health" or "the right to health." The WHO is subject to the direction of member states, and as such, it can reflect geopolitical concerns in spite of the independence of its secretariat. From the mid-twentieth century until the 1990s, however, the WHO followed a radically different approach to development than did nation-states: The WHO chose to emphasize the social and health dimensions of development over the economic dimensions. The organization has always placed emphasis on poor people and health over profitability (Chorev 2012). As some observers have argued, it has developed an expansive role for itself in the emergency governance of pandemics (Hanrieder and Kreuder-Sonnen 2014).

Public health interventions in COVID-19

The implications of the 1918 influenza pandemic for today's COVID-19 pandemic are limited in part because the viruses at issue differ markedly in their transmissibility, age distribution among the ill, and acute and prolonged effects on the body (Petersen, Koopmans, Go, Hamer, Petrosillo, Castelli, Storgaard, Al Khalili, and Simonsen 2020; Morawska and Cao 2020; Carfi, Bernabei, and Landi 2020; Tenforde, Kim, and Lindsell 2020). Wartime conditions and limited infectious disease knowledge in 1918 constrained the response at that time to palliative care for those who were ill and nonpharmaceutical interventions (NPIs) for transmission prevention (Jester, Uyeki, and Jernigan 2018). NPIs employed during the 1918 pandemic included familiar techniques such as isolation and quarantine, school closures, and mass-gathering bans. As a class of disease responses, NPIs run the gamut from hand washing to face covering recommendations to isolating sick patients.

The comparison to 1918 is limited, however, not least of all because of the establishment of the WHO in 1948. As the UN agency charged with leading global health policy and programs (Chorev 2012), its official mission is "building a better, healthier future for people all over the world" (World Health Organization 2020b). According to its own constitution, all people have the fundamental right to health; the WHO has thus worked since its founding to promote the idea of a rights-based approach to health, which more explicitly draws on other human rights to realize the right to health (World Health Organization 2020a). The organization acts as the directing and coordinating authority for global health work, promoting and conducting health research and providing technical assistance and information in the area of health (World Health Organization 2006).

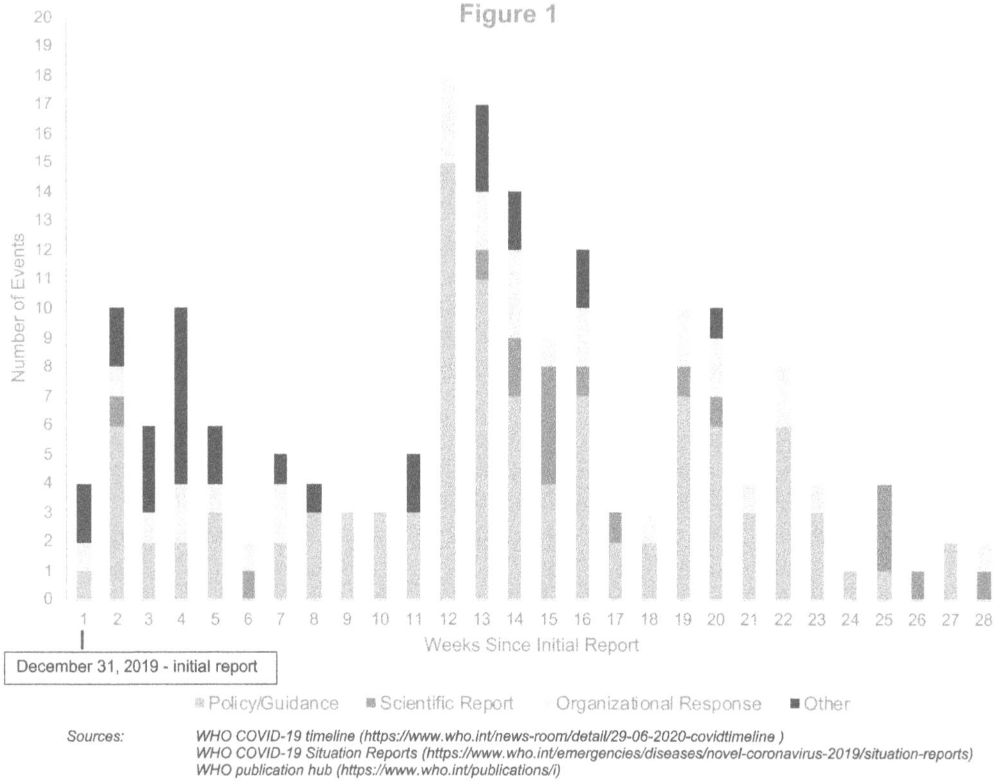

Figure 1. Types of WHO response in the weeks following the initial reporting of the cluster of pneumonia cases from Wuhan, China. Events were adapted from WHO timeline, WHO daily Situation Reports, and WHO publication hub. Events were categorized by Policy/Guidance (published interim or draft guidance, reports, briefs, rapid advice guides, and other technical guidance); Scientific Report (scientific briefs or announcements of summary of current scientific understanding); Organizational Response (establishment of teams or groups in response to COVID-19, field visits and deployment of teams, convening of committees, forums, organization of international studies and awareness campaigns, coordination of supplies, call for donors); Other (significant events acknowledged by WHO, responses from UN or non-WHO actors, press briefings and statements by Director-General, tweets from WHO or regional offices). Figure does not include WHO R&D Blueprints, epidemiological protocols, or tools. "Number of Events" are number of events occurring within a week distinguished by type of event (color), "Weeks Since Initial Report" are relative to initial report of cluster of pneumonia cases (Week 1). Figure only captures events between December 31, 2020 – June 30, 2020, each week analyzed ranged from 1-18 events.
Sources: WHO COVID-19 timeline (https://www.who.int/news-room/detail/29-06-2020-covidtimeline), WHO COVID-19 Situation Reports (https://www.who.int/emergencies/diseases/novel-coronavirus-2019/situation-reports), WHO publication hub (https://www.who.int/publications).

On the one hand, the WHO has an expansive mission; on the other, it has limited funds to achieve its massively ambitious portfolio—just $6.27 billion for 2018–2019, which was the same amount people in the United States spent on Black Friday in 2019 (Youde 2020). The organization is constrained because it cannot compel member states to do anything: For example, some states ignored WHO advice during the H1N1 pandemic and imposed travel restrictions (Worsnop 2017). It is largely an information hub and global coordinator of state activity during pandemics (Busby 2020), with few operational abilities (Wenham 2017; Youde 2020).

As an oversight institution, the WHO has published a multitude of guidelines and protocols for governments to produce their own strategic preparedness for disease epidemics, especially anticipating another major influenza pandemic. The pandemic preparedness plans emphasized surveillance and epidemiology, healthcare system preparedness, reducing disease in communities through medical countermeasures or NPIs, and effective communication (World Health Organization 2018). Consideration of the ethical implementation of these strategies also runs through these documents, with potential ethical issues during infectious disease outbreaks further explored in multiple WHO documents (World Health Organization 2007a, 2008, 2015, 2016, 2017b). Two key components for the pandemic preparedness plans—public health surveillance and NPIs that restrict movement (e.g., travel restrictions and quarantine)—are highlighted in these ethics documents as posing potential ethical dilemmas because of the tension between individual rights to privacy and freedom of movement versus the collective good of containing and preventing infections. The Siracusa Principles, which were written to protect human rights when a government may limit individual rights during emergency situations, are emphasized within the WHO's ethical considerations, particularly in situations of isolation, quarantine, border control, and social-distancing measures. The principles afford particular attention to those most vulnerable to discrimination, stigmatization, or isolation (World Health Organization 2007a, 2008, 2016).

Despite all of these tools to protect the right to health, and human rights more generally, the WHO has been relatively silent on human rights during the COVID-19 pandemic. The pandemic has put the WHO's years of pandemic planning to the test: The newest pandemic has not been caused by another iteration of influenza but, rather, by a novel coronavirus with no effective vaccine or known epidemiology. Analysis of the WHO's timeline of events and actions in Figure 1 suggest that the WHO was quick to react to the COVID-19 pandemic through early draft guidance, organizational responses such as field visits to the disease epicenter, and communication with the public. With little information about the new disease outbreak, however, initial guidance from the WHO (Figure 1: Week 2) was based on previous guidance developed in relation to the SARS and MERS outbreaks, focusing on infection prevention and control in clinical settings, without public health recommendations beyond standard contact precautions and surveillance preparation. In February 2020 (see Figure 1: Week 7), the WHO built on its initial guidelines concerning surveillance, government preparedness, and communication, but offered no large-scale community public health response advice (World Health Organization 2020d).

Meanwhile, the first impacted country, China, quickly tried to contain and control the community spread of SARS-CoV-2 in Wuhan. In the absence of any medical countermeasures, the only available tools were NPIs, and for China, these included implementing severe NPI measures of months-long "stay-at-home" orders, suspension of public gatherings, and travel bans, in addition to application of modern big data and artificial intelligence techniques to strengthen contact tracing. A press conference of the WHO-China Joint Mission on February 24 (Figure 1: Week 8) emphasized the enormous cost and sacrifices made by the Chinese government and people in order to take an "all-of-government, all-of-society" approach to controlling COVID-19 (World Health Organization 2020f).

Although the mission team leaders acknowledged that similar aggressive tactics would not likely work in all contexts, they recommended that other countries employ NPI measures such as isolation, medical observation, social distancing, personal protection, and prevention. The full report issued as a reference for other countries (Figure 1: Week 9) further emphasized that NPI measures are the only proven methods to break the transmission of SARS-CoV-2, with proactive public health surveillance and public engagement (World Health Organization 2020g). Although ethical and scientific considerations of these NPI measures had been compiled in the WHO's guidance for influenza, these crucial considerations were not emphasized in the organization's recommendations related to COVID-19 (World Health Organization 2019).

Following these recommendations, the WHO increased its focus on releasing technical guidance (see Figure 1). Although some of the subsequent documents and media statements acknowledged human rights and the difficulties faced by vulnerable populations, the WHO did not explicitly guide countries to consider the human rights implications of its technical recommendations. The WHO also did not remind states of the need to uphold Siracusa Principles, nor did it emphasize the importance of reciprocity and proportionality when employing aggressive NPI measures. Further, none of the WHO's recommendations were accompanied by guidance on remedies or the consequences of using blunt tools.

Much later (Figure 1: Week 17), in "Addressing Human Rights as Key to the COVID-19 Response," the WHO identified several key human rights concerns (including gender, vulnerable populations, and discrimination based on race), but it did not provide significant background or guidance on how to address these possible COVID-19-related rights infringements (World Health Organization 2020c). The WHO finally published comprehensive considerations for these public health and social measures weeks after the initial recommendations (Figure 1: Week 20; World Health Organization 2020e).

With 2.6 billion people living under some sort of NPI movement restriction by the end of March 2020 (Jankowicz 2020), these blanket public health policies were implemented around the world without guidance or consideration for those most vulnerable—such as people burdened by food and housing insecurity, mental health issues, domestic abuse situations, or comorbidities. This has taken place despite the WHO's focus on ensuring ethical health policy decisions are made and human rights implications are considered. Given the urgency of stopping a novel infectious disease with no known medical interventions, the ethical and human rights components of a public health response became an afterthought.[1]

Discussion and conclusion

Are these severe public health measures employed during COVID-19 worth the sacrifices made by the individual for the collective good? The evidence is mixed. Recent studies of physical distancing and other NPIs during the current pandemic have shown that they may decrease the incidence and mortality of COVID-19 (Yehya, Venkataramani, and Harhay 2020; Pei, Kandula, and Shaman 2020; Nazrul, Sharp, Chowell, Shabnam, Kawachi, Lacey, Massaro, D'Agostino, and White 2020; Lai, Ruktanonchai, Zhou, Prosper, Luo, Floyd, Wesolowski, Santillana, Zhang, Du, Yu, and Tatem 2020). In looking back at whether NPIs were helpful during the 1918 influenza pandemic, Markel, Lipman, Navarro, Sloan, Michalsen, Stern, and Cetron (2007) found that NPIs in combination reduced the total mortality burden. Correia, Luck, and Verner (2020) further showed that these interventions from the 1918 pandemic did not negatively affect the economy, and regions that took earlier, more aggressive actions recovered faster economically. A less invasive NPI, such as universal facemask wearing, may be sufficiently effective to stop transmission of SARS-CoV-2 even in high-risk places like hair salons and healthcare facilities (Wang, Ferro, Zhou, Hashimoto, and Bhatt 2020; Hendrix, Walde, Findley, and Trotman 2020).

However, despite the potential benefits of NPIs during the 1918 influenza pandemic, the biological, social, and economic context of the 1918 flu are different from current COVID-19 pandemic, making it unclear how well 1918 techniques travel (Markel, Stern, Navarro, Michalsen, Monto, and Digiovanni 2006; Markel et al. 2007; Correia et al. 2020). Furthermore, Matrajt and Leung (2020) showed through modeling of different social distancing practices that NPIs like social distancing alone will not be enough to control the pandemic, delaying but not preventing the spread of COVID-19. Similarly, another modeling study showed that NPIs provide a temporary suppression, with likely rebounds and perhaps even larger, later epidemics in the absence of vaccination (Ferguson, Laydon, Nedjati-Gilani, Imai, Ainslie, Baguelin, Bhatia, Boonyasiri, Cucunuba, Cuomo-Dannenburg, Dighe, Dorigatti, Fu, Gaythorpe, Green, Hamelt, Hinsley, Okell, Van Elsland, Thompson, Verity, Volz, Wang, Wang, Walker, Walters, Winskill, Whittaker, Donnelly, Riley, and Ghani 2020).

Perhaps blanket policies like NPIs are all we have against the microscopic foe SARS-CoV-2. Using NPIs in extreme ways, however, can create human rights quandaries and upend safeguards that human rights are designed to protect. Public health guidance, such as the Siracusa Principles, emphasizes the use of evidence-based policies proportionate to health need. Invasive NPIs that limit other rights or exacerbate underlying societal inequities were always intended to be short-term. Yet the balance of the right to health *vis-à-vis* other rights has been difficult to maintain for multiple reasons, as we have demonstrated in relation to the WHO's work.

Realizing the right to health hinges on a whole gamut of other rights, this interdependence is a primary reason that in the emergency responses to COVID-19 we saw either neglect or truncation of other rights in favor of preventing sickness. Other reasons, however, are linked to the difficulty IGOs face in spearheading global efforts to stop a global disease and to the disconnect between human rights and global politics, on the one hand, and public health and medicine, on the other. In order to protect health and human rights, emphasizing the effects on recipients of health policy is just as critical as understanding the profile of a disease and anticipating its spread (Directorate-General for Research and Innovation et al. 2020).

Note

1. Due to the evolving nature of the pandemic and public health response, this analysis of the public health and human rights response during COVID-19 is only updated as of August 1, 2020.

Acknowledgments

Thanks to Katie Houston and Laila Khoshkar for research assistance, and to Alexandra Logue for editorial comments.

Funding

This work was supported by the Canada Research Chairs (Canada Research Chair in Global Governance and Civil Society).

References

ABDUL-JABBAR, Kareem. (2020) Kareem Abdul-Jabbar: Don't Understand the Protests? What You're Seeing is People Pushed to the Edge. *Los Angeles Times*, 30 May. [Online.] Available: https://www.latimes.com/opinion/story/2020-05-30/dont-understand-the-protests-what-youre-seeing-is-people-pushed-to-the-edge [12 July 2020].

AMON, Joseph J., GIRARD, François, and KESHAVJEE, Salmaan. (2009) *Limitations on Human Rights in the Context of Drug-resistant Tuberculosis: A Reply to Boggio et al.* [Online.] Available: https://www.hhrjournal.org/2009/10/limitations-on-human-rights-in-the-context-of-drug-resistant-tuberculosis-a-reply-to-boggio-et-al/ [12 July 2020].

ARTHUR, Bruce. (2020) We say we're all in this together, but are we? *The Star*, 29 April. [Online]. 29 April. Available: https://www.thestar.com/opinion/star-columnists/2020/04/29/we-say-were-all-in-this-together-but-the-vulnerable-are-getting-hit-hardest-by-the-pandemic.html [20 July 2020].

BACKMAN, Gunilla, HUNT, Paul, KHOSLA, Rajat, JARAMILLO-STROUSS, Camilla, FIKRE, Belachew Mekuria, RUMBLE, Caroline, PEVALIN, David, PÁEZ, David Acurio, PINEDA, Mónica Armijos, FRISANCHO, Ariel, TARCO, Duniska, MOTLAGH, Mitra, FARCASANU, Dana, and VLADESCU, Cristian. (2008) Health systems and the right to health: An assessment of 194 countries. *The Lancet*, 372(9655), 2047–2085.

BAYER, Ronald. (2007) The continuing tensions between individual rights and public health. *European Molecular Biology Organisation*, 8(12), 1099–1103. doi:10.1038/sj.embor.7401134

BOGGIO, Andrew, ZIGNOL, Matteo, JARAMILLO, Ernesto, NUNN, Paul, PINET, Geneviève, and RAVIGLIONE, Mario. (2008) *Limitations on Human Rights: Are they Justifiable to Reduce the Burden of TB in the Era of MDR- and XDR-TB?* [Online]. Available: https://sites.sph.harvard.edu/hhrjournal/2013/09/limitations-on-human-rights-are-they-justifiable-to-reduce-the-burden-of-tb-in-the-era-of-mdf-and-xdr-tb/ [12 July 2020].

BROBERG, Morton, and SANO, Hans-Otto. (2017) Strengths and weaknesses in a human rights-based approach to international development—An analysis of a rights-based approach to development assistance based on practical experiences. *The International Journal of Human Rights*, 22(5), 664–680.

BUSBY, Joshua W. (forthcoming) Understanding the anemic global response to COVID-19. *Journal of Health Politics, Policy and Law.*

BUSBY, Joshua. (2020) *What International Relations Tells us About COVID-19.* [Online]. Available: https://www.e-ir.info/2020/04/26/what-international-relations-tells-us-about-covid-19/ [21 July 2020].

BUSSMANN, Margit, and SCHNEIDER, Gerald. (2015) A porous humanitarian shield: The laws of war, the Red Cross, and the killing of civilians. *The Review of International Organization*, 11(3), 337–359.

CARFI, Angelo, BERNABEI, Roberto, and LANDI, Francesco. (2020) Persistent symptoms in patients after acute COVID-19. *JAMA*, 324(6), 603–604.

CHOREV, Nitsan. (2012) *The World Health Organization Between North and South* (Ithaca, NY: Cornell University Press).

COLGROVE, James, and BAYER, Ronald. (2005) Manifold restraints: Liberty, public health, and the legacy of *Jacobson v. Massachusetts*. *American Journal of Public Health*, 95(4), 571–576.

CORREIA, Sergio, LUCK, Stephan, and VERNER, Emil. (2020) *Pandemics Depress the Economy, Public Health Interventions Do Not: Evidence from the 1918 Flu.* [Online]. Available: https://ssrn.com/abstract=3561560 [31 July 2020].

DANIELSON, Roxie. (2020) For the homeless, the coronavirus crisis is untenable—But so is the physical-distancing response. *The Globe and Mail*, 24 April. [Online]. Available: https://www.theglobeandmail.com/opinion/article-for-the-homeless-both-the-coronavirus-crisis-and-the-social/ [12 July 2020].

DAVIES, Sarah E. (2008) Securitizing infectious disease. *International Affairs*, 84(2), 295–313. doi:10.1111/j.1468-2346.2008.00704.x

DAVIES, Sarah E. (2017) Infectious disease outbreak response: Mind the rights gap. *Medical Law Review*, 25(2), 270–292. doi:10.1093/medlaw/fwx011

DIRECTORATE-GENERAL FOR RESEARCH AND INNOVATION (EUROPEAN COMMISSION), EUROPEAN GROUP ON ETHICS IN SCIENCE AND NEW TECHNOLOGIES (EUROPEAN COMMISSION), GROUP OF CHIEF SCIENTIFIC ADVISORS (EUROPEAN COMMISSION), PIOT PETER. (2020) *COVID-19 Pandemic: Statement on Scientific Advice to European Policy Makers During the COVID-19 Pandemic.* [Online]. Available: https://op.europa.eu/en/publication-detail/-/publication/346c8eaf-ba79-11ea-811c-01aa75ed71a1/language-en/format-PDF/source-139601691 [21 July 2020].

ELBE, Stefan, ROEMER-MAHLER, Anne, and LONG, Christopher. (2014) Security circulation pharmaceutically: Antiviral stockpiling and pandemic preparedness in the European Union. *Security Dialogue*, 45(5), 440–457. doi: 10.1177/0967010614530072

FADEN, Ruth, BERNSTEIN, Justin, and SHEBAYA, Sirine. (2020) *Public Health Ethics.* [Online]. Available: https://plato.stanford.edu/archives/fall2020/entries/publichealth-ethics/ [31 July 2020].

FARRELL, Henry, and NEWMAN, Abraham L. (2019) Weaponized interdependence: How global economic networks shape state coercion. *International Security*, 44(1), 42–79. doi:10.1162/isec_a_00351

FAZAL, Tanisha. (2020) Health diplomacy in pandemical times: Drifting toward bilateralism? *International Organization*, 1–20. doi:10.1017/S0020818320000326

FERGUSON, Neil, LAYDON, Daniel, NEDJATI-GILANI, Gemma, IMAI, Natsuko, AINSLIE, Kylie, BAGUELIN, Marc, BHATIA, Sangeeta, BOONYASIRI, Adhiratha, CUCUNUBA, Zulma, CUOMO-DANNENBURG, Gina, DIGHE, Amy, DORIGATTI, Ilaria, FU, Han, GAYTHORPE, Katy, GREEN, Will, HAMELT, Arran, HINSLEY, Wes, OKELL, Lucy C., VAN ELSLAND, Sabine, THOMPSON, Hayley, VERITY, Robert, VOLZ, Erik, WANG, Haowei, WANG, Yuanrong, WALKER, Patrick, WALTERS, Caroline, WINSKILL, Peter, WHITTAKER, Charles, DONNELLY, Christl, RILEY, Steven, and GHANI, Azra. (2020) *Report 9: Impact of Non-Pharmaceutical Interventions (NPI) to Reduce COVID-19 Mortality and Healthcare Demand. Imperial College COVID-19 Response Team.* [Online]. Available: https://doi.org/10.25561/77482 [21 July 2020].

FORMAN, Lisa. (2017) What do human rights bring to discussions of power and politics in health policy and systems? *Global Public Health*, 14(4), 489–502. doi:10.1080/17441692.2017.1405457

FORMAN, Lisa. (2020) The evolution of the right to health in the shadow of COVID-19. *Health and Human Rights Journal*, 22(1), 375–378.

GADARIAN, Shana, and ALBERTSON, Bethany. (2014) Ebola Will Make Americans More Likely to Give up Civil Liberties. *The Washington Post*, 24 October. [Online]. Available: https://www.washingtonpost.com/news/monkey-cage/wp/2014/10/24/ebola-will-make-americans-more-likely-to-give-up-civil-liberties/ [1 August 2020].

GRUSKIN, Sofia, AHMED, Shahira, BOGECHO, Dina, FERGUSON, Laura, HANEFELD, Johanna, MACCARTHY, Sarah, RAAD, Zyde, and STEINER, Riley. (2012) Human rights in health systems frameworks: What is there, what is missing, and why does it matter? *Global Public Health*, 7(4), 337–351. doi:10.1080/17441692.2011.651733

GRUSKIN, Sofia, and DICKENS, Bernard. (2006) Human rights and ethics in public health. *American Journal of Public Health*, 96(11), 1903–1905. doi:10.2105/AJPH.2006.099606

GRUSKIN, Sofia, MILLS, Edward J., and TARANTOLA, Daniel. (2007) History, principles, and practice of health and human rights. *The Lancet*, 370(9585), 449–455.

GUILLEN, Mauro F. (forthcoming) *The Politics of Pandemics: Democracy, State Capacity, and Economic Inequality. Working Paper.* [Online]. Available: https://knowledge.wharton.upenn.edu/article/politics-pandemics-countries-respond-better-others/ [28 September 2020].

GULATI, Gautam, DUNNE, Colum P., and KELLY, Brendan D. (2020) *Do COVID-19 Responses Imperil the Human Rights of People with Disabilities?* [Online]. Available: https://www.hhrjournal.org/2020/06/do-covid-19-responses-imperil-the-human-rights-of-people-with-disabilities/ [12 July 2020].

HANRIEDER, Tine, and KREUDER-SONNEN, Christian. (2014) WHO decides on the exception? Securitization and emergency governance in global health. *Security Dialogue*, 45(4), 331–348. doi:10.1177/0967010614535833

HELFER, Laurence R., and VOETEN, Erik. (2013) International courts as agents of legal change: Evidence from LGBT rights in Europe. *International Organization*, 68(1), 77–110.

HENDRIX, Michael J., WALDE, Charles, FINDLEY, Kendra, and TROTMAN, Robin. (2020) *Absence of Apparent Transmission of SARS-CoV-2 from Two Stylists After Exposure at a Hair Salon with a Universal Face Covering Policy—Springfield, Missouri, May 2020.* [Online]. Available: doi:http://dx.doi.org/10.15585/mmwr.mm6928e2 [31 July 2020].

HOROWITZ, Jason, and BUBOLA, Emma. (2020) Isolating the Sick at Home, Italy Stores up Family Tragedies. *The New York Times*, 24 April. [Online]. Available: https://www.nytimes.com/2020/04/24/world/europe/italy-coronavirus-home-isolation.html?action=click&module=Top%20Stories&pgtype=Homepage [31 July 2020].

INSTITUTE OF MEDICINE (US) COMMITTEE FOR THE STUDY OF THE FUTURE OF PUBLIC HEALTH. (1988) A history of the public health system. In *The Future of Public Health* (Washington, DC: National Academies Press).

JANKOWICZ, Mia. (2020) *More People are Now in 'Lockdown' Than Were Alive During World War II.* [Online]. Available: https://www.sciencealert.com/one-third-of-the-world-s-population-are-now-restricted-in-where-they-can-go [21 July 2020].

JESTER, Barbara, UYEKI, Timothy, and JERNIGAN, Daniel. (2018) Readiness for responding to a severe pandemic 100 years after 1918. *American Journal of Epidemiology*, 187(12), 2596–2602. doi:10.1093/aje/kwy165

KRUG, Etienne G., DAHLBERG, Linda L., MERCY, James A., ZWI, Anthony V., and LOZANO, Rafael (eds.). (2002) *World Report on Violence and Health.* [Online]. Available: https://www.who.int/violence_injury_prevention/violence/world_report/en/ [12 July 2020].

LAI, Shengjie., RUKTANONCHAI, Nick W., ZHOU, Liangcai, PROSPER, Olivia, LUO, Wei, FLOYD, Jessica R., WESOLOWSKI, Amy, SANTILLANA, Mauricio, ZHANG, Chi, DU, Xiangjun, YU, Hongjie, and TATEM, Andrew J. (2020) *Effect of Non-Pharmaceutical Interventions to Contain COVID-19 in China.* [Online]. Available: doi:https://doi.org/10.1038/s41586-020-2293-x[31 July 2020].

LONDON, Leslie. (2008) What is a human-rights based approach to health and does it matter? *Health and Human Rights*, 10(1), 65–80.

LONDON, Leslie, and SCHNEIDER, Helen. (2012) Globalisation and health inequalities: Can a human rights paradigm create space for civil society action? *Social Science and Medicine*, 74(1), 6–13. doi:10.1016/j.socscimed.2011.03.022

MAHDAWI, Arwa. (2020) For Some People, Social Distancing Means Being Trapped Indoors with an Abuser. *The Guardian*, 21 March. [Online]. Available: https://www.theguardian.com/commentisfree/2020/mar/21/coronavirus-domestic-violence-week-in-patriarchy [12 July 2020].

MARKEL, Howard, LIPMAN Harvey B., NAVARRO, J. Alexander, SLOAN, Alexandra, MICHALSEN, Joseph R., STERN, Alexandra Minna, and CETRON, Martin S. (2007) *Nonpharmaceutical Interventions Implemented by US Cities During the 1918–1919 Influenza Pandemic.* [Online]. Available: doi:10.1001/jama.298.6.644 [31 July 2020].

MARKEL, Howard, STERN, Alexandra M., NAVARRO, J. Alexander, MICHALSEN, Joseph R., MONTO, Arnold S., and DIGIOVANNI, Cleto. (2006) Nonpharmaceutical influenza mitigation strategies, US communities, 1918–1920 pandemic. *Emerging Infectious Diseases*, 12(12), 1961–1964. doi:10.3201/eid1212.060506

MATRAJT, Laura, and LEUNG, Tiffany. (2020) Evaluating the effectiveness of social distancing interventions to delay or flatten the epidemic curve of coronavirus disease. *Emerging Infectious Diseases*, 26(8), 1740–1748.

MEIER, Benjamin Mason, EVANS, Dabney P., KAVANAGH, Matthew M., KERALIS, Jessica M., and ARMAS-CARDONA, Gabriel. (2018) Human rights in public health: Deepening engagement at a critical time. *Health and Human Rights*, 20(2), 85–91.

MORAWSKA, Lidia, and CAO, Junji. (2020) Airborne transmission of SARS-CoV-2: The world should face the reality. *Environment International*, 139, 105730.

NAZRUL, Islam, SHARP, Stephen J., CHOWELL, Gerardo, SHABNAM, Sharmin, KAWACHI, Ichiro, LACEY, Ben, MASSARO, Joseph M., D'AGOSTINO, Ralph B. Sr., and WHITE, Martin. (2020) Physical distancing interventions and incidence of coronavirus disease 2019: Natural experiment in 149 countries. *The BMJ*, 370(m2743), 1–10.

OOMS, Gorik, KEYGNAERT, Ines, and HAMMONDS, Rachel. (2019) The right to health: From citizen's right to human right (and back). *Public Health*, 172, 99–104.

PEI, Sen, KANDULA, Sasikiran, and SHAMAN, Jeffrey. (2020) *Differential Effects of Intervention Timing on COVID-19 Spread in the United States*. [Online]. Available: https://www.medrxiv.org/content/10.1101/2020.05.15.20103655v2 [31 July 2020].

PEREHUDOFF, Katrina, and FORMAN, Lisa. (2019) What constitutes 'reasonable' state action on core obligations? Considering a right to health framework to provide essential medicines. *Journal of Human Rights Practice*, 11(1), 1–21. doi:10.1093/jhuman/huz013

PETERSEN, Eskild, KOOPMANS, Marion, GO, Unyeong, HAMER, Davidson H., PETROSILLO, Nicola, CASTELLI, Francesco, STORGAARD, Merete, AL KHALILI, Sulien, and SIMONSEN, Lone. (2020) Comparing SARS-CoV-2 with SARS-CoV and influenza pandemics. *The Lancet*, 20(9), 238–244.

RODRÍGUEZ-GARAVITO, César. (2017). *A Human Right to a Healthy Environment? Moral, Legal, and Empirical Considerations*. [Online]. Available: doi:http://dx.doi.org/10.2139/ssrn.2955357 [26 August 2020].

RUBENSTEIN, Leonard, and DECAMP, Matthew. (2020) *Revisiting Restrictions of Rights After COVID-19*. [Online]. Available: https://www.hhrjournal.org/2020/06/revisiting-restrictions-of-rights-after-covid-19/ [12 July 2020].

SAIZ, Ignacio. (2004) Bracketing sexuality: Human rights and sexual orientation—A decade of development and denial at the UN. *Health and Human Rights*, 7(2), 48–80. doi:10.2307/4065348

SILVA, Diego S., and SMITH, Maxwell J. (2015) Commentary: Limiting rights and freedoms in the context of Ebola and other public health emergencies: How the principle of reciprocity can enrich the application of the Siracusa Principles. *Health and Human Rights*, 17(1), 52–57. doi:10.2307/healhumarigh.17.1.52

SIMMONS, Beth A. (2009) *Mobilizing Human Rights: International Law in Domestic Politics* (Cambridge, UK: Cambridge University Press).

SMITH-CANNOY, Heather. (2012) *Insincere Commitments: Human Rights Treaties, Abusive States, and Citizen Activism* (Washington, DC: Georgetown University Press).

SOHRABI, Catrin, ALSAFI, Zaid, O'NEILL, Niamh, KHAN, Mehdi, KERWAN, Ahmed, AL-JABIR, Ahmed, IOSIFIDIS, Christos, and AGHA, Riaz. (2020) World Health Organization declares global emergency: A review of the 2019 novel coronavirus (COVID-19). *International Journal of Surgery*, 76, 71–76.

TAUBENBERGER, Jeffery K., and MORENS, David M. (2006) 1918 influenza: The mother of all pandemics. *Emerging Infectious Diseases*, 12(1), 15–22. doi:10.3201/eid1201.050979

TENFORDE, Mark W., KIM, Sara S., LINDSELL, Christopher J., et al. (2020) Symptom duration and risk factors for delayed return to usual health among outpatients with COVID-19 in a multistate health care systems network—United States, March–June 2020. *Morbidity and Mortality Weekly Report*, 69(3), 993–998. doi: 10.15585/mmwr.mm6930e1

TODRYS, Katherine W., HOWE, Erin, and AMON, Joseph J. (2013) Failing Siracusa: Governments' obligations to find the least restrictive options for tuberculosis control. *Public Health Action*, 3(1), 7–10. doi:10.5588/pha.12.0094

TOEBES, Brigit. (2015) Human rights and public health: Towards a balanced relationship. *The International Journal of Human Rights*, 19(4), 488–504. doi:10.1080/13642987.2015.1044814

WANG, Xiaowen, FERRO, Enrico G., ZHOU, Guohai, HASHIMOTO, Dean, and BHATT, Deepak L. (2020) *Association Between Universal Masking in a Health Care System and SARS-CoV-2 Positivity Among Health Care Workers*. [Online]. Available: doi:10.1001/jama.2020.12897 [31 July 2020].

WENHAM, Clare. (2017) What we have learnt about the World Health Organization from the Ebola outbreak. *Philosophical Transactions of the Royal Society B*, 371(1721). doi:10.1098/rstb.2016.0307

WENHAM, Clare, and FARIAS, Deborah B. L. (2019) Securitizing Zika: The case of Brazil. *Security Dialogue*, 50(5), 398–415. doi:10.1177/0967010619856458

WORLD HEALTH ORGANIZATION. (2006) *Constitution of the World Health Organization*. [Online]. Available: https://www.who.int/governance/eb/who_constitution_en.pdf [23 July 2020].

WORLD HEALTH ORGANIZATION. (2007a) *Ethical Considerations in Developing a Public Health Response to Pandemic Influenza*. [Online]. Available: https://www.who.int/csr/resources/publications/WHO_CDS_EPR_GIP_2007_2/en/ [21 July 2020].

WORLD HEALTH ORGANIZATION. (2007b) *WHO Guidance on Human Rights and Involuntary Detention for xdr-tb Control*. [Online]. Available: https://www.who.int/tb/features_archive/involuntary_treatment/en/ [12 July 2020].

WORLD HEALTH ORGANIZATION. (2008) *Addressing Ethical Issues in Pandemic Influenza Planning: Discussion Papers*. [Online]. Available: https://apps.who.int/iris/handle/10665/69902 [21 July 2020].

WORLD HEALTH ORGANIZATION. (2015) *Global Health Ethics: Key Issues*. [Online]. Available: https://apps.who.int/iris/bitstream/handle/10665/164576/9789240694033_eng.pdf?sequence=1 [12 July 2020].

WORLD HEALTH ORGANIZATION. (2016) *Guidance for Managing Ethical Issues in Infectious Disease Outbreaks.* [Online]. Available: https://apps.who.int/iris/handle/10665/250580 [21 July 2020].

WORLD HEALTH ORGANIZATION. (2017a) *Human Rights and Health.* [Online]. Available: https://www.who.int/news-room/fact-sheets/detail/human-rights-and-health [31 July 2020].

WORLD HEALTH ORGANIZATION. (2017b) *WHO Guidelines on Ethical Issues in Public Health Surveillance.* [Online]. Available: https://www.who.int/ethics/publications/public-health-surveillance/en/ [21 July 2020].

WORLD HEALTH ORGANIZATION. (2018) *A Checklist for Pandemic Influenza Risk and Impact Management: Building Capacity for Pandemic Response—2018 Update.* [Online]. Available: https://www.who.int/influenza/preparedness/pandemic/influenza_risk_management_checklist_2018/en/ [21 July 2020].

WORLD HEALTH ORGANIZATION. (2019) *Non-pharmaceutical Public Health Measures for Mitigating the Risk and Impact of Epidemic and Pandemic Influenza.* [Online]. Available: https://www.who.int/influenza/publications/public_health_measures/publication/en/ [21 July 2020].

WORLD HEALTH ORGANIZATION. (2020a) *A Human Rights-based Approach to Health.* [Online]. Available: https://www.who.int/hhr/news/hrba_to_health2.pdf [21 July 2020].

WORLD HEALTH ORGANIZATION. (2020b) *About WHO.* [Online]. Available: https://www.who.int/about [21 July 2020].

WORLD HEALTH ORGANIZATION. (2020c) *Addressing Human Rights as Key to the COVID-19 Response.* [Online]. Available: https://www.who.int/publications/i/item/addressing-human-rights-as-key-to-the-covid-19-response [21 July 2020].

WORLD HEALTH ORGANIZATION. (2020d) *Operational Planning Guidance to Support Country Preparedness and Response.* [Online]. Available: https://www.who.int/docs/default-source/coronaviruse/covid-19-sprp-unct-guidelines.pdf?sfvrsn=81ff43d8_4 [31 July 2020].

WORLD HEALTH ORGANIZATION. (2020e) *Overview of Public Health and Social Measures in the Context of COVID-19.* [Online]. Available: https://www.who.int/publications/i/item/overview-of-public-health-and-social-measures-in-the-context-of-covid-19 [31 July 2020].

WORLD HEALTH ORGANIZATON. (2020f) *Press Conference of WHO–China Joint Mission on COVID-19.* [Online]. Available: https://www.who.int/docs/default-source/coronaviruse/transcripts/joint-mission-press-conference-script-english-final.pdf?sfvrsn=51c90b9e_10 [21 July 2020].

WORLD HEALTH ORGANIZATION. (2020g) *Report of the WHO–China Joint Mission on Coronavirus Disease 2019* (COVID-19). [Online]. Available: https://www.who.int/publications/i/item/report-of-the-who-china-joint-mission-on-coronavirus-disease-2019-(covid-19). [21 July 2020].

WORSNOP, Catherine Z. (2017) Domestic politics and the WHO's international health regulations: Explaining the use of trade and travel barriers during disease outbreaks. *Review of International Organizations*, 12(3), 365–395.

YAMIN, Alicia Ely. (2017) Taking the right to health seriously: Implications for health systems, courts, and achieving universal health coverage. *Human Rights Quarterly*, 39(2), 341–368. doi:10.1353/hrq.2017.0021

YEHYA, Nadir, VENKATARAMANI, Atheendar, and HARHAY, Michael O. (2020) Statewide interventions and COVID-19 mortality in the United States: An observational study. *Clinical Infections Diseases.* doi:https://doi.org/10.1093/cid/ciaa923[31 July 2020].

YOUDE, Jeremy. (2020) Trump wants to review the WHO's actions. These are its key roles and limitations. *The Washington Post,* 16 April. [Online]. Available: https://www.washingtonpost.com/politics/2020/04/16/trump-wants-review-whos-actions-these-are-its-key-roles-limitations/ [21 July 2020].

Contesting power and control

Legal empowerment approaches in the context of COVID-19

Sukti Dhital and Tyler Walton

ABSTRACT
Emerging data reveals the COVID-19 pandemic's disproportionate impact on historically marginalized communities. Drawing on in-depth interviews with legal empowerment practitioners, this article explores case studies of three communities (in Argentina, India, and the United States) that highlight a grassroots approach to tackling injustice during COVID-19. The article finds lasting insights for human rights practitioners and scholars, with the concepts of translation, trust, and transformation integral to disrupting power structures and creating pathways for communities to become the authors of their own justice and liberation.

Introduction

The COVID-19 pandemic has triggered chaos across the globe, with governments struggling to reduce the spread of the virus amid rising challenges to human rights (Human Rights Watch 2020). Emerging data reveal the pandemic's disproportionate impact on the historically marginalized communities of black and brown people, Dalits and indigenous peoples, women, and people with disabilities (Devakumar, Bhopal, and Shannon 2020). These disparities are fueled by structural inequalities that deny people their human rights, including a right to access justice.[1] In 2019, a staggering 5.1 billion people were found to lack meaningful access to justice (Taskforce on Justice 2019). COVID-19 exacerbates this justice gap, with marginalized communities experiencing a pandemic within a pandemic of inequality and oppression.

In the midst of this devastating challenge, a grassroots approach to justice offers hope. Legal empowerment—a rights-based methodology that centers people in their own fight for justice—creates opportunities for people to "know, use, and shape" the laws that impact their lives (Satterthwaite forthcoming). These methods are a form of community immunity against injustice—parallel to the sought-after herd immunity to COVID-19 (Kwok, Lai, Wei, Wong, and Tang 2020).

In this article, we seek to understand how legal empowerment approaches to tackle injustice during COVID-19 may yield lasting insights for human rights scholars and practitioners. We open with a background on legal empowerment and human rights. Next, we explore the concepts of translation, trust, and transformation through three case studies carried out during the time of the COVID-19 pandemic, with informal settlement communities in Buenos Aires, Argentina, in New Delhi, India, and among undocumented communities in Chicago, the United States. The case studies are based on in-depth interviews[2] with members of three legal empowerment organizations and analysis of their resources: the Asociación Civil por la Igualdad y la Justicia (ACIJ) in Argentina, Nazdeek in India, and Organized Communities Against Deportation (OCAD) in Chicago. The case studies reveal that in both ethos and practice, the organizations remain rooted to acts of translation, trust, and transformation as essential drivers for building grassroots power and advancing justice.

This article is based on the spirit, labor, and dedication of these resilient communities; we highlight this work with humility and gratitude (Hung 2017).

Legal empowerment and human rights

Institutions regularly empower formal experts (such as lawyers, academics, or policymakers) to make decisions that impact the human rights of communities without their meaningful participation. Legal empowerment strives for a different world, one in which power structures are contested and disrupted, and directly impacted people become the authors of their own justice and liberation (Dhital 2018). Proponents of this approach believe that those closest to a problem are closest to a solution, and recognize lived experience as essential expertise (Dhital 2018). Lawyers and other formally trained individuals are seen as valuable partners in the fight for justice, with communities driving the decision-making process.[3] Legal empowerment takes many forms, including community paralegal programs, know-your-rights workshops, accompaniment programs, community-driven litigation, and community-driven campaigning efforts (JusticePower 2020a).

The field has iterated and evolved, drawing insights from trade union (Levi 2003) and feminist movements (Ackerly 2018), which saw the "emancipatory power of popular education and therefore embedded rights awareness with self-reflection and collective action" (Feruglio 2017: 6). It also finds roots in anti-apartheid movements, in which women community paralegals partnered with lawyers, NGOs, and churches to document violations, provide legal assistance, and bear witness to the injustice endured by communities of color (Dugard and Drage 2013).

Legal empowerment emerged as a principal strategy to increase access to justice and achieve sustainable development (Golub 2003; Gisselquist 2019). The term gained prominence with the 2008 UN Commission on Legal Empowerment of the Poor (CLEP),[4] which defined legal empowerment as "the process through which the poor become protected and are enabled to use the law to advance their rights and their interests" (2008: 26). CLEP anchored legal empowerment in the "basic principles of human rights articulated in the 1948 Universal Declaration of Human Rights (UDHR)—and the subsequent universal and regional international human rights conventions" (2008: 20). It underlined that all people have the right to access justice without discrimination, and that states must take positive steps to make this promise real for all (CLEP 2008). Meaningful participation was seen as essential to protecting this right, with former Special Rapporteur for Extreme Poverty and Human Rights Magdalena Sepulveda linking the right to participation with empowerment, and describing it as a "key human rights goal and principle" (2012: 6). Legal empowerment was thus understood as both a means of realizing human rights and an end in itself (US Agency for International Development 2007).

Today more than 2,300 organizations are part of a global network dedicated to legal empowerment (Namati 2020), with a growing community of organizations moving beyond an approach to providing "access to justice" in conventional terms, toward embracing grassroots power as key to achieving social transformation.

Three case studies: Translation, trust, and transformation

During the COVID-19 pandemic, we sought to explore how legal empowerment organizations were responding to the justice crisis. What strategies did they use to build power and advance justice as marginalized communities suffered under the weight of SARS-CoV-2? Did their work pivot in response to new and old forms of discrimination fueled by state and social responses to the virus? Through in-depth case studies with organizations in Buenos Aires, New Delhi, and

Chicago, we found remarkable levels of symmetry despite varying social, economic, political, and cultural contexts. Central to all of the work was community partnerships grounded in acts of translation, trust, and transformation. We argue that these components are foundational to shifting power, building individual and collective agency, and protecting human rights.

Translation flows: It democratizes laws and legal systems into a language that communities can understand, while also creating pathways for communities to share their lived realities and demand justice. Trust is a practice of vulnerability: It is an act of inclusive decision making and is foundational to thriving relationships between organizations and community partners. Transformation is both present and future: It is an active process through which individuals and communities reclaim their power, and in so doing reimagine and rebuild systems that work for everyone. Although all three organizations practice translation, trust, and transformation, the case studies explore each practice through the lens of a single organization.

Translation: *Asociación Civil por la Igualdad y la Justicia*

Founded in 2002 and based in Buenos Aires, ACIJ is an organization of lawyers, researchers, and activists dedicated to defending the rights of marginalized people and developing participatory and deliberative practices of democracy in Argentina. It engages in grassroots legal education, strategic litigation, action-research, and advocacy, and works with communities living in *villas*—informal settlements in Buenos Aires. The *villas* have a long history of political and social mobilization, with social movements organizing for public policies and a right to stay for nearly a century (Blaustein 2001). Today, people in the *villas* face profound housing insecurity and lack basic amenities such as water, electricity, and internet infrastructure (Mesel and Vitale 2019). Essential supplies are provided through *referentes sociales*—social leaders of local organizations who obtain public and private support to provide food and promote community health and solidarity (Mesel and Vitale 2019).

The first case of COVID-19 in Argentina was recorded on March 3, 2020 (*Buenos Aires Times*, 2020). In the weeks to follow, the virus spread rapidly in the *villas*, with cases doubling every seven days, compared to every 10 days in the city at large (Buenos Aires Ciudad 2020). Although *villas* make up only 10 percent of the city's population, at one point 46.8 percent of total COVID-19 cases were from the *villas*, with some neighborhoods within the *villas* reporting 70 percent positivity rates (Buenos Aires Ciudad 2020). Elena was one of these diagnoses. A social leader and member of *Bajo Autopista*—a collective of women resisting relocation as a result of the city's urbanization plan—Elena saw fear, hunger, and sickness escalate without an adequate government response. There was a breakdown in communication and translation was necessary. *Bajo Autopista* reached out to ACIJ for support.

Translation in action

Translation spans the literal act of translating words from one language to another to the "vernacularization" (Merry 2006) of the law into a language that is accessible, and the "localization" of concepts (Mattingly 2019) to connect them to the lived experiences of a community. Translation is an essential piece of ACIJ's work, as exemplified by the legal empowerment course involving social leaders across the *villas*. Known as the School of Human Rights: Villas (Slums) and Legal Empowerment Strategies, this four-month course covers the social and political history of the *villas*, human rights of *villa* dwellers, and strategies to protect those rights. The course translates laws and policies into a language that is understandable to members of the community and draws on lived expertise to craft resistance strategies. A WhatsApp group created at the end of the course encourages ongoing exchange and collaboration.

Once COVID-19 hit the *villas*, the WhatsApp group became more active, with social leaders sharing public health information and government responses to the pandemic. ACIJ, in conversation with the community, saw the need for urgent translation. The organization pivoted and held five virtual webinars on COVID-19 with more than 70 community members. These interdisciplinary trainings covered public health and sanitation measures, rights and benefits linked to COVID-19, and legal tools to address rights violations. ACIJ also created a resource that outlined rights connected specifically to the pandemic, such as a moratorium on evictions and entitlements to specific social security benefits for families during the crisis.

Translation does not only flow to community, it also flows out from community. As Felipe Mesel (2020), a lawyer with ACIJ reflected, "With legal empowerment, communities seize the right to translate." Community data justice projects are one such example. In these projects, communities collect, analyze, and translate data that lay the foundation for individual and systemic demands (Davis 2020). These efforts have been described as "community resilience, the power of collecting and sharing our stories, and the possibilities of community self-defense" (Our Data Bodies 2019). ACIJ recognizes that data are a "contested terrain in a political debate over who counts, who does the counting, and who gets counted" (Davis 2017: 1145), and that people who are "uncounted" are rendered invisible, creating "a data paradox, in which invisibility reinforces lack of resources and services" (Davis 2017: 1157).

People living in the *villas* suffer from invisibility, with a lack of data on their conditions reinforcing exclusion and, in turn, a denial of basic services (Castro 2014; Petty, Saba, Lewis, Gangadharan, and Eubanks 2018). ACIJ, in partnership with the community, saw an opening to change this, by creating a way for small data to "draw … on the problems faced by real people" in order to "help identify the problems that matter to a community" and to "shape the best ways to address those problems" (Burnett and Walker 2018).

In 2014, ACIJ launched the *Caminos de la Villa* project, a participatory mapping effort of the *villas*. ACIJ later approached Google, which added a functionality to enable communities to collect data and upload the information onto Google Street View.[5] The resulting maps were incorporated into official maps, and community members felt legitimated and seen, a crucial step toward recognition within the public agenda.

In the next phase, community members began documenting the lack of public services on the participatory map. The data were used for litigation, human rights documentation, and advocacy. The project also mapped the city's urbanization plans. Whereas the government of Buenos Aires had described the plans as a vehicle for getting formal services into informal settlements, *Caminos de la Villa* demonstrated that urbanization was only occurring in areas where property value was high (ACIJ 2020a). This participatory data-gathering exercise also served as a vital truth-telling tool.

Once COVID-19 hit the *villas*, ACIJ saw the power of using *Caminos de la Villa* to highlight the disparate impact of the virus within the city. Relying on official government statistics, the site shows the disproportionate number of cases within the *villas* as compared to other parts of the city (ACIJ 2020b). *Caminos de la Villa* reveals a broken system, with the map itself (created by and for community) enabling the visualization of discrimination and exclusion.

Trust: Nazdeek

Founded in 2012 and based in New Delhi, Nazdeek fuses grassroots legal education, community monitoring, legal remedies, research, and advocacy to bring justice closer to marginalized communities in South Asia. The organization is a collective of women activist-lawyers, researchers, and community paralegals—community justice workers who act as a bridge between the legal system and the community. Nazdeek focuses its work in the urban settlements of New Delhi, tea plantations of Assam, and garment factories of Tamil Nadu, with the aim of advancing the rights of indigenous and Dalit communities.

Baprola is one of these settlements. Baprola sits on the outskirts of Delhi and was selected by the government as a site for relocation of thousands of families evicted from their *basti* or slum (Misra 2019). Despite the law and government plans mandating otherwise, these disproportionately poor and Dalit families were relocated from the city center to an area without schools, hospitals, ration shops (local food distribution centers that provide government-subsidized food grains to poor people), or employment opportunities (Misra 2019).

Members of Nazdeek learned of Baprola in 2015, while working in a nearby informal settlement, and approached community members to explore a legal empowerment project. Since then, Nazdeek has trained more than 25 women paralegals on rights-based frameworks, helping to build their skills to document, monitor, and file complaints. Nazdeek has also partnered with community members to file strategic litigation and has offered advocacy support. Together, they have pressured the government of India to set up a local health clinic and nutritional centers, to improve water and sanitation delivery, and to appoint community health workers.

Trust in action

In spring 2020, Seema was the first community paralegal to call Nazdeek. She said there was a food emergency in Baprola due to the lockdown issued by the Indian government as the COVID-19 pandemic ensued. Families were hungry and scared, and she wondered if Nazdeek could step in. Just days before, as the number of confirmed COVID-19 cases in India reached approximately 500, the entire country was ordered into a sudden, complete shutdown (Gettleman and Schultz 2020). Indian police authorities enforced the lockdown with use of force (Gettleman and Schultz 2020). Hundreds of thousands of daily-wage migrant workers in Delhi became jobless and began walking home to their villages across the country (Pandey 2020). Hunger skyrocketed, with numerous ration shops suddenly shuttered without warning; the few open were unable to meet the increased demand (*The Wire* 2020). Although Seema knew that Nazdeek did not itself carry out relief work, she also knew that the organization was driven by community needs.

Nazdeek's work is rooted in trust. Developing and maintaining trust is essential for communities and organizations to work together to advance justice (Schoorman, Mayer, and Davis 2007). Trust is built and fostered through open and shared decision making (Colquitt and Rodell 2011). Lawyers and other formal practitioners must recognize their privilege and power, and open up space for communities to engage and ultimately lead decision-making processes.

Lam Ho, the founder and director of the US-based legal empowerment organization Beyond Legal Aid, describes the trust-building process as a "willingness to be vulnerable" that involves a "depowering of lawyers," along with an "un-learning" of roles and "admit[ting] what we do not know" (JusticePower 2020b). Nazdeek similarly strives to address these dynamics, although caste and class hierarchies render this a continual work in progress. As an organization with lawyers and researchers (some of whom are not directly impacted by the same risks faced by community members), Nazdeek's staff recognize the asymmetries of power and the need to center community expertise. This is where trust comes in.

Based on community demands, Nazdeek pivoted in the wake of the COVID-19 lockdown in India and contacted donors to secure funds to deliver emergency relief kits. The relief work ran from March to May 2020, involving intensive planning and coordination with partner organizations: Ultimately, nearly 20,000 people received essential supplies. By mid-May, once ration shops and health clinics began reopening due to civil society pressure, Nazdeek again pivoted to address legal issues arising from the pandemic. This time the call was from Geeta, another paralegal in Baprola. She shared that the community had registered its first confirmed COVID-19 case. She stressed the attendant lack of information and fear of spread due to the settlement's dense population. Nazdeek decided to conduct a remote training that would cover public health safety measures as well as pandemic-related rights and resources.

Nazdeek held the training on July 2, 2020, with six community paralegals and two community organizers. Several test runs of the video technology were carried out to ensure adequate video and audio quality, and to help members download and navigate the tool. Before the training, members of Nazdeek sent a PowerPoint presentation, shared YouTube videos on public health measures, and purchased data packages to ensure that everyone could join and download materials onto their devices. The training was interactive and impactful, blending substantive law with hypothetical scenarios and role-play activities, in which participants were asked to identify rights violations and legal strategies.

Nazdeek also continued to seek accountability for rights violations spurred by COVID-19. India's longstanding challenges with backlogged courts and unresponsive administrative grievance mechanisms made these mechanisms largely inaccessible (Gauri 2010; Hertel 2016). Despite this, Nazdeek filed complaints and petitions to record the structural violence caused by a failing system and obtain redress (Gupta 2012). The organization also shared community-collected data to highlight challenges in accessing COVID-19-related benefits.

All of these efforts grew from trust developed and strengthened by centering communities in the decision-making process. Rather than doing the work for communities, Nazdeek works with communities to determine their goals and demands. During a pandemic, the practice of trusting community members to decide what they needed remained steady. Although Nazdeek as an organization had never carried out relief work, trust in partnership and process led the way. The organization's steadfast gaze on exploiting legal mechanisms also signaled to the Indian government, as well as to community partners, that Nazdeek will keep fighting for a more just future. Shreya Sen, senior program officer with Nazdeek explained, "We want to tell the true story of how COVID is impacting a dysfunctional state. Systems—like the health and justice system—are failing. Even if the system fails, we will continue to demand a response" (Poddar, Satpute, and Sen 2020).

Transformation: Organized Communities Against Deportation

OCAD is a group of "undocumented, unapologetic, and unafraid organizers building a resistance movement against deportations and the criminalization of immigrants and people of color" (OCAD 2020). The organization is based in Chicago, a city with an estimated 450,000 undocumented immigrants, the majority of whom are Latinx, Asian, and black (Tribune Graphics 2017).

Many of Chicago's immigrants live and work in the shadows because of their citizenship status. Perceptions of "illegality" tend to rely on national origin, social class, and criminal background rather than actual legal status (Flores and Schachter 2018), placing immigrants at the intersection of this perceived "illegality" and structural racism, classism, and discrimination. OCAD fights to change these terrorizing systems and "create an environment for our communities to work, organize, and thrive with happiness and without fear" (OCAD 2020). Members engage in community-driven campaigns, litigation, grassroots legal education, and mutual aid to build individual and collective power.

The organization is "undocumented-led" and guided by community input and direction, garnered through *asambleas* (community assemblies). Before the COVID-19 pandemic, the assemblies were held twice a month with around 50 members who discussed information on active immigration cases, explored organizing actions, identified strategic actions, and shared a collective meal. OCAD is led by Lxs Luchadorxs, a committee of about 10 members who have faced their own deportation proceedings.

Transformation in action

In spring of 2020, OCAD received worried reports of expanded COVID-19 surveillance measures by Immigration and Customs Enforcement (ICE), justified on public health grounds and enacted in conjunction with broad emergency powers. Related measures included contact tracking using cell phone data and facial recognition technology, body temperature tracking, electronic anklet monitoring, and predictive modeling based on big data (Just Futures Law 2020). Prior to the pandemic, ICE regularly targeted undocumented immigrants for deportation through the use of surveillance technology (Funk 2019). This technology has become more sophisticated, as corporations including Palantir, Clearview, Google, and Amazon have begun to sell facial-recognition software, data, and analytics services to public agencies, police departments, and ICE (Garvie and Moy 2019; Mac, Haskins, and McDonald 2020). OCAD members were particularly concerned that surveillance in response to the COVID-19 pandemic would increase risks of deportation.

Challenging surveillance was not new for OCAD; the organization was a founding member of a coalition committed to the elimination of the gang database used by the Chicago Police Department to surveil, harass, target, and deport people from black and brown communities (OCAD 2020). But surveillance during the COVID-19 pandemic felt new and more dangerous (Just Futures Law 2020). OCAD was approached by Just Futures Law, a legal organization focused on transformative and innovative immigration lawyering, to discuss surveillance trends and explore a community-based litigation project. Before making a decision, OCAD emphasized the need to present the project to the assemblies and Lxs Luchadorxs.

OCAD works to catalyze the transformation of undocumented communities into holders of knowledge and agents of change. Leadership is a learned skill that OCAD cultivates through sharing knowledge, organizing behind common goals, and activating members into collective political action. Transformation is often viewed as a goal of legal empowerment work. As Domingo and O'Neil observed, "Legal empowerment occurs when poor or marginalised people use the law, legal systems, and justice mechanisms to improve or transform their social, political or economic situations" (2014: 4).

Toward this goal, organizations use a "range of tools driven by the communities with which they work, including information, organizing, advocacy, and litigation" (Chapman 2018: 183). These efforts create space for communities to learn and dream. They also seek to activate institutions through individual and collective claims, with a goal of social transformation. Satterthwaite (forthcoming) has described this work as "critical legal empowerment," a "practice and a lens, making visible the work communities and movements are doing to transform legal systems."

Transformation is also a personal practice through which individuals see themselves as "bearers of rights" and "agents capable of action" who are able to build individual and collective agency (Maru and Gauri 2018: 1). As Antonio Gutierrez of OCAD explained:

> We organize the community so that they tap into the collective power. We believe in the autonomy and self-determination of the communities in which we work. This involves waking the social and political conscience of the community, bringing them from the inactivity pressed upon them by systemic racism and xenophobia, and into a state of wakefulness and activity that is essential to movement building and achieving just outcomes. We believe in collective learning, knowledge, and healing. We are what we need. (2020)

Central to this work is the power generated by being together in one space. And yet, the need to physically distance during the pandemic made these efforts near impossible. Recognizing the integral role of *asambleas* as transformative spaces for community leadership, OCAD transitioned its assemblies online. This shift was done with intention, taking into account accessibility and tech literacy: OCAD shared instructional videos with members detailing how to download and set up the Zoom videoconference platform, and narrated the tutorial in Spanish.

During the digital assemblies, members discussed individual cases, existing campaigns, and the proposal to partner with Just Futures Law on a COVID-19 surveillance project. OCAD created a presentation that translated the proposal from Just Futures Law into Spanish and broke down the concepts of laws and rights into a language that spoke to members' experiences.

Surveillance plays an active role in the lives of many OCAD members; the presentation resonated with their experiences of ankle bracelets, regular ICE check-ins, and the Chicago gang database that regularly shares information with ICE. Members also raised additional privacy concerns, including images taken by traffic cameras and license plate readers. These conversations were part of the regular practice of coming together to share experiences and connecting those experiences to broader systems. Members felt empowered to discuss the information presented to them, as well as add issues they saw as integral to challenging dehumanizing systems. In this case, it was concerns around data collected by traffic cameras; in other projects, it was pushing lawyers to file motions as an organizing tactic.

Ultimately, OCAD's membership agreed to partner on the surveillance project. They have filed Illinois Freedom of Information Act (FOIA) requests for records on how government agencies are using technology to expand data surveillance during the COVID-19 pandemic.[6] As of this writing, the organizations await responses from the city of Chicago and other government agencies after filing. They plan to use the information elicited through the FOIA requests to build a community-led campaign against surveillance.

Conclusion

The COVID-19 pandemic thrust already marginalized communities into a deeper justice crisis. Legal empowerment organizations leaned into their work of translation, trust, and transformation as strategies for power contestation and rights claiming. As evident from the three case studies analyzed in this article, this form of human rights practice offers enduring insights into how to breathe justice into social and legal systems while enabling communities to rebuild a just, transformed future.

Notes

1. The right to access justice is essential to the protection of many human rights and is also a human right itself. Access to justice is protected under the International Covenant on Civil and Political Rights (ICCPR; UN General Assembly 1966: Article 14) as clarified by General Comment No. 32 to the ICCPR (Human Rights Committee 2007).
2. We conducted in-depth interviews with Felipe Mesel of ACIJ (Mesel 2020); Tripti Poddar, Jayshree Satpute, and Shreya Sen of Nazdeek (Poddar, Satpute, and Sen 2020); and Antonio Gutierrez of OCAD (Gutierrez 2020). These interviews occurred via phone and video-conferencing, with additional correspondence via email, from July 6, 2020, to August 6, 2020. All quotes attributed to Mesel, Poddar, Satpute, Sen, and Gutierrez were provided by and verified by the person to which they are attributed. Pseudonyms were used when referencing community members to protect their identities and security. We are deeply indebted to the organizations whose work is highlighted.
3. Experts play an important role in the development of policy responses to COVID-19, and problems arise when governments contradict public health experts, but even when governments listen to experts, "questions remain about how to mitigate … inequalities to support the world's most vulnerable" (Weible, Nohrstedt, Cairney, Carter, Crow, Durnová, Heikkila, Ingold, McConnell, and Stone 2020). This article focuses on that question.
4. The International Commission on Legal Empowerment of the Poor (CLEP) was hosted by the United Nations Development Programme (UNDP) in 2005; it was formed to focus on the link between exclusion, poverty, and the law. CLEP's final report, *Making the Law Work for Everyone* (2008), was adopted by the UN General Assembly (2008) and was followed up with a report by the UN Secretary-General on "legal empowerment of the poor and eradication of poverty" (2009).
5. Images collected by the community can be viewed on the Google Maps Street View website. For an example of an image taken in Villa 31 in November 2016, see https://www.google.com/maps/@-34.585301,-58.3776946,2a,75y,100.37h,102t/data=!3m6!1e1!3m4!1sgvEz-qtevT7sftAbRrVqZg!2e0!7i13312!8i6656 [18 August 2020].

6. FOIA requests were made to the Chicago Police Department (Non-Commercial Police FOIA Request: P585877-061420), Mayor Lori Lightfoot, and the Chicago Department of Public Health via email on 11 June 2020.

References

ACKERLY, Brooke. (2018) *Just Responsibility: A Human Rights Theory of Global Justice* (New York, NY: Oxford University Press).

ASOCIACIÓN CIVIL POR LA IGUALDAD Y LA JUSTICIA (ACIJ). (2020a) *Caminos de la Villa.* [Online]. Available: https://caminosdelavilla.org [18 August 2020].

ASOCIACIÓN CIVIL POR LA IGUALDAD Y LA JUSTICIA (ACIJ). (2020b) *Situación de las Villas ante COVID-19.* [Online]. Available: https://www.covid-19.caminosdelavilla.org [18 August 2020].

BLAUSTEIN, Eduardo. (2001) *Prohibido Vivir Aquí. Una Historia de los Planes de Erradicación de las Villas de la Última Dictadura.* [Online]. Available: http://cidac.filo.uba.ar/sites/cidac.filo.uba.ar/files/revistas/adjuntos/UNIDAD%2015%20-%20MUROS%20SIGLOS.pdf [August 2020].

BUENOS AIRES CIUDAD. (2020) *Actualización de los Casos de Coronavirus en la Ciudad.* [Online]. Available: https://www.buenosaires.gob.ar/coronavirus/noticias/actualizacion-de-los-casos-de-coronavirus-en-la-ciudad-buenos-aires [18 August 2020].

BUENOS AIRES TIMES. (2020) *Argentina Confirms First Case of COVID-19 Coronavirus.* [Onine]. Available: https://www.batimes.com.ar/news/argentina/argentina-confirms-first-case-of-covid-19-coronavirus.phtml [18 August 2020].

BURNETT, Matthew, and WALKER, Tom. (2018) *How Small Data Can Improve Access to Justice for the Poor.* [Online]. Available: https://www.opensocietyfoundations.org/voices/how-small-data-can-improve-access-justice-poor [18 August 2020].

CASTRO, Daniel. (2014) *The Rise of Data Poverty in America.* [Online]. Available: http://www2.datainnovation.org/2014-data-poverty.pdf [18 August 2020].

CHAPMAN, Peter. (2018) The legal empowerment movement and its implications. *Fordham Law Review Online*, 87(30), 183–185.

COLQUITT, Jason A., and RODELL, Jessica B. (2011) Justice, trust, and trustworthiness: A longitudinal analysis integrating three theoretical perspectives. *Academy of Management Journal*, 54(6), 1183–1206. doi:10.5465/amj.2007.0572

DAVIS, Sara L. M. (2017) The uncounted: Politics of data and visibility in global health. *International Journal of Human Rights*, 21(8), 1144–1163. doi:10.1080/13642987.2017.1348707

DAVIS, Sara L. M. (2020) *The Uncounted: Politics of Data in Global Health* (New York, NY: Cambridge University Press).

DEVAKUMAR, Delan, BHOPAL, Sunil S., and SHANNON, Geordan. (2020) COVID-19: The great unequaliser. *Journal of the Royal Society of Medicine*, 113(6), 234–235. doi:10.1177/0141076820925434

DHITAL, Sukti. (2018) *Reimagining Justice: Human rights Through Legal Empowerment.* [Online]. Available: https://www.openglobalrights.org/Reimagining-justice-human-rights-through-legal-empowerment/ [18 August 2020].

DOMINGO, Pilar, and O'NEIL, Tam. (2014) *The Politics of Legal Empowerment: Legal Mobilisation Strategies and Implications for Development.* [Online]. Available: https://www.odi.org/sites/odi.org.uk/files/odi-assets/publications-opinion-files/9008.pdf [18 August 2020].

DUGARD, Jackie, and DRAGE, Katherine. (2013) *'To Whom Do the People Take Their Issues?' The Contribution of Community-Based Paralegals to Access to Justice in South Africa (English).* Justice and Development Working Paper Series, no. 21 (Washington, DC: World Bank Group).

FERUGLIO, Francesca. (2017) *Do More Empowered Citizens Make More Accountable States? Power and Legitimacy in Legal Empowerment Initiatives in Kenya and South Africa.* [Online]. Available: http://opendocs.ids.ac.uk/opendocs/handle/123456789/13172 [18 August 2020].

FLORES, Rene D., and SCHACHTER, Ariela. (2018) Who are the 'illegals'? The social construction of illegality in the United States. *American Sociological Review*, 83(5), 839–868. doi:10.1177/0003122418794635

FUNK, McKenzie. (2019) How ICE picks its targets in the surveillance age. *The New York Times*, 20 October. [Online]. Available: https://www.nytimes.com/2019/10/02/magazine/ice-surveillance-deportation.html [18 August 2020].

GARVIE, Clare, and MOY, Laura M. (2019) *America Under Watch: Face Surveillance in the United States*. [Online]. Available: https://www.americaunderwatch.com [18 August 2020].

GAURI, Varun. (2010) Fundamental rights and public interest litigation in India: Overreaching or underachieving? *Indian Journal of Law & Economics*, 3(1), 71–93.

GETTLEMAN, Jeffrey, and SCHULTZ, Kai. (2020) Modi orders 3-week total lockdown for all 1.3 billion Indians. *The New York Times*, 24 March.

GISSELQUIST, Rachel M. (2019) Legal empowerment and group-based inequality. *Journal of Development Studies*, 55(3), 333–347. doi:10.1080/00220388.2018.1451636

GOLUB, Stephen. (2003) *Beyond the Rule of Law Orthodoxy: The Legal Empowerment Alternative*. [Online]. Available: https://carnegieendowment.org/files/wp41.pdf [18 August 2020].

GUPTA, Akhil. (2012) *Red Tape: Bureaucracy, Structural Violence, and Poverty in India* (Durham, NC: Duke University Press).

GUTIERREZ, Antonio. (2020) Interview by the authors, July 8–August 6.

HERTEL, Shareen. (2016) A new route to norms evolution: Insights from India's right to food campaign. *Social Movement Studies*, 15(6), 610–621. doi:10.1080/14742837.2016.1213161

HUMAN RIGHTS WATCH. (2020) *Human Rights Dimensions of COVID-19 Response*. [Online]. Available: https://www.hrw.org/news/2020/03/19/human-rights-dimensions-covid-19-response [18 August 2020].

HUNG, Betty. (2017) Movement lawyering as rebellious lawyering: Advocating with humility, love, and courage. *Clinical Law Review*, 23(2), 663–669.

JUST FUTURES LAW. (2020) *Surveillance during COVID-19*. Available: https://justfutureslaw.org/wp-content/uploads/2020/04/COVID.SURVEILLANCE.JFLv4_.pdf [August 2020].

JUSTICEPOWER. (2020a) *Legal Empowerment Strategies*. [Online]. Available: Justicepower.org [18 August 2020].

JUSTICEPOWER. (2020b) *Webinar: JusticePower—Community Driven Litigation*. [Online]. Available via: https://justicepower.org/community-driven-litigation/ [18 August 2020].

KWOK, Kin On, LAI, Florence, WEI, Wan In, WONG, Samuel Yueng Shan, and TANG, Julian W. T. (2020) Herd immunity—Estimating the level required to halt the COVID-19 epidemics in affected countries. *Journal of Infection*, 80(6), E32–E33. doi:10.1016/j.jinf.2020.03.027

LEVI, Margaret. (2003) Organizing power: The prospects for an American labor movement. *Perspectives on Politics*, 1(1) 45–68. doi:10.1017/S1537592703000045

MAC, Ryan, HASKINS, Caroline, and MCDONALD, Logan. (2020) *Clearview's Facial Recognition App Has Been Used by the Justice Department, ICE, Macy's, Walmart, and the NBA*. [Online]. Available: https://www.buzzfeednews.com/article/ryanmac/clearview-ai-fbi-ice-global-law-enforcement [18 August 2020].

MARU, Vivek, and GAURI, Varun. (2018) *Community Paralegals and the Pursuit of Justice* (New York, NY: Cambridge University Press).

MATTINGLY, David. (2019) *Thirteen Insights from the Front Lines of Human Rights Activism*. [Online]. Available: https://www.opendemocracy.net/en/frontline-insights/13-insights-front-lines-human-rights-activism/ [18 August 2020].

MERRY, Salle Engle. (2006) Transnational human rights and local activism: Mapping the middle. *American Anthropologist*, 108(1), 38–51. doi:10.1525/aa.2006.108.1.38

MESEL, Felipe, and VITALE, Pablo. (2019) *La Villa 31 y 31 Bis: La Larga Luchador la Reurbanización. Ciclos de Movilización Jurídica y Política*. [Online]. Available: https://acij.org.ar/wp-content/uploads/2019/10/Empoderamiento-jur%C3%ADdico-y-abogac%C3%ADa-comunitaria-en-latinoamérica-digital-baja-1.pdf [18 August 2020].

MESEL, Felipe. (2020) Interview by the authors, July 6– August 6.

MISRA, Kiran. (2019) *'Did they Send us Here to Die?' Housing Rights at a Crossroads in India's Capital*. [Online]. Available: https://pulitzercenter.org/reporting/did-they-send-us-here-die-housing-rights-crossroads-indias-capital [18 August 2020].

NAMATI. (2020) *Member Directory*. [Online]. Available: https://namati.org/network/members/ [18 August 2020].

ORGANIZED COMMUNITIES AGAINST DEPORTATIONS (OCAD). (2020) *About Us*. [Online]. Available: https://www.organizedcommunities.org/about [18 August 2020].

OUR DATA BODIES. (2019) *Our Data Bodies Playbook Is out!* [Online]. Available: https://www.alliedmedia.org/news/2019/02/07/our-data-bodies-playbook-out [August 2020].

PANDEY, Vikas. (2020) *Coronavirus Lockdown: The Indian Migrants Dying to Get Home*. [Online]. Available: https://www.bbc.com/news/world-asia-india-52672764 [18 August 2020].

PETTY, Tawana, SABA, Mariella, LEWIS Tamika, GANGADHARAN, Seeta Peña, and EUBANKS, Virginia. (2018) *Reclaiming Our Data—Interim Report: Detroit*. [Online]. Available: http://eprints.lse.ac.uk/89638/1/Gangadharan_Reclaiming-our-data_Published.pdf [18 August 2020].

PODDAR, Tripti, SATPUTE, Jayshree, and SEN, Shreya. (2020) Interview by authors, July 9– August 6.

SATTERTHWAITE, Margaret L. (forthcoming) Critical legal empowerment for human rights. In *Legal Mobilization for Human Rights: Collected Courses of the Academy of European Law*, Grainne de Búrca (ed.) (New York, NY: Oxford University Press).

SCHOORMAN, F. David, MAYER, Roger C., and DAVIS, James H. (2007) An integrative model of organizational trust: Present, past, and future. *Academy of Management Review*, 32(2) 344–354. doi:10.5465/amr.2007.24348410

SEPULVEDA, Magdalena. (2012) *Report of the Special Rapporteur on Extreme Poverty and Human Rights.* UN Doc. A/67/278, Aug. 9 (New York, NY: United Nations).

TASKFORCE ON JUSTICE. (2019) *Justice for All: Final Report.* [Online]. Available: https://www.justice.sdg16.plus/ [18 August 2020].

THE WIRE. (2020). *HC Tells Delhi Govt to Keep Ration Shops Open, Disburse Food to All.* [Online]. Available: https://thewire.in/government/hc-tells-delhi-govt-to-keep-ration-shops-open-disburse-food-to-all [18 August 2020].

TRIBUNE GRAPHICS. (2017) *Estimating the Chicago Area's Undocumented Immigrant Population.* [Online]. Available: https://www.chicagotribune.com/news/ct-met-undocumented-immigrants-gfx-20170103-htmlstory.html [18 August 2020].

UNITED NATIONS COMMISSION ON LEGAL EMPOWERMENT OF THE POOR (CLEP). (2008) *Making the Law Work for Everyone, Volume 1: Report of the Commission on Legal Empowerment of the Poor.* [Online]. Available: https://www.un.org/ruleoflaw/files/Making_the_Law_Work_for_Everyone.pdf [18 August 2020].

UNITED NATIONS GENERAL ASSEMBLY. (1966) *International Covenant on Civil and Political Rights: United Nations Treat Series*, vol. 99, p. 171, 16 December. (New York, NY: United Nations).

UNITED NATIONS GENERAL ASSEMBLY. (2008) *Legal Empowerment of the Poor and Eradication of Poverty: United Nations General Assembly.* A/RES/63/142, 11 December (New York, NY: United Nations).

UNITED NATIONS HUMAN RIGHTS COMMITTEE. (2007) *General Comment no. 32, Article 14, Right to Equality Before Courts and Tribunals and to Fair Trial.* CCPR/C/GC/32, 23 August (Geneva, Switzerland: UNHRC).

UNITED NATIONS SECRETARY-GENERAL. (2009) *Legal Empowerment of the Poor and Eradication of Poverty: United Nations General Assembly.* A/64/133 (New York, NY: United Nations).

US AGENCY FOR INTERNATIONAL DEVELOPMENT. (2007) *Legal Empowerment of the Poor: From Concepts to Assessment.* [Online]. Available: http://pdf.usaid.gov/pdf_docs/Pnadm500.pdf [18 August 2020].

WEIBLE, Christopher M., NOHRSTEDT, Daniel, CAIRNEY, Paul, CARTER, David P., CROW, Deserai A., DURNOVÁ, Anna P., HEIKKILA, Tanya, INGOLD, Karin, MCCONNELL, Allen, and STONE, Diane. (2020) COVID-19 and the policy sciences: Initial reactions and perspectives. *Policy Sciences* (April 18), 1–17.

Freedom of movement, migration, and borders

Jaya Ramji-Nogales and Iris Goldner Lang

ABSTRACT
COVID-19 policies in the European Union and the United States have severely restricted free movement, migration, and asylum rights, in particular putting into jeopardy the human rights of refugees. This article addresses these implications while indicating the particularities of anti-COVID-19 mobility measures on both sides of the Atlantic. The article will disclose that COVID-19 mobility measures represent extraordinary challenges to fundamental principles of both the European Union and the United States; free movement of persons without border controls is a central reason for the existence of the European Union, and protection of individuals fleeing persecution has been a core commitment of the United States since its founding. The human rights implications of all of these border closures are alarming, putting at grave risk vulnerable populations who are ostensibly protected by these domestic and international legal obligations.

Introduction

COVID-19 policies in the European Union and the United States have severely restricted free movement, migration, and asylum rights, in particular putting into jeopardy the human rights of refugees. This article addresses these implications, while indicating the particularities of anti-COVID-19 mobility measures on both sides of the Atlantic. The discussion will show that the effects of these measures in the European Union were most visible on the internal plane, where free movement rights of EU citizens suffered due to the reintroduction of intra-Schengen border controls and the imposition of travel restrictions and bans on entry and exit to and from EU member states' territories. On top of this, EU member states closed all external borders, banning entry to all nonessential travel from third countries and imposing a number of restrictions, which led to a temporary halt in the registration and lodging of asylum applications in a number of member states. On the other hand, in the United States, the impact of COVID-19 mobility policies was predominantly felt on the external plane by non-US citizens, as the country closed its borders to asylum seekers and banned entry of nationals from 31 countries. These measures have had devastating human rights consequences.

Although all of these measures were justified in the name of public health, in both the European Union and the United States we see the COVID-19 pandemic being used as a convenient rationale for restrictions on movement – a rationale that disguises other, less salutary, motivations. Additionally, some restrictions appear disproportionate, given that public health could have been protected by less restrictive means and without such substantial interference with human rights. This article will address these issues by discussing the situation in the United States and the European Union, followed by concluding remarks, summarizing the main findings for both sides of the Atlantic.

Shutting down the southern border: The Trump administration and COVID-19

> Hiring manythousands [sic] of judges, and going through a long and complicated legal process, is not the way to go – will always be disfunctional [sic]. People must simply be stopped at the Border and told they cannot come into the U.S. illegally. Children brought back to their country. (Trump 2018)

In the United States, the Trump administration has used the COVID-19 pandemic to achieve its core immigration policy goal of closing the border to asylum seekers. As a populist who believes that harsh restrictions on immigration were key to his election and will be key to his reelection, Trump has worked since his inauguration to "build the wall" and destroy the asylum system. Drawing from the toolkit of its previous nationality bans and border restrictions, the administration has constructed a web of presidential proclamations that accomplish the unthinkable: expelling all noncitizens who arrive at the border without even the chance to lodge a claim for protection under the UN Convention Relating to the Status of Refugees or the UN Convention Against Torture and Other Cruel, Inhuman, or Degrading Treatment or Punishment, both of which the United States has bound itself to follow.[1]

While the "Muslim ban" he issued his first week in office garnered outrage, protests, and lawsuits, less attention was paid to the blueprints Trump had issued two days earlier to dismantle the asylum system. After the US Supreme Court upheld the third iteration of the Muslim ban in June 2018, the administration turned its destructive gaze to the asylum program. After Trump's first asylum ban at the border was enjoined in December 2018, the Department of Homeland Security (DHS) began implementing the "Migrant Protection Protocols," returning to Mexico all undocumented non-Mexicans arriving at the southern land border pending their immigration hearings. In July 2019, the administration issued its second ban on asylum seekers, this time rendering ineligible for asylum individuals who transited through a third country in which they did not apply for protection from persecution or torture prior to entering the United States at the southern land border. This rule was enjoined in June 2020, but by that time, the border restrictions justified by the COVID-19 pandemic were already in place, preventing asylum seekers from accessing protection at the southern border.

Using the COVID-19 pandemic as justification, the Trump administration has banned nationals from 31 countries from entering the United States. The first ban went into effect on February 2, 2020, through a presidential proclamation that barred many noncitizens traveling to the United States from China.[2] This order aligned with the racialized rationales behind the Muslim ban, as did the February 29 order implementing a nearly identical ban with respect to Iran (Kritzman-Amir and Ramji-Nogales 2019). The surprise came on March 11, when Trump issued a ban on travelers from Schengen Area,[3] and three days later, the United Kingdom and the Republic of Ireland, on similar terms (Trump 2020a). These bans, which are currently in effect, have no end date; the current public health emergency has been used to justify permanent bans. Moreover, although each of these bans appears to contain an exception for asylum seekers,[4] it is hard to understand how asylum seekers who are now ineligible for a visa will be able to lodge a claim for protection in the United States.

At the same time, the administration was closing down the southern border even to asylum seekers. On March 20, the DHS, using the risk of spreading the COVID-19 virus as justification, shut the land border with Mexico to a group of noncitizens that includes most if not all asylum seekers[5] (US Department of Homeland Security, US Customs and Border Protection 2020a). Guidance provided to Customs and Border Protection agents did not instruct them to ask whether migrants had a fear of return, as they are normally required to do in order to provide asylum seekers with access to the asylum system. The only group of migrants who are not subject to the ban are those who make an "affirmative, spontaneous, and reasonably believable claim that they fear being tortured in the country they are being sent back to" Lind (2020). This policy hinges human rights protections on the migrant's ability to raise and specify a torture claim, an approach that does not comport with the obligations of the Convention Against Torture, not to mention the Refugee Convention. A group of leading public health experts challenged the health rationale for the ban and offered guidance on safely processing asylum seekers at the border. Ignoring this advice, the Trump administration instead extended this 30-day order four times, using "prolonged temporariness" to normalize a radical assault on the human rights of asylum seekers (Kritzman-Amir and Ramji-Nogales 2019).

Yet one pandemic-justified ban was not sufficient for the Trump administration, which has thrown every toy in its cart at the border closure, particularly targeting asylum seekers. The executive added two more bans, one relying on the economy for its rationale and the other making permanent the ability of the administration to close the border to asylum seekers for overly broad "health" reasons. First, on April 22, using the "risk to the US labor market during the economic recovery following the COVID-19 outbreak" as his justification, Trump banned the entry of most immigrants into the United States (Trump 2020b). This labor market ban on immigrant visas, which was originally in place for 60 days, has been extended through December 31 and has been expanded to include nonimmigrants arriving on particular visas for skilled and temporary workers (Trump 2020c). On the heels of several other devastating executive restrictions on the asylum process, on July 9, the Trump administration issued a proposed regulation that adds as a bar to asylum and protection under the Convention Against Torture "symptoms consistent with … any contagious or infectious disease[,] … contact with such a disease[,] … or coming from a country … where such disease is prevalent or epidemic" and that disease poses a public health emergency or danger. When this rule becomes final, it will achieve Trump's goal of closing the border to asylum seekers (US Department of Homeland Security and US Department of Justice 2020a). In the meantime, a final rule effective October 13 authorizes the Director of the Centers for Disease Control and Prevention, by issuing an order, to expel non-citizens at the border or within the United States from a "designated foreign [country, as necessary] . . . to avert the serious danger of the introduction of a quarantinable communicable disease." (US Department of Homeland Security and US Department of Justice 2020).

As in the European Union, the Trump administration's approach to temporary labor migration highlights the flimsiness of the COVID-19 rationale for closing the border to asylum seekers. On March 20, the US Department of State announced that it would temporarily suspend all routine visa processing at its embassies and consulates abroad. Six days later, the State Department designated both agricultural and nonagricultural temporary work visas as "mission critical" and a "national security priority," and announced that it would continue processing these visas, eliminating the requirement of an in-person interview in some cases (US Department of State 2020). Trump's labor market ban on immigrant visas creates an exception for, "any alien seeking to enter the United States to provide temporary labor or services essential to the United States food supply chain." In short, the COVID-19 pandemic is invoked as a justification to keep out asylum seekers but brushed aside when it comes to temporary migrant workers, who are essential to the economic engine of the United States.

The human rights consequences of Trump's COVID-19 policies at the border have been dire. Relying on these bans, US Customs and Border Protection (CBP) has expelled nearly 70,000 migrants at the southern border, using expedited processes so summary that they took only an estimated 96 minutes to review claims and deport applicants (US Department of Homeland Security 2020b). The COVID removals included more than a thousand unaccompanied children, some as young as 10 years old. Many asylum seekers pushed back into Mexico are unable to access adequate shelter, necessary medical care, and sufficient food. All face escalating violence at the hands of cartels; kidnappings and murders in Mexico rose in March 2020 (Human Rights First 2020).

The situation for detained migrants during the COVID-19 pandemic is similarly dire. By late July 2020, nearly 4,000 immigration detainees had tested positive for COVID-19; 941 of them remained in custody (US Immigration and Customs Enforcement 2020). It is difficult if not impossible to ensure social distancing and other safety practices in immigration detention centers. The health of all detainees, and especially those with underlying conditions that make them more vulnerable, is at serious risk; the Trump administration's decision to detain them for entering without documents is inhumane. Moreover, The Trump administration has used the COVID-19 pandemic to launch a second family separation initiative, this time offering parents the "binary choice" of remaining in detention with their minor children in the face of the pandemic or being separated from their children, who would be released from detention (Amnesty International 2020).

Free movement of EU citizens, migration, and EU borders in the time of COVID-19

In this section, we will discuss restrictions to free movement of persons that have been adopted by EU member states as a response to the COVID-19 pandemic and the implications these have had on EU citizens and third-country nationals. First, we will address the implications of anti-COVID-19 measures on mobility of EU citizens within the European Union and on the functioning of internal Schengen border controls. We will briefly lay out EU rules on free movement of EU citizens and on Schengen, and outline the types of national restrictions adopted as a response to the pandemic. We will pay particular attention to their compliance with the EU principles of nondiscrimination and proportionality, which underpin EU free movement rules, with a particular focus on the requirements of necessity and proportionality *stricto sensu*. Finally, we will examine the implications of anti-COVID-19 measures for the external EU borders, in particular for migrants and refugees.

Anti-COVID-19 measures and free movement of EU citizens

In March 2020 almost all EU member states unilaterally adopted a number of anti-COVID-19 measures, drastically restricting free movement of persons in the EU. They also enforced lockdowns, which included restrictions on intrastate nonessential movements, and temporarily closed their external borders toward third countries for most nonresidents. Never in the history of the European integration, which is based on the idea of a single market, has the European Union been confronted with such a magnitude of restrictive measures, which have called into question the viability of the internal market. The European Commission, which was initially reluctant to reintroduce internal border controls and travel restrictions/bans, soon yielded under pressure to the reality of unilateral national restrictions implemented across the Union and began adopting a set of soft law measures aimed at coordinating national measures.[6]

Restrictive measures in most EU member states that limited several aspects of the right to free movement can be categorized into two groups. First, by July 15, 2020, 17 Schengen states reintroduced internal border controls on their intra-Schengen borders.[7] Additionally, non-Schengen EU member states strengthened their border controls toward neighboring member states. Consequently, in the spring of 2020, the entire European territory stopped being a border-control-free area, which was a strong blow to what has always been considered as one of the most notable achievements of European integration. Interestingly, even though the Schengen Borders Code does not expressly mention the reintroduction of internal border controls in case of threats to public health, the European Commission accepted member states' restrictions by suggesting that, in an extremely critical situation, a risk posed by a contagious disease can be equated to a public policy or internal security threat.[8]

The second type of anti-COVID-19 measures restricting free movement of persons in the European Union were various travel restrictions, suspending different forms of passenger transportation – such as flights, trains, buses, and maritime transport – and bans on entry and exit of persons to and from national territories.[9] The difference in scope and rigidity of national travel restrictions and bans resulted in a spectrum of diverse and sometimes inconsistent restrictions across the Union. As an example, most entry bans to national territories contained exceptions for domestic nationals and residents: Some provided exceptions for nationals, residents, and persons confirmed negative for COVID-19, whereas others offered exceptions to nationals, residents, and persons entering the national territory for "valid reasons."

Member states justified all travel restrictions – including entry and exit bans to and from national territories – on public health grounds. Unlike the Schengen Borders Code, the EU Treaty and secondary law rules on free movement of EU citizens explicitly allow states to justify national restrictions for public health reasons, provided these restrictions are applied to all EU citizens in a nondiscriminatory and proportionate manner.

According to the Citizens' Rights Directive, public health grounds can be relied on only for diseases with epidemic potential, as defined by the WHO, and for other infectious or contagious parasitic diseases if they are the subject of protection provisions applying to nationals of the host member state.[10] There is no doubt that COVID-19 satisfies these parameters, meaning that public health grounds can be invoked as a legitimate justification for national travel restrictions and entry/exit bans.

However, national travel restrictions and bans are admissible under EU law only if they do not discriminate against nationals of other member states who are residents in the host member state, in comparison to domestic nationals, and if they satisfy the principle of proportionality. Consequently, exemptions to entry bans applicable exclusively to domestic nationals and not to resident EU citizens from other member states, as well as bans on transit of EU citizens and residents who are returning home to their member state, would be contrary to EU law.[11]

The fulfillment of the principle of proportionality is particularly problematic in relation to anti-COVID-19 measures restricting free movement of persons. Evaluating whether a particular restrictive measure, such as an introduction of border controls or a travel ban, is proportionate to the level of protection of human health it affords is particularly difficult when faced with a high degree of scientific uncertainty associated with COVID-19. Even though travel restrictions/bans and border controls are obviously suitable for the protection of public health, as they contribute to the reduction of the number of SARS-CoV-2 virus infections by minimizing the number of personal contacts and transmissions, it is much more difficult to determine whether they satisfy the criteria of necessity and proportionality *stricto sensu*. At the time when most EU member states decided to introduce rigorous travel restrictions and bans, the level of knowledge about COVID-19 was (and still is) not sufficient and conclusive enough to judge with certainty that no alternative, less restrictive measure would protect public health interests just as effectively (criterion of necessity). Scientific knowledge about COVID-19 was not sufficient to determine with certainty whether the same result would have been achieved just as effectively through mass screening and testing at all border control points and through increased contact tracing and better public health communication.

In addition, the creation of special border corridors for thousands of seasonal workers, which were set up by some member states, significantly departed from the general idea that free movement of persons should be temporarily sacrificed for the benefit of public health. The way such mobility corridors were arranged, without sufficient regard to public health precautions (Bejan 2020), can be viewed as inconsistent with other anti-COVID-19 measures, thus challenging the suitability of those measures. On the other hand, if it was possible to organize such mobility corridors while respecting all public health standards, one cannot but wonder why it would not be possible to do the same on a wider scale, which calls into question the necessity of COVID-19 restrictive measures.

In addition, there are different views as to whether travel restrictions and bans are reasonable, considering other competing interests – that is, whether they justify the degree of interference to free movement in the EU (proportionality *stricto sensu*). The answer to this question might vary depending on how wealthy a society is and how long it can withstand the economic consequences of lockdowns. This explains why in the summer of 2020 a number of EU member states whose economies depend on tourism decided to ease travel restrictions and bans, despite the fact that some of them are faced with a higher number of SARS-CoV-2 infections than in winter/spring 2020. It also means that, if the European Union is faced with another wave of COVID-19 infections in autumn and winter of 2020–2021, this may not result in the same degree and type of travel restrictions and bans as the ones in effect during the winter and spring of 2020.

Rights of migrants and refugees in the European Union in the time of COVID-19

Member states' temporary closure of external borders with third countries has had significant implications for all third-country nationals nonresident in the European Union. The closure of external borders was accompanied by a spectrum of national measures restricting migrants' and refugees' rights and leading to a temporary halt in the registration and lodging of asylum applications and the right to move in and out of reception centers in a number of member states.[12] For example, in March 2020 Hungary indefinitely suspended admission of migrants to its transit zones, thus effectively suspending access to asylum. Prime Minister Viktor Orbán justified this suspension by claiming there was a clear link between illegal migration and the COVID-19 outbreak (Hungary Today 2020). Greece and Cyprus also temporarily suspended asylum applications, whereas Italy and Malta announced that their ports cannot be classified as "safe places." Belgium closed its arrival centers for newly arriving asylum seekers, whereas Spain suspended all second interviews, thus temporarily suspending the processing of asylum applications. France also suspended all registration activities, which, in effect, led to the suspension of all asylum procedures. In addition, member states, the UN High Commissioner for Refugees, and the International Organization for Migration temporarily suspended resettlement operations (European Commission 2020d).

The situation in reception centers proved particularly critical due to the fact that many reception facilities in different member states were overcrowded and not properly equipped to put in place adequate preventive measures. For this reason, once SARS-CoV-2 virus entered a reception center, it spread easily in the center, and all of its users were forced to remain locked down in the center to prevent further transmission. Such a SARS-CoV-2 virus infection occurred in a German reception center, where half of 600 people tested positive and all of the people in the center were placed in lockdown (Nielsen 2020).

The limited access to EU member states' asylum systems and processing was reflected in the number of asylum claims, which hit the lowest level since 2008 and represented an 87 percent decrease from pre-COVID-19 levels in January and February 2020 (European Asylum Support Office [EASO] 2020b). All these measures made it even more challenging for these highly vulnerable individuals to reach the EU territory and seek asylum there. Most of these measures were imposed for public health reasons, but one wonders whether in some instances COVID-19 was used to justify restrictions that were motivated by other reasons, such as in the case of Hungary. Additionally – and similar to travel bans for EU citizens – it is questionable whether some of the restrictions applicable to asylum seekers were disproportionate – that is, whether public health could have been protected by less restrictive means and whether these measures were reasonable, considering the level of interference with human rights.

There were also some positive developments. In some member states, detention regimes were eased. For example, in Belgium almost half of detainees without criminal records were released due to the interruption of return procedures, whereas in Sweden the total number of spaces in detention centers was significantly reduced to avoid overcrowding. Additionally, some member states, such as Portugal, improved asylum seekers' access to healthcare.

Conclusion

Both the European Union and the United States have locked down their borders in response to the COVID-19 pandemic. At least some aspects of these closures violate international law, and all raise the question of whether public health is an adequate legal justification for the measures taken in the name of the COVID-19 pandemic that restrict the human rights of migrants, including asylum seekers. The border closures also raise the question of whether public health is the actual reason for restricting entry, or whether it is merely a vehicle for disguising otherwise unlawful political choices.

The responses of the European Union and the United States to the COVID-19 pandemic put serious pressure on the international refugee law regime. Although the European Union has historically taken its human rights obligations seriously, many states suspended access to the asylum process temporarily. Perhaps less surprisingly, given that the United States views its relationship to international law as exceptional, the Trump administration closed external borders to Canada and Mexico even to asylum seekers, and banned entry by travelers from numerous countries. This policy appears more permanent than the EU restrictions. Moreover, the United States continued to detain asylum seekers despite the risks posed by the pandemic, whereas some EU nations eased their detention policies. The human rights consequences of the external border shutdowns are deeply concerning, as are US detention practices, and their repercussions may outlast the pandemic.

Choices about which borders to close reveal fundamental differences between the European Union and the United States. The United States has been a federal nation for nearly 250 years; although some state governors raised the specter of closing internal borders, the strongest measures taken to date have been quarantines imposed on travelers from other states. The European Union, which has been working toward an ever-more-perfect union since 1958, faced a serious threat to that goal, as EU states closed internal borders within and beyond the Schengen zone and implemented travel restrictions and entry and exit bans on nonnationals.

It is not clear whether public health emergencies are an adequate legal justification for border closures in either legal regime. In each case, the use of the COVID-19 pandemic as justification to exclude certain individuals has been belied by exceptions created for seasonal workers needed to keep economies working. In Europe, travel restrictions and entry and exit bans have been relaxed to enable the summer tourist season, but may return with another wave of infections.

All of these border closures were unprecedented, undermining regional EU treaty commitments and violating international legal obligations under the UN Refugee Convention. These closures also represent extraordinary challenges to fundamental principles of each union; free movement of people without border control is a central reason for the existence of the European Union, and protection of individuals fleeing persecution has been a core commitment of the United States since its founding. The human rights implications of all of these border closures are alarming, putting at grave risk vulnerable populations who are ostensibly protected by these domestic and international legal obligations.

Notes

1. The United States did not ratify the Refugee Convention but did ratify the Refugee Protocol, which incorporates the obligations of the Convention. UN Protocol Relation to the Status of Refugees, 606 U.N.T.S. 267 (1967; ratified by the United States on Nov. 1, 1968); UN Convention Relation to the Status of Refugees, 189 U.N.T.S. 150 (1951); UN Convention Against Torture and Other Cruel, Inhuman, or Degrading Treatment or Punishment, U.N. Doc. A/39/51 (1987; ratified by the United States on Oct. 21, 1994).
2. The ban does not apply to permanent residents or their spouses, parents, children, and siblings, as well as a few other groups.
3. The Schengen Area comprises 26 European states: Austria, Belgium, Czech Republic, Denmark, Estonia, Finland, France, Germany, Greece, Hungary, Iceland, Italy, Latvia, Liechtenstein, Lithuania, Luxembourg, Malta, Netherlands, Norway, Poland, Portugal, Slovakia, Slovenia, Spain, Sweden, and Switzerland.
4. Section 2(b) of these bans states, "Nothing in this proclamation shall be construed to affect any individual's eligibility for asylum, withholding of removal, or protection under the regulations issued pursuant to the legislation implementing the Convention Against Torture and Other Cruel, Inhuman or Degrading Treatment or Punishment, consistent with the laws and regulations of the United States."
5. This ban does not apply to permanent residents and other select groups of noncitizens with visas to study or work.
6. For the overview of the Commission's measures, European Commission (2020a).
7. For the full list of EU member states' notification of temporary reintroduction of internal border controls, see European Commission (2020b). For a detailed account of national measures reintroducing internal border controls, see Carrera and Chun (2020). For one of the first legal appraisals of travel bans, see Thym (2020).
8. See point V.18 of *Commission COVID-19 Guidelines* for border management measures to protect health and ensure the availability of goods and essential services, C(2020) 1753 final, 16.3.2020: "Member States may reintroduce temporary border controls at internal borders if justified for reasons of public policy or internal security. In an extremely critical situation, a Member State can identify a need to reintroduce border controls as a reaction to the risk posed by a contagious disease. Member States must notify the reintroduction of border controls in accordance with the Schengen Borders Code."
9. For the list of national restrictions impacting mobility and transport for each member state separately, see European Commission (2020c).
10. Article 29(1) of Directive 2004/38 on the right of citizens of the Union and their family members to move and reside freely within the territory of the member states.
11. See point V.21 of the *European Commission COVID-19 Guidelines* for border management measures to protect health and ensure the availability of goods and essential services, C(2020) 1753 final, 16.3.2020: "A Member State must not deny entry to EU citizens or third-country nationals residing on its territory and must facilitate transit of other EU citizens and residents that are returning home. Member States can, however, take appropriate measures such as requiring persons entering their territory to undergo self-isolation or similar measures upon return from an area affected by Covid-19 provided they impose the same requirements on their own nationals." From this perspective, the Hungarian entry ban applicable to all EEA citizens apart from permanent residents (those with minimum five years of legal residence in Hungary) is a discriminatory measure that is not suitable for attainment of public health.
12. For a list of anti-COVID-19 measures affecting migration and asylum in the EU, see EASO (2020a) and ECRE (2020).

References

AMNESTY INTERNATIONAL. (2020) *Family Separation 2.0: 'You Aren't Going to Separate Me from My Only Child.'* [Online]. Available: https://www.amnestyusa.org/wp-content/uploads/2020/04/Amnesty-International-USA-Family-Separation-2.0_May-21-2020-.pdf. [9 October 2020].

BEJAN, Raluca. (2020) *COVID-19 and Disposable Migrant Workers.* [Online]. Available: https://verfassungsblog.de/covid-19-and-disposable-migrant-workers/ [15 July 2020].

CARRERA, Sergio, and CHUN, Luk. (2020) *Love Thy Neighbour? Coronavirus Politics and Their Impact on EU Freedoms and Rule of Law in the Schengen Area.* [Online]. Available: https://www.ceps.eu/wp-content/uploads/2020/04/LSE2020-04_Love-thy-neighbour.pdf [15 July 2020].

DIRECTIVE 2004/38/EC OF THE EUROPEAN PARLIAMENT AND OF THE COUNCIL OF 29 APRIL 2004 ON THE RIGHT OF CITIZENS OF THE UNION AND THEIR FAMILY MEMBERS TO MOVE AND RESIDE FREELY WITHIN THE TERRITORY OF THE MEMBER STATES AMENDING REGULATION (EEC) NO 1612/68 AND REPEALING DIRECTIVES 64/221/EEC, 68/360/EEC, 72/194/EEC, 73/148/EEC, 75/34/EEC, 75/35/EEC, 90/364/EEC, 90/365/EEC AND 93/96/EEC, Official Journal L 158, 30.4.2004, pp. 77–123.

EUROPEAN ASYLUM SUPPORT OFFICE (EASO). (2020a) *COVID-19 Emergency Measures in Asylum and Reception Systems.* [Online]. Available: https://www.easo.europa.eu/sites/default/files/covid19-emergency-measures-asylum-reception-systems.pdf [15 July 2020].

EUROPEAN ASYLUM SUPPORT OFFICE (EASO). (2020b) *Record Low Number of Asylum Applications Lodged in EU.* [Online]. Available: https://www.easo.europa.eu/news-events/record-low-number-asylum-applications-lodged-eu [15 July 2020].

EUROPEAN COMMISSION. (2020a) *Overview of the Commission's Response.* [Online]. Available: https://ec.europa.eu/info/live-work-travel-eu/health/coronavirus-response/overview-commissions-response_en [15 July 2020].

EUROPEAN COMMISSION. (2020b) *Member States' Notifications of the Temporary Reintroduction of Border Control at Internal Borders Pursuant to Article 25 and 28 et seq. of the Schengen Borders Code.* [Online]. Available: https://ec.europa.eu/home-affairs/sites/homeaffairs/files/what-we-do/policies/borders-and-visas/schengen/reintroduction-border-control/docs/ms_notifications_-_reintroduction_of_border_control_en.pdf [15 July 2020].

EUROPEAN COMMISSION. (2020c) *Coronavirus Response.* [Online]. Available: https://ec.europa.eu/transport/coronavirus-response_en [15 July 2020].

EUROPEAN COMMISSION. (2020d) *Communication from the Commission COVID-19: Guidance on the Implementation of Relevant EU Provisions in the Area of Asylum and Return Procedures and on Resettlement.* 2020/C 126/02, C/2020/2516, OJ C 126, 17.4.2020, pp. 12–27. [Online]. Available: https://ec.europa.eu/info/sites/info/files/guidance-implementation-eu-provisions-asylum-retur-procedures-resettlement.pdf [9 October 2020].

EUROPEAN COUNCIL ON REFUGEES AND EXILES (ECRE). (2020) *Information Sheet 5 May 2020: Covid-19 Measures Related to Asylum and Migration across Europe.* [Online]. Available: https://www.ecre.org/wp-content/uploads/2020/05/COVID-INFO-5-May-.pdf [15 July 2020].

HUMAN RIGHTS FIRST. (2020) *Pandemic as Pretext: Trump Administration Exploits COVID-19, Expels Asylum Seekers and Children to Escalating Danger.* [Online]. Available: https://www.humanrightsfirst.org/sites/default/files/PandemicAsPretextFINAL.pdf [9 October 2020].

HUNGARY TODAY. (2020) *Orbán to EU Counterparts: Clear Link between Coronavirus and Illegal Migration.* [Online]. Available: https://hungarytoday.hu/orban-to-eu-counterparts-clear-link-between-coronavirus-and-illegal-migration/ [15 July 2020].

KRITZMAN-AMIR, Tally, and RAMJI-NOGALES, Jaya. (2019) Nationality bans. *Illinois Law Review*, 2019(2), 563–613.

LIND, Dara. (2020) *Leaked Border Patrol Memo Tells Agents to Send Migrants back Immediately – Ignoring Asylum Law.* [Online]. Available: https://www.propublica.org/article/leaked-border-patrol-memo-tells-agents-to-send-migrants-back-immediately-ignoring-asylum-law

NIELSEN, Nikolaj. (2020) *Half of Refugees at German Camp Test Covid-19 Positive.* [Online]. Available: https://euobserver.com/coronavirus/148072 [15 July 2020].

THYM, Daniel. (2020) *Travel Bans in Europe: A Legal Appraisal (Parts I and II).* [Online]. Available: http://eumigrationlawblog.eu/travel-bans-in-europe-a-legal-appraisal-part-i/ [15 July 2020].

TRUMP, Donald J. (2018) (@realDonaldTrump), Twitter. [Online]. Available: https://twitter.com/realDonaldTrump/status/1011228265003077632 [25 June 2018, 5:43 AM].

TRUMP, Donald J. (2020a) *Proclamation on the Suspension of Entry as Immigrants and Nonimmigrants of Certain Additional Persons who Pose a Risk of Transmitting Coronavirus.* [Online]. Available: https://www.whitehouse.gov/presidential-actions/proclamation-suspension-entry-immigrants-nonimmigrants-certain-additional-persons-pose-risk-transmitting-coronavirus-2/?utm_source=link [14 March 2020].

TRUMP, Donald J. (2020b) *Proclamation Suspending Entry of Immigrants Who Present Risk to the U.S. Labor Market During the Economic Recovery Following the COVID-19 Outbreak.* [Online]. Available: https://www.whitehouse.gov/presidential-actions/proclamation-suspending-entry-immigrants-present-risk-u-s-labor-market-economic-recovery-following-covid-19-outbreak/ [22 April 2020].

TRUMP, Donald J. (2020c) *Proclamation Suspending Entry of Immigrants Who Present Risk to the U.S. Labor Market During the Economic Recovery Following the COVID-19 Outbreak.* [Online]. Available: https://www.whitehouse.gov/presidential-actions/proclamation-suspending-entry-aliens-present-risk-u-s-labor-market-following-coronavirus-outbreak/?utm_source=link [14 March 2020].

UNITED NATIONS. (1951) *Convention Relating to the Status of Refugees: 189 UNTS 150* (New York, NY: United Nations).

UNITED NATIONS. (1967) *Protocol Relating to the Status of Refugees: 606 UNTS 267* (New York, NY: United Nations).

UNITED NATIONS. (1987) *Convention Against Torture and Other Cruel, Inhuman, or Degrading Treatment or Punishment.* U.N. Doc. A/39/51 (New York: United Nations).

US DEPARTMENT OF HEALTH AND HUMAN SERVICES (2020) *Control of Communicable Diseases; Foreign Quarantine: Suspension of the Right To Introduce and Prohibition of Introduction of Persons Into United States From Designated Foreign Countries or Places for Public Health Purposes, 85 Fed. Reg. 56424* (Washington DC: US Dept. of Health and Human Services).

US DEPARTMENT OF HOMELAND SECURITY AND DEPARTMENT OF JUSTICE. (2020) *Proposed Rule: Security Bars and Processing: 85 Fed. Reg. 41201* (Washington, DC: US Dept. of Homeland Security and DOJ).

US DEPARTMENT OF HOMELAND SECURITY, U.S. CUSTOMS AND BORDER PROTECTION. (2020a) *Notification of Temporary Travel Restrictions Applicable to Land Ports of Entry and Ferries Service Between the United States and Mexico: 85 Federal Register 31057* (Washington, DC: US Dept. Of Homeland Security and US Customs and Border Protection).

US DEPARTMENT OF HOMELAND SECURITY, U.S. CUSTOMS AND BORDER PROTECTION. (2020b) *Nationwide Enforcement Actions: Title 8 Enforcement Actions and Title 42 Expulsions.* [Online]. Available: https://www.cbp.gov/newsroom/stats/cbp-enforcement-statistics/title-8-and-title-42-statistics [9 October 2020].

US DEPARTMENT OF STATE, BUREAU OF CONSULAR AFFAIRS. (2020) *Important Announcement on H2 Visas.* [Online]. Available: https://travel.state.gov/content/travel/en/News/visas-news/important-announcement-on-h2-visas.html [26 March 2020].

US IMMIGRATION AND CUSTOMS ENFORCEMENT. (2020) *ICE Guidance on COVID-19, ICE Detainee Statistics.* [Online]. Available: https://www.ice.gov/coronavirus#main-content [29 July 2020].

OPEN ACCESS

State surveillance and the COVID-19 crisis

Kristine Eck and Sophia Hatz

ABSTRACT

The outbreak of COVID-19 has ushered in a global rise in state surveillance. In an effort to trace the spread of the disease and to enforce lockdowns, governments in democracies and autocracies alike have turned to surveillance technologies such as contact tracing apps. Governments have also tightened their hold on communication flows in other ways, through censorship and information manipulation. These kinds of government actions are not new: States have long recognized the value of controlling information in times of crisis. In this article, we consider these tactics in the context of the COVID-19 pandemic, in which, unlike most other security threats, the threat posed is not endogenous to governance and applies to all countries. We consider how observations from this context prompt future research and reflect on the implications of information control for civil liberties.

Introduction

In April 2020, the Norwegian Institute of Public Health (NIPH) launched a mobile app called *Smittestopp* ("infection stop") designed to collect users' geolocated movement data in order to help authorities trace the spread of COVID-19. This app was described by Amnesty International (2020) as one of the most invasive COVID-19 contact tracing apps in the world, alongside those in countries like Bahrain and Kuwait. By June, the Norwegian data oversight agency warned the NIPH that it would stop it from handling data collected through the app (Agence France-Presse 2020).

Norway's *Smittestopp* exemplifies an unexpected byproduct of the COVID-19 pandemic: a global rise in state surveillance. Since the outbreak of COVID-19, governments in country after country have turned to surveillance as a means of tracing the spread of the disease and enforcing lockdowns. Autocratic countries like China and Singapore were quick to adapt and extend existing digital surveillance technologies to monitor COVID-19. And democratic countries followed suit: In a matter of months, more than 34 countries enacted surveillance measures; 22 of them were full democracies (OneZero 2020).[1]

Governments have also responded to a rapid outpouring of misinformation in social media outlets. Rumors and falsehoods about the origins, symptoms, and remedies for COVID-19 became so widespread that in February 2020 the World Health Organization (WHO) deemed the situation an "infodemic"—weeks before it declared a pandemic.[2] In this context, governments have taken measures such as the censorship of online content and the criminalization of "fake news." But some governments themselves have also contributed to this infodemic by deliberately misrepresenting information about the disease.

These kinds of government actions are not new: States have long recognized the value of controlling information in times of crisis. Scholars will recognize the measures implemented by governments during the COVID-19 pandemic as examples of surveillance, censorship, and information manipulation. Previous research has described how governments use these tactics to contain domestic political threats: Surveillance allows for the detection of dissent and for the targeted application of repression (Gohdes 2019); censorship enables states to restrict criticism of the government, to cut communication necessary for collective action, and to silence reports of abuse (Gunitsky 2015); and information manipulation can serve as a tool for distracting the public, for discourse framing, and for countermobilization (Gunitsky 2015; King, Pan and Roberts 2017). Although a pandemic is a different context than contentious politics, we have seen an analogous tendency of states to ramp up personal data collection and to tighten their control over information.[3]

In this article, we begin by defining surveillance, censorship, and information manipulation, and anchoring these concepts in the existing literature. Although researchers tend to study these tactics separately, we observe that these practices often cooccur. We suggest that jointly considering the array of information control tactics governments have at their disposal may provide insights into how states adjudicate between them. We probe this idea in the context of the COVID-19 pandemic, which prompted a global rise in information-control practices, especially state surveillance. We conclude by reflecting on the implications of information control during COVID-19 for the protection of civil liberties.

Surveillance, censorship, and information manipulation

We view surveillance, censorship, and information manipulation as distinct tactics that are components of a more general strategy, which we label *information control*. Information control tactics differ in the means by which control is achieved, as well as in the types of information that are controlled. A government may use these tactics individually or in tandem, and it may change its strategy over time.

State surveillance involves the monitoring, collecting, and/or processing of personal data by a government. This can include the monitoring of online activity, location tracking via Bluetooth or Global Positioning System (GPS), tracking financial transactions, video surveillance, facial scans, and the collection of biometric data. The kinds of information states have the capacity to collect and connect is vast, precise, and often private in nature. Foundational works in sociology, economics, and philosophy consider state surveillance as fundamental to both governance and social control: It is a method of identifying individuals, ordering society, and ensuring discipline.[4]

State surveillance received renewed scholarly attention with the advent of the internet and other advanced information and communications technology (ICT). ICT massively increases the power, reach, and capacity of governments to monitor their populations (Lyon 2007; Marx 2015). Within political science, much research on surveillance has come to focus on its application by authoritarian regimes, as a tool to counter domestic political threats (e.g., Kuran 1997; Jiang and Yang 2016), as surveillance allows for the detection of dissent and the extraction of intelligence, which enables the targeted application of repression (Gohdes 2019).

State censorship involves a government blocking or altering communication in order to control the information individuals disseminate to one another. For example, states can place filters to restrict the results returned by online search engines, remove specific online content and block websites, disable social media, remove leaks by whistleblowers,[5] and shut down the internet. Like most recent research on surveillance, contemporary studies of censorship take ICT as a point of departure and tend to focus on authoritarian regimes (e.g., Roberts 2018; Gohdes 2019; Gläßel and Paula 2020). ICT has facilitated the spread of popular sentiments and provided new tools for collective action, but it has also bolstered governments' capacities to intervene in communications and social networks (Weidmann and Rød 2019). By deleting information from the public eye, states are able to restrict criticism of the government, silence reports of abuse, limit communication necessary for the coordination of collective action, and curtail the dissemination of information the public uses to form policy opinions (Hayes and Reineke 2007; King, Pan, and Roberts 2013; Gunitsky 2015). Governments may also cut digital communication completely; when information flows may be too great to selectively censor, governments may resort to internet shutdowns.

States do not only censor information, however: They also actively engage in *state information manipulation,* which is the manipulation, fabrication, or cooptation of information for strategic purposes (Gunitsky 2015).[6] Examples include a government's production of fake news, fabrication of social media posts, dissemination of propaganda or libel, and restriction of access to governmental data. For example, the Chinese government hires internet commentators to post large numbers of fabricated social media comments as if they were the genuine opinions of ordinary Chinese people, a tactic aimed at distracting the public and shifting focus (King et al. 2017; Roberts 2018). Other scholars have pointed to how states disseminate propaganda or false information for purposes such as shaping the political attitudes of citizens (Geddes and Zaller 1989) and for countermobilization of a regime's support base (Gunitsky 2015).

Although some research contains an implicit recognition that states employ an array of tactics to collect and control information (e.g., Geddes and Zaller 1989), the field more often tends to silo these different tactics. For instance, although the monitoring of individuals and of communications is necessary for their silencing, studies of state censorship rarely account for ongoing state surveillance, theoretically or empirically. In practice, state uses of surveillance, censorship, and information manipulation often occur in tandem.

Information control in the context of the COVID-19 pandemic

The COVID-19 pandemic provides a unique setting for understanding state information control as, unlike most other security threats, the threat posed by the disease is not endogenous to governance and is applicable to all countries.[7] Because information control is routine in most autocracies, we focus particularly on consolidated democracies, where new information control practices risk undermining established civil liberties.

Surveillance

Surveillance is the tactic that has been most readily embraced by democratic governments, which they have seemingly adopted with the same energy as their autocratic counterparts. The types of surveillance measures adopted in response to the COVID-19 pandemic include public surveillance of population movements under lockdown through closed-circuit television (CCTV), drones, mobile phone usage data, and biometric tracker bracelets.[8] But the most prominent form of surveillance has been the adoption of mobile applications that allow for COVID-19 tracking. The basic premise is to scale up traditional contact tracing by leveraging digital technology. Yet there is a tension in the digital utopianism that sees mobile phones as a means by which to help protect from disease and fears of privacy invasion. Concerns about digital overreach in democracies are not new, but the high stakes of the COVID-19 pandemic have seen official state surveillance efforts fast-tracked and securitized in a way that is new to the digital landscape.

There is no single approach to these surveillance apps, and they vary depending on whether they are the result of public or private initiatives,[9] what sort of technology is used to track contact between individuals,[10] whether data storage is centralized or decentralized, whether the app is voluntary, whether limitations are placed on data collection, whether there are provisions for destroying the data, whether the data is anonymized, and whether the app is transparent (e.g.,

Table 1. Government-sponsored Covid-19 Tracking Apps in Europe

Country	Govt app	Country	Govt app
United Kingdom	in development	Macedonia	yes
Ireland	in development	Croatia	in development
Netherlands	no	Montenegro	no
Belgium	no	Slovenia	no
Luxembourg	no	Greece	no
France	in development	Cyprus	yes
Switzerland	in development	Bulgaria	yes
Spain	Basque region only	Moldova	no
Portugal	no	Romania	no
Germany	yes	Estonia	in development
Poland	yes	Latvia	yes
Austria	yes	Lithuania	yes
Hungary	yes	Armenia	no
Czech Republic	yes	Georgia	yes
Slovak Republic	yes	Finland	in development
Italy	yes	Sweden	no
Albania	no	Norway	yes
Kosovo	no	Denmark	yes
Serbia	no		

Sources: MIT Technology Review, Digital Trights Tracker, individualized online searches.

through open-source code). All of these technologies raise questions not only of privacy infringement but also of whether they are even effective to begin with (Stanley and Granick 2020).

Most democratic governments have reiterated their commitment to ensuring privacy in this context, but concerns remain. Anonymized data, for example, are at risk of reidentification (De Montjoye, Hidalgo, Verleysen and Blondel 2013), and although data may be stored on users' phones rather than centralized in order to minimize privacy concerns, there are fears that the data can be hacked. Citizens have generally allowed governments a wide berth in responding to the pandemic, but privacy activists have raised questions about the extent to which these surveillance measures are truly "extraordinary," as opposed to extensions of already ongoing moves by democratic states to engage in domestic surveillance.

Importantly, we see variation across democratic governments in terms of the extent to which they have sought to ensure that encroachments on civil liberties are necessary, effective, and proportionate. If we consider the Norwegian example, the benefits of the app were ultimately deemed insufficient to warrant its overreach into citizen privacy. Indeed, numerous governments' own oversight bodies have pushed back in relation to the design of contact tracing apps. Slovakia, for example, fast-tracked several amendments to its telecommunications act that expanded telecom companies' obligations to retain individual location data. These measures were challenged at the Slovakian Constitutional Court and were subsequently suspended due to their "vagueness and insufficient safeguards against misuse" (Electronic Frontier Foundation 2020).

Table 1 shows the development of COVID-19 tracking apps across European democracies as of June 19, 2020. Fifteen countries had already launched COVID-19 tracking apps. They were in development in an additional seven countries, whereas 14 countries had opted against the apps for the time being. There are likely to be numerous and heterogeneous reasons for this cross-national variation, but eyeballing the data, it is evident that it is not only a question of feasibility: Many countries that have the technological resources to quickly develop an app have opted not to do so. Similarly, many countries that are famously concerned with personal privacy protection, such as Germany, have been forerunners in adopting apps.

This variation in surveillance is evident not only in Europe but across the globe. In India, for example, the government and many major private employers are requiring employees to download the official, ostensibly voluntary COVID-19 tracking app. India has no national data privacy law, and critics have pointed out that it is not clear who has access to data from the app and in what situations (O'Neill 2020).

There are certainly reasons to fear mission creep—that governments will not be willing abandon the new surveillance opportunities these apps offer and that personal data will be collected indefinitely and used for unanticipated ends. In the United Kingdom, the government plans to retain the data it collects for up to 20 years and denies individuals an absolute right to have their data deleted upon request (Hern 2020). Rights groups have raised fears that the data may be used for other purposes, and have pointed out that the government has failed to conduct a legally mandated data protection impact assessment (Sabbagh and Hern 2020). There are precedents for these fears. For example, the US Patriot Act, passed in 2001 in response to the terrorist attacks of September 11, 2000, gave the government broad surveillance powers with limited oversight. It remains in place today, despite the lack of any indication there is an immediate threat of a foreign attack on US soil.

Censorship and information manipulation

During the COVID-19 pandemic, censorship has primarily been justified as a response to the infodemic. The spread of rumors, falsehoods, and conspiracy theories, primarily on social media, rapidly became a serious threat to governments' efforts to contain the disease. The WHO has warned that false and misleading information by nonhealth actors has dangerous consequences for individuals' health and undermines trust in health authorities (WHO 2020). In this context, governments have imposed various measures of censorship, including regulating online content and criminalizing "fake news."

Autocratic countries with existing censorship regimes were quick to tune their filters to COVID-19-related content. For example, as Chinese citizens began to share information about a mysterious disease in Wuhan, online posts and hashtags related to disease were quickly deleted and the users' accounts blocked (Shiji 2020). In democracies, governments have taken a less top-down approach, often collaborating with the private sector to remove falsehoods from the internet (Goldsmith and Woods 2020). Tech companies such as Facebook, Twitter, and Google have used human censors and computer algorithms to remove pandemic-related falsehoods, ban events in contradiction of social distancing directives, and alert users who have been exposed to content later found to be misleading.[11]

In more extreme cases, the regulation of COVID-related content has involved prohibiting information not attributable to the government or a public health authority.[12] This has primarily taken place in authoritarian countries, where states have tighter controls over the media; but it has also occurred in democracies. In March 2020, Armenia introduced legislation requiring any dissemination of information regarding the disease to draw on information provided by a special emergency office under the prime minister (International Center for Not-for-Profit Law/ ICNL 2020).

Another, more extreme form of censorship that has arisen in the context of COVID-19 has been the criminalization of misinformation. This has been widespread across both autocracies and democracies. At least 24 countries have passed laws or orders restricting or punishing the dissemination of false information,[13] and in 15 of these countries, the dissemination of false information is punishable with prison time. Although Hungary is the only EU member to have passed laws on fake news, there have been calls within the European Commission to go beyond the current self-regulatory nature of online media (Stolton 2020).

Even as governments have taken steps to contain the spread of COVID-related misinformation, governments have also participated in the manipulation of information themselves. The most obvious examples come from countries with low levels of expressive freedoms to begin with, but well-known examples of government information manipulation have taken place in consolidated democracies, as well. Most notably, US President Donald Trump initially dismissed the virus as a "hoax" and has continuously promoted the drug chloroquine as a remedy for COVID-19, even though experts have refuted these claims (Haberman 2020).

Aside from distributing false information, many countries have restricted access to official information.[14] In Georgia, regulations introduced in connection with the containment of COVID-19 extended the timeframe for government responses to requests for public information, essentially exempting the government from ordinary deadlines set by law. Similar exemptions to the Freedom of Information Act were passed in some US states (e.g., New Jersey and Washington, DC). The Brazilian government has stopped releasing counts of COVID-19 cases and deaths (ICNL 2020), and Sweden has concealed from the public certain government communications and information concerning preparedness for the virus (Rudbäck 2020).

Discussion

Although much of what know about state information control comes from the literature on authoritarian regimes, during the Covid-19 pandemic we have witnessed a dramatic rise in information control among democracies and autocracies alike. The rise among democracies is particularly troubling, as democracy rests on principles such as freedom of expression and the right to privacy, and democratic countries have become the cornerstones of international efforts toward protection of human rights (Beutz 2003).

The empirics of the COVID-19 pandemic illustrate that states can deploy different means of informational control. During the pandemic, surveillance has dominated as the information control tactic of choice. Indeed, surveillance is often a necessary first step toward censorship and information manipulation; in order to control information, communications must first be monitored. On the other hand, some forms of censorship have not increased or may have even lessened during the COVID-19 pandemic. The critical necessity to access information during the pandemic makes it difficult for governments to justify internet shutdowns on the grounds of public order or national security (UN 2020b). The empirics also illustrate that different tactics of information control often co-occur and reinforce each other; in some countries, laws criminalizing fake news and granting governments special privileges to surveil have been packaged together under emergency orders passed in response to the pandemic (ICNL 2020).

Information control has been a priority for governments, even relative to other modes of crisis response. But states' intentions behind information control are difficult to infer, even when explicitly deployed in the name of a public health emergency. Although many countries have justified censorship on the basis of the infodemic, this is not the only possible chronology. Rumors on social media may have arisen in response to perceived information vacuums or due to discrepancies between official figures and experiences on the ground. If this is true, states may have had other motives for censorship and information manipulation, including as a pretext to silence critics and consolidate political power (Roth 2020).

Observations such as these prompt questions for future research. Scholars will need to tackle the question of explaining variation in information control. Why have some democratic countries adopted surveillance measures while others have not? How do we explain the differences in privacy protections? Why do some countries use multiple information control tactics while others do not? In the longer term, researchers will also be able to examine which countries dismantled information control apparatuses after the pandemic and which retained them.

The COVID-19 pandemic also indicates that different types of existential threats may prompt different types of government intervention and, as a consequence, regimes may adjust their expectations of the political costs of information control. For example, as the pandemic hit Israel, Prime Minister Benjamin Netanyahu revealed the existence of a secret national database containing private personal data on all Israeli citizens, their daily movements, transactions, and social contacts. The pandemic, Netanyahu inferred, provided a good moment for the revelation of these data and their overt deployment (Silverstein 2020). To understand how state leaders adjudicate between tactics, researchers will need to consider how different securitization processes may face different levels of contention.

Researchers will also need to study the consequences of information control measures adopted during the COVID-19 pandemic. How do citizens assess whether the government has their welfare in mind or ulterior motives? How do preexisting levels of trust impact the citizen–state relation as a consequence of the pandemic, in both the short term and the long term? A growing body of research indicates that states' efforts to control information may have profound effects on individuals' political attitudes and behaviors, and that these effects can run in multiple directions (Penney 2016; Stoycheff 2016; Brayne 2017; Eck, Hatz, Crabtree and Tago, forthcoming). Will the information control responses adopted in response to COVID-19 shift citizen attitudes relating to trust and legitimacy and, if so, in which direction?

In addition to the COVID-19 pandemic and the infodemic, the United Nations has warned of a third "parallel epidemic of authoritarian and repressive measures" (UN 2020b). Not only are falsehoods spread by nonstate actors dangerous, individuals are jeopardized when states withhold information, when they have diminished trust in public authorities, and when official statements contain propaganda and disinformation (UN 2020b). This third trend has the potential to be endemic: Activists across the globe have articulated fears that the COVID-19 pandemic may have ushered in a new era of normalized state surveillance. For states to mitigate these fears requires extraordinary levels of transparency and oversight to ensure the new information control measures are being used to promote the safety and security of citizens and not to strengthen government control. The United Nations has warned that the potential for abuse is high and that "what is justified during an emergency now may become normalized once the crisis has passed. … All measures must incorporate meaningful data protection safeguards, be lawful, necessary, and proportionate, time-bound and justified by legitimate public health objectives" (UN 2020a). Whether governments heed these admonitions to ensure and protect civil liberties will be a major post-pandemic issue.

Notes

1. We identified democracies as a score of 6 or above on the Polity2 variable (see https://www.systemicpeace.org/csprandd.html).
2. The WHO declared a *Public Health Emergency of International Concern* on January 30, 2020, referred to the "infodemic" on February 15, and declared a pandemic on March 11 (see www.who.int and www.euro.who.int).
3. We focus on government actions, as these have the clearest implications for civil liberties under international human rights law. We discuss private efforts when they are undertaken at the behest of, or are promoted by, governments. Although many surveillance apps have been developed by private actors, such as companies or universities, governments have encouraged or even mandated their use. Also, when it comes to online content regulation, much private action can be viewed as action by the state, as states often impose obligations to regulate communication and information (Land 2019).
4. See Marx (2015) and Lyon (2007) for overviews of the literature on surveillance.
5. We restrict our definitions to state policies and practices that target information, rather than people. For this reason, we consider the removal of information leaked by whistleblowers and the removal of media content as examples of censorship, whereas we bracket the targeting of whistleblowers and journalists.
6. What we will define as "information manipulation" is referred to by various terms, such as "flooding" (Roberts 2018), "propaganda" (Geddes and Zaller 1989), "false news" (Gläßel and Paula 2020), "astroturfing" and "reverse censorship" (King et al. 2017), and "social media co-option" (Gunitsky 2015). Other terms popular during the COVID-19 pandemic are "misinformation" and "disinformation."
7. Although the scope of the threat may be perceived by countries differently, depending on the quality of their healthcare systems or demographic characteristics, the pandemic was arguably understood as a threat by every country.
8. Adopted in Lichtenstein, Bahrain, and Hong Kong (OneZero 2020).

9. Notably, the rare Apple–Google partnership allows governments to use its open-source application programming interface (API) to develop national apps. Some governments have opted to adopt this technology, whereas others have developed their own apps. There have been extensive debates about how to ensure privacy protections in these mobile apps. In many of these discussions, companies have been less willing than governments to encroach on personal privacy (McGee, Murphy, and Bradshaw 2020), although they have not gone far enough for many privacy activists. Some government officials have criticized the stranglehold companies have on countries' ability to design surveillance apps (Ilves 2020). The complicated relationships between public and private interests in digital surveillance is a promising avenue for future research.
10. Bluetooth technology records what other phones an individual has come into proximity with, whereas geolocation technology records locations where the phone has been physically. For reasons relating to both accuracy and privacy protection, the Bluetooth approach is typically favored by privacy advocates.
11. These measures include responses to misinformation from government officials; corporate measures have occurred both in collaboration with and in opposition to governments.
12. Here it becomes clear how censorship differs from fact-checking.
13. Argentina, Algeria, Azerbaijan, Bolivia, Bosnia and Herzegovina, Botswana, China, Ethiopia, Hungary, India, Lesotho, Malaysia, North Macedonia, Philippines, Russia, Solomon Islands, South Africa, Thailand, United Arab Emirates, the United States (Puerto Rico), Uzbekistan, Vietnam, and Zimbabwe (ICNL 2020).
14. We view this as information manipulation, as the information targeted is produced by the government rather than the populace, as in censorship.

References

AGENCE FRANCE-PRESSE. (2020) Norway suspends virus-tracing app due to privacy concerns, *The Guardian*, 15 June. [Online]. Available: https://www.theguardian.com/world/2020/jun/15/norway-suspends-virus-tracing-app-due-to-privacy-concerns [28 July 2020].

AMNESTY INTERNATIONAL. (2020) *Bahrain, Kuwait and Norway Contact Tracing Apps Among Most Dangerous for Privacy*. [Online]. Available: https://www.amnesty.org/en/latest/news/2020/06/bahrain-kuwait-norway-contact-tracing-apps-danger-for-privacy/ [18 June 2020].

BEUTZ, Molly. (2003) Functional democracy: Responding to failures of accountability. *Harvard International Law Journal*, 44(2), 387–432.

BRAYNE, Sarah. (2017) Big data surveillance: The case of policing. *American Sociological Review*, 82(5), 977–1008. doi:10.1177/0003122417725865

DE MONTJOYE, Yves-Alexandre, HIDALGO, César A., VERLEYSEN, Michel, and BLONDEL, Vincent D. (2013) Unique in the crowd: The privacy bounds of human mobility. *Scientific Reports*, 3, 1376.

ECK, Kristine, HATZ, Sophia, CRABTREE, Charles, and TAGO, Atsushi. (forthcoming) Evade and deceive? Citizen responses to surveillance. *Journal of Politics*.

ELECTRONIC FRONTIER FOUNDATION. (2020) *International Proposals for Warrantless Location Surveillance to Fight COVID-19*. [Online]. Available: https://www.eff.org/deeplinks/2020/05/global-contact-tracing-international-proposals-track-COVID-19 [14 July 2020].

GEDDES, Barbara, and ZALLER, John. (1989) Sources of popular support for authoritarian Regimes. *American Journal of Political Science*, 33(2), 319–347.

GLÄßEL, Christian, and PAULA, Katrin. (2020) Sometimes less is more: Censorship, news falsification, and disapproval in 1989 East Germany. *American Journal of Political Science*, 64(3), 682–698.

GOHDES, Anita R. (2019) Repression technology: Internet accessibility and state violence. *American Journal of Political Science*, 64(3), 488–503.

GOLDSMITH, Jack, and WOODS, Andrew Keane. (2020) Internet speech will never go back to normal, *The Atlantic*, 25 April. [Online]. Available: https://www.theatlantic.com/ideas/archive/2020/04/what-covid-revealed-about-internet/610549/ [28 July 2020].

GUNITSKY, Seva. (2015) Corrupting the cyber-commons: Social media as a tool of autocratic stability. *Perspectives on Politics*, 13(1), 42–54. doi:10.1017/S1537592714003120

HABERMAN, Maggie. (2020) Trump has given unusual leeway to Fauci, but aides say he's losing his patience, *The New York Times*, 23 March. [Online]. Available: https://www.nytimes.com/2020/03/23/us/politics/coronavirus-trump-fauci.html [28 July 2020].

HAYES, Andrew F, and REINEKE, Jason B. (2007) The effects of government censorship of war-related news coverage on interest in the censored coverage: A test of competing theories. *Mass Communication & Society*, 10(4), 423–438.

HERN, Alex. (2020) Public Health England will keep personal data of people with coronavirus for 20 years, *The Guardian*, 28 May. [Online]. Available: https://www.theguardian.com/world/2020/may/28/nhs-will-keep-personal-data-of-people-with-coronavirus-for-20-years–uk-test-and-trace-programme [28 July 2020].

ILVES, Ieva. (2020) Why are Google and Apple dictating how European democracies fight coronavirus?, *The Guardian*, 16 June. [Online]. Available: https://www.theguardian.com/commentisfree/2020/jun/16/google-apple-dictating-european-democracies-coronavirus [14 July 2020].

INTERNATIONAL CENTER FOR NOT-FOR-PROFIT LAW (ICNL). (2020) *COVID-19 Civic Freedom Tracker*. [Online]. Available: https://www.icnl.org/COVID19tracker [28 July 2020].

JIANG, Junyan, and YANG, Dali L. (2016) Lying or believing? Measuring preference falsification from a political purge in China. *Comparative Political Studies*, 49(5), 600–634. doi:10.1177/0010414015626450

KING, Gary, PAN, Jennifer, and ROBERTS, Margaret E. (2013) How censorship in China allows government criticism but silences collective expression. *American Political Science Review*. 107(2), 326–343. doi:10.1017/S0003055413000014

KING, Gary, PAN, Jennifer, and ROBERTS, Margaret E. (2017) How the Chinese government fabricates social media posts for strategic distraction, not engaged argument. *American Political Science Review*, 111(3), 484–501. doi:10.1017/S0003055417000144

KURAN, Timur. (1997) *Private Truths, Public Lies: The Social Consequences of Preference Falsification* (Cambridge, MA: Harvard University Press).

LAND, Molly K. (2019) Regulating private harms online: Content regulation under human rights law. In *Human Rights in the Age of Platforms*, Rikke Frank Jørgensen (ed.) (Cambridge, MA: MIT Press).

LYON, David. (2007) *Surveillance Studies: An Overview* (Cambridge, UK: Polity Press).

MARX, Gary T. (2015) Surveillance studies. In *International Encyclopedia of the Social & Behavioral Sciences* (2nd ed.), James D. Wright (ed.) (Cambridge, MA: Elsevier Academic Press).

MCGEE, Hannah, MURPHY, Patrick, and BRADSHAW, Tim. (2020) Coronavirus apps: The risk of slipping into a surveillance state, *Financial Times*, 27 April. [Online]. Available: https://www.ft.com/content/d2609e26-8875-11ea-a01c-a28a3e3fbd33 [28 July 2020].

ONEZERO. (2020) *We Mapped How the Coronavirus is Driving New Surveillance Programs Around the World*. [Online]. Available: https://onezero.medium.com/the-pandemic-is-a-trojan-horse-for-surveillance-programs-around-the-world-887fa6f12ec9 [18 June 2020].

O'NEILL, Patrick Howell. (2020) *India is Forcing People to Use Its COVID App, Unlike Any Other Democracy*. [Online]. Available: https://www.technologyreview.com/2020/05/07/1001360/india-aarogya-setu-COVID-app-mandatory/ [18 June 2020].

PENNEY, Jonathon W. (2016) Chilling effects: Online surveillance and Wikipedia use. *Berkeley Technology Law Journal*, 31(1), 117–182.

ROBERTS, Margaret E. (2018) *Censored: Distraction and Diversion Inside China's Great Firewall* (Princeton, NJ: Princeton University Press).

ROTH, Kenneth. (2020) *How Authoritarians Are Exploiting the Covid-19 Crisis to Grab Power*. [Online]. Available: https://www.nybooks.com/daily/2020/03/31/how-authoritarians-are-exploiting-the-covid-19-crisis-to-grab-power/ [28 July 2020].

RUDBÄCK, Johana. (2020) *Minskad Insyn Hos FHM—Mötesanteckningar Hålls Hemliga* [Reduced transparency at the Public Health Agency—Meeting Notes are Kept Secret]. [Online]. Available: https://www.svt.se/nyheter/inrikes/minskad-insyn-hos-fhm-motesanteckningar-halls-hemliga [28 July 2020].

SABBAGH, Dan, and HERN, Alex. (2020) Privacy group prepares legal challenge to NHS test-and-trace scheme, *The Atlantic*, 31 May. [Online]. Available: https://www.theguardian.com/world/2020/may/31/privacy-campaigners-prepare-legal-challenge-to-uks-test-and-trace-scheme [28 July 2020].

SHIJI, Da. (2020) *The Truth About 'Dramatic Action.'* [Online]. Available: https://chinamediaproject.org/2020/01/27/dramatic-actions/ [28 July 2020].

SILVERSTEIN, Richard. (2020) Israel is militarising and monetising the COVID-19 pandemic, *The Wire*, 20 April. [Online]. Available: https://thewire.in/world/israel-is-militarising-and-monetising-the-covid-19-pandemic [28 July 2020].

STANLEY, Jay, and GRANICK, Jennifer Stiusa. (2020) *The Limits of Location Tracking in an Epidemic*. [Online]. Available: https://www.aclu.org/report/aclu-white-paper-limits-location-tracking-epidemic [18 June 2020].

STOLTON, Samuel. (2020) *Regulation Against Fake News 'Very Important,' Reynders Says*. [Online]. Available: https://www.euractiv.com/section/digital/news/regulation-against-fake-news-very-important-reynders-says/ [28 July 2020].

STOYCHEFF, Elizabeth. (2016) Under surveillance: Examining Facebook's spiral of silence effects in the wake of NSA internet monitoring. *Journalism & Mass Communication Quarterly*, 93(2), 296–311.

UNITED NATIONS. (2020a) *COVID-19 and Human Rights: We Are All in This Together*. [Online]. Available: https://www.un.org/en/un-coronavirus-communications-team/we-are-all-together-human-rights-and-covid-19-response-and [28 July 2020].

UNITED NATIONS. (2020b) *Disease Pandemics and the Freedom of Opinion and Expression*. UN Doc. A/HRC/44/49. [Online]. Available: https://www.ohchr.org/EN/Issues/FreedomOpinion/Pages/ReportDiseasePandemics.aspx [17 August 2020].

WEIDMANN, Nils B, and RØD, Espen Geelmuyden. (2019) *The Internet and Political Protest in Autocracies* (Oxford, UK: Oxford University Press).

WORLD HEALTH ORGANIZATION (WHO). (2020) *Working Together to Tackle the 'Infodemic.'* [Online]. Available: https://www.euro.who.int/en/health-topics/Health-systems/pages/news/news/2020/6/working-together-to-tackle-the-infodemic [28 July 2020].

Hazardous confinement during the COVID-19 pandemic: The fate of migrants detained yet nondeportable

Didier Fassin

ABSTRACT
As the French government decided on a lockdown of the population to prevent the spread of COVID-19, it soon appeared that, in an apparent paradox, two forcibly confined categories were particularly at risk: prisoners and detainees. Confronted with multiple mobilizations from civil society, authorities reacted in two distinct ways, significantly reducing the demographic of correctional facilities to allow for protective measures, but refusing to temporarily close detention centers, despite their insalubrious conditions and the impossibility of organizing deportations. These differential policies reveal an implicit moral hierarchy, in which undocumented migrants occupy the lower segment of the social scale, as well as a politics of indifference, which inculcates in them the illegitimacy of their presence and the unworthiness of their lives. Rebellions, self-harm, and hunger strikes are attempts to denounce and resist this intolerable situation.

"We'd rather die of hunger than from this shit!" wrote the migrants of the Lesquin Detention Center, in the North of France, on March 15, in a distressed public call. A case of infection by the novel coronavirus had been diagnosed among them two days earlier, leading several to stop going to the dining room for fear of being contaminated; as consequence, they had not gotten their meals for three days.[1] They were soon followed by others facing similar conditions at the Mesnil-Amelot Detention Center, near the Roissy airport, but those migrants made it clear this time, in an anguished statement published on March 30, that they were definitely on a hunger strike:

> We demand our immediate liberation and the closing of the center. We are afraid of being contaminated by the coronavirus. There are still new arrivals. Here there is no hygiene. There are no flights. Nothing. Why are we still here? There are guys who cut themselves to get out of here. The police are violent toward us.[2]

Several such protests, sometimes accompanied with gestures of despair including self-mutilations or with rebellions punished by prison sentences, took place in various detention centers where undocumented migrants were being held at the height of the pandemic. Alarm was palpable, but incomprehension as well. Why were they detained, as staying in these centers was supposed to be the prelude to their deportation, which the situation rendered impossible? Most countries had closed their borders, flights were cancelled. The centers themselves were progressively deserted. Visits from relatives and friends were no longer authorized. Nongovernmental organizations (NGOs) that had been granted presence to assist migrants in their legal files and bear witness to their conditions of detention were not sending their members anymore because of the risk incurred. Only the police were still there, as well as the minimal staffing from the private companies in charge of catering, while the personnel responsible for cleaning had exercised their right to opt out.

With the expansion of the epidemic across the country, the number of detainees had significantly decreased after the liberation of many, but as the justice system itself was partially shut down, hearings with liberty and custody judges were often postponed, not allowing for those who remained to have their situations examined as provided by law. For them, the risk of being infected could come either from police officers or from newly detained migrants. They knew this and dreaded it. Calls to temporarily close all detention centers multiplied from various sides, but the Minister of the Interior and the prefects remained unmoved.

In this article, I want to question the way French authorities treat undocumented migrants in the context of the pandemic. Although the imposed but voluntary confinement of the general population was intended to protect it from the risk of being infected, the forcible lockdown of detainees has exposed them to this very risk due to the poor conditions of their detention, the lack of preventative measures, the absence of testing, the unfeasibility of isolation, and the delay in diagnosis and treatment of patients. The government was alerted by multiple institutions, organizations, unions, and intellectuals not only to the potential danger for the migrants under these circumstances but also to the absurdity and illegality of detaining them in anticipation of their deportation when there was no chance of conducting such an operation.

This dual paradox—a forcible lockdown with predictable results the opposite of those intended as the outcome of the voluntary confinement, and a senseless measure supposedly to prepare expulsions but actually impossible to carry out—is only one on the face of it (Fassin 2019). In fact, exposing undocumented migrants to such a deadly threat pertains to the same politics of life as exposing them to even deadlier threats in the Mediterranean and the Alps as they attempt to reach the European, or more specifically French, territory. It is a politics of indifference (Herzfeld 1993).

In that regard, it is revealing that the other locked-up population, prisoners, received more attention from the government during the health crisis. The contrast between the policies toward migrants whose only crime was to be undocumented and the policies toward individuals who have been accused of or sentenced for an offense is indicative of implicitly established moral hierarchies. In contemporary society, exiles—those being called undocumented migrants who may also be asylum seekers—often occupy the lower segment of the social scale, even more disgraced than criminals. The French case is certainly not an exception in this respect (De Genova and Peutz 2010). It can be regarded as exemplary of the more general condition of those who flee their home countries because of war, persecution, hardship, and a dire future.

Based on research carried out in May and June 2020 in the Paris region through interviews, observation, and collection of data, I will first recount how the government reacted to the pandemic, emphasizing the situation of prisoners and detainees. I will then focus on the political mobilization to protect these populations from infection, and the differential response provided by the authorities. I will finally show that the health crisis did not provoke the crisis in the detention centers but, instead, uncovered their appalling ordinary reality.

The forgotten

The first case of the novel coronavirus infection in France was diagnosed on January 24, 2020, but it was later discovered that several patients presenting typical symptoms and who subsequently tested positive were already present in the country as early as mid-December 2019. Yet, only at the end of February were several clusters identified in three different regions, with initial patients having returned from Wuhan or Lombardy.

On March 7, despite a rapid doubling of cases and deaths every 48 hours, President Emmanuel Macron ostensibly went to the theater with his wife, stating that people should continue to live normally; on March 15, when the incidence of the infection had been multiplied by 28 and its mortality by 42 in only two weeks, the French government decided to uphold the municipal elections. However, the next day, a strict shelter-in-place order with the slogan, "Save lives, stay home," was announced for a period of two weeks, which was later extended for a total of almost two months.[3] Only essential workers could go on with their activities, even though face masks remained unavailable for several weeks. In an awkward justification for their worrying shortage, two successive health ministers asserted at the time that these masks were actually useless for the general public.

To enforce the measures taken to fight the epidemic, notably the confinement, a state-of-emergency law was enacted on March 24, giving special powers to the executive branch and the police.[4] The violation of the prohibition of being outside, except with the appropriate document authorizing it, was sanctioned by a $160 fine, increased to $1,800 in cases of repeated offenses and even up to $4,500 with up to six months of imprisonment in cases of continued recidivism. In two months, more than 20 million checks were conducted and more than a million tickets issued, disproportionately to people belonging to ethno-racial minorities in disadvantaged neighborhoods, accompanied sometimes by violent interactions with the police.[5] Even homeless people were occasionally fined for not abiding by the law. In sum, to make up for their lack of preparedness in the crisis foretold and for their ignorance of its early signs, the authorities turned to sanitary policing, imposing a rigorous confinement to protect the population from the spread of the infection.

But although confinement was presented as the best response to the expansion of the epidemic, it soon appeared that in two specific contexts where it was by definition implemented in the strictest way—in correctional facilities and detention centers—it threatened to produce the opposite of the desired effect. In the former—more specifically, in short-stay prisons, which house people awaiting trial and those who are sentenced to less than two years imprisonment—overcrowding reached unprecedented levels, two or even frequently three inmates being locked up 23 hours a day in the 100 square feet of a supposedly individual cell.[6] In the latter, all activities, including meals, were collective and, as people could circulate freely within the centers, social distancing was impossible to respect, even less so as information regarding preventative measures was rarely available.[7] In both situations, there were constant new arrivals of prisoners and migrants, respectively, and whereas visits had been forbidden, the personnel, either prison guards or police officers who came from outside, had frequent unprotected interactions with those locked up. Besides, although clear recommendations had been issued by the Ministry of Health for both institutions in the first days of the national confinement, hand sanitizer was lacking and masks were not provided. Finally, in the absence of testing, it was difficult to know whether people were infected by the coronavirus when they presented fever, cough, or other symptoms.

In the prison where I conducted my study, the physician in charge considered that inmates who complained about a loss of smell or taste were actually trying to manipulate her, and she therefore did not acknowledge them as probable cases. In detention centers, only severe forms of coronavirus infection were tested and isolated, thus ignoring a majority of clinical forms with little or no symptoms, particularly frequent among young men. In these circumstances, it was predictable that it would not take much to render the epidemiological situation critical and the atmosphere explosive in these institutions. It should, however, be noted from the start that during the five months following the declaration of national confinement, only one death was reported among the more than 70,000 inmates who were present at the beginning of the epidemic—that of a 74-year-old man who had been sentenced and incarcerated while already sick—and none has been reported in detention centers. The fact that there are very few individuals beyond the age of 60 in these facilities certainly accounts for this absence of fatality. As for the number of cases during that period, there are no reliable statistics, making it possible to establish it, as there has been no systematic testing in these facilities.

Difference

As the health crisis was looming, the awareness of the vulnerability of both populations rapidly gave rise to a broad mobilization.[8] Researchers and intellectuals wrote opinion pieces asking whether, in the President's solemn address to the nation on March 16, his call for "a 'sense of responsibility and solidarity' stopped at the doors of correctional facilities and detention centers" (Fassin 2020).

On March 17, the Controller General of Facilities of Deprivation of Liberty, Adeline Hazan, wrote to the Minister of Justice, Nicole Belloubet, asking her "to reduce the carceral population to a level not above the actual capacity of the prison system" as the inmates' safety was "not guaranteed anymore," and to the Minister of the Interior, Christophe Castaner, asking him "to proceed immediately to the temporary closure of administrative detention centers" as "the prospect of deportations was slim, if not illusory."[9]

On March 19, the Defender of Rights, Jacques Toubon, also questioned the government on the situation of undocumented migrants, affirming that, in consideration of the situation, "the lockup lacked legal grounds" because they could not be deported, and even if they could, their expulsion to another country could "facilitate the spread of the virus contrary to the recommendations of the World Health Organization."[10]

On March 21, the Controller and the Defender along with the president of the National Consultative Commission for Human Rights, Jean-Marie Burguburu, signed an opinion editorial in the main French newspaper urging the government to take measures to protect undocumented migrants (Toubon, Hazan, and Burguburu 2020). In parallel, NGOs, including the International Observatory of Prisons and the Observatory of the Detention of Foreigners, and justice professional associations, such as the French Union of Lawyers and the National Bar Council, multiplied initiatives with the same ends but distinct means.

Regarding the prison system, a petition asking for the liberation of incarcerated persons with short sentences or near the end of their sentence was signed by a thousand judges, lawyers, social scientists, and health professionals.[11] Regarding the detention centers, legal actions were taken at the local, national and international levels, liberty and custody judges, and courts of appeal were seized for the release of individuals, while the Council of State and the European Court of Human Rights were requested to rule on the general principle of a temporary closure.[12] All these convergent actions were conducted in less than two weeks.

The response of the authorities was very different with respect to the treatment of the two populations. Whereas the Ministry of Justice took measures to reduce significantly the carceral population, the Ministry of the Interior refused to close the detention centers. The joint requests of official independent bodies, human rights organizations, professionals, and intellectuals were heard in regard to the condition of prisoners but not that of migrants. The fact that the latter came from the so-called Global South (particularly from the African continent and the Middle East) suggests a racial dimension in these policies, which is confirmed by the existence of systemic discrimination deeply ingrained in French law-enforcement institutions, and complaints by detainees about racist slurs coming from the police.

In correctional facilities, the population decreased by 19 percent in less than three months. There were 72,575 inmates on March 16 and 58,874 on June 11.[13] During that period, the density of short-stay prisons declined from 140 to 108 percent, suggesting that the objective of one inmate per cell determined by an 1875 law, which had not been respected for decades, was almost reached. However, due to cells being rehabilitated or remaining dedicated to other functions, the actual density was higher than official statistics indicated. This evolution was hailed by the Union of Wardens, which demanded that what had been achieved because of the health crisis, thus demonstrating that single cell housing was possible, could become the norm. This remarkable result was attributable to the combination of a reduction in new incarcerations, partially due to the *quasi*-shutdown of the justice system and to the acceleration of the release—often with ankle monitoring—of inmates approaching the end of their sentence, as ordered in a decree by the Ministry of Justice. A series of other measures was adopted to compensate for the loss of visits and activities, such as the granting of free access to television and a $50 telephone card to call families, and the organization of regular meetings between the personnel and the inmates to improve the understanding of the plan implemented.

As for the detention centers, they remained open, with new migrants incessantly arriving over time. Surely, some did close after the liberty and custody judge freed the occupants, for instance in Strasbourg and Nice, or after the prefect decided to transfer those to another center, notably in Hendaye and Plaisir, with sometimes contrary arbitrations by the judge who released detainees and the prefect who added new ones, as was the case at the Spanish border. But the majority of them—especially the larger ones, such as Mesnil-Amelot near Roissy, Vincennes near Paris, Oissel near Rouen, and Coquelles near Calais—kept a large portion of their detainees.[14] For those, the resistance to their closure came from both judges and prefects (Muchielli 2020). The former had the discretionary power to release or not as a function of their assessment of the infectious risk and, probably even more, of their ideological inclination. The latter opposed more specifically the release of migrants just liberated from prison with the argument that they could cause public disorder, although in most cases the offense for which they had been sentenced was relatively minor. Nevertheless, on the whole, the number of undocumented migrants detained in the centers substantially waned.

Although the government does not systematically publish statistics on this topic, which renders comparisons difficult, Cimade, an NGO present in detention centers since 1985, did produce some figures based on voluntary workers' observations on the ground. A year before the beginning of the epidemic, the number of persons detained was 878. At the time of the confinement, it was 343. Ten days later, 154. Seven centers had no detainees, nine had less than ten, five had eleven or more.[15] This contraction of the population, which was limited in time, as the number of those detained began to increase again in April, served as a justification for the dismissal by the Council of State of the application for interim relief filed by several human rights and justice professional organizations that requested the closure of detention centers. For the highest French administrative court, the drop in the demographic rendered protection measures possible.

Had they visited detention centers, its members might have thought otherwise. Commenting on this decision, the NGOs that had initiated the case wrote that the court was providing "protection on the cheap for the migrants."[16] A representative who visited the center of Cornebarrieu, near Toulouse on April 3 described in his report the absence of masks, the lack of cleaning products, and the nonrespect of social distancing for both detainees and personnel. Similar observations were made on April 17 by the Controller General of Facilities of Deprivation of Liberty for the centers of Mesnil-Amelot and Vincennes, where eight cases were then officially reported.[17] Although there was little testing, which did not allow for a precise estimation of the epidemiological situation, detainees who had symptoms and were confirmed as COVID-19 patients were supposed to be sent to the special medical centers established by the Regional Health Agency. However, this institution refused those just liberated from prison with the justification that they could disturb public order. Consequently, they ended up staying in isolation in the detention center.

The difference in the treatment of correctional facilities and detention centers by the authorities is not, however, only a question of numbers. After all, both significantly reduced their population so as to render its protection theoretically possible. It is also a question of management and commitment. The administration of correctional institutions devoted considerable efforts to ensure the protection of their inmates and personnel, designing protocols with the Health Ministry, coordinating with the local criminal courts, setting regional weekly videoconferences between wardens, involving guards in the prevention plans, and—to a certain degree—explaining the measures to the prisoners. There was nothing comparable for the detention centers, which are under the distant authority of the prefect and whose personnel is composed of police officers with little interest in serving as custodians of people who have not committed crimes.

As their reactions proved, inmates and migrants made no mistake about the difference. There were few protests in the correctional facilities, and with one exception, these were limited to peaceful collective refusals to leave the yard and return to the cell until some specific demands were heard by the warden. They were disciplined by the prisons' special units without excessive use of force, although those considered to be the leaders were transferred to other facilities.

Conversely, in detention centers, there were multiple incidents, including hunger strikes and desperate revolts that were ignited by a climate of fear of coronavirus infection and of anger at the apathy of the authorities. Thus, the starting point for the riot in Vincennes was the rebuff of detainees' demand to have sick migrants taken care of in a hospital. Instead, the authorities sent police officers who used tear gas and violence to put down the disorder and transferred the migrants involved in the protests to other centers, purposely without their belongings—"like homeless people," one of them said. But such treatment was nothing new in detention centers. Rather than having generated these situations, the pandemic has simply unveiled them. It has been a catalyst and revealer of structural inequities.

Indifference

The detention centers were created in 1981 by the newly elected Socialist government to confine foreigners on the brink of being deported.[18] They replaced a previous informal system whose infamous legacy was a warehouse in Arenc, near Marseille, where tens of thousands of Algerians were detained before being sent back to their country in the 1960s and 1970s. Once legalized, their development was parallel to the hardening of immigration policies from the 1980s onward, when the rise of the National Front moved these issues to the center of the public debate. Instead of denouncing this ideology, the Conservatives' and even the Socialists' and Communists' responses contributed to the legitimation of xenophobia. Thus, in 1984, the Prime Minister of a leftist coalition government, Laurent Fabius, stated that "the far-right has wrong answers to good questions."[19]

But it was in the 2000s that Minister of the Interior and later President Nicolas Sarkozy spectacularized the statistics of deportation, announcing and boasting about the numbers annually as his political signature, thus giving detention centers a crucial role and unprecedented visibility.[20] Two phenomena contributed to their rapid expansion. First, there was an increase in the number of individuals being detained every year: 14,000 at the end of the 1990s; 36,000 a decade later; more than 45,000 today. Second, there was an extension of the maximum duration of detention: it was seven days in 1981; it became nine days in 1999, 32 days in 2003, and 45 days in 2011; finally, in 2019, it doubled to reach 90 days.[21] In other words, both flows and stocks have progressed rapidly, generating a need for more space.

The most substantial expansion of the system occurred after the vote for the law extending the maximum duration of detention to three months: There were 1,069 places in 2017, 1,549 in 2018, and 1,814 in 2019, an increase of 70 percent in two years, with 2,341 personnel and police mobilized. The official reason for the legislation was that it gave the administration more time to expedite the examination of cases and therefore made it be more effective in terms of deportations as the *laissez-passer* delivered by the corresponding foreign consulates were often delayed. Yet, a Senate report had demonstrated the previous year that only 6 percent of these *laissez-passer* were sent beyond the 45th day of detention (Buffet 2017). More than anything else, the law was supposed to show strength. However, the actual productivity of this policy and its cost effectiveness were rarely questioned. An analysis conducted by two representatives of the National Assembly shows that in 2018, out of 105,084 orders to leave the country delivered by the police and residence bans decided by judges in the metropolitan territory, only 15,677 deportations (that is, 15 percent) have been executed. More specifically, among the migrants who had been housed in detention centers, the proportion of those actually deported was 40 percent. The average cost of each deportation was estimated at $16,250 (Januel 2019).

This may seem a high price for such a modest outcome, and even more so, considering the invisible cost of suffering for the more than 45,000 individuals detained for increasingly long periods of time—25,000 in the metropolitan territory and 20,000 overseas—as well as their families. Many of them are separated from their spouses and children, who have legal status or, for some, French citizenship. Besides, 14 percent are asylum seekers are caught under the so-called Dublin Regulation, which requires that a file must be examined in the country where the fingerprints of the applicant were initially registered—that is, often the one they entered first.[22] The insistence of the Ministry of the Interior to not close the detention centers must therefore be analyzed in light of these poor results and high costs.

That this system has mostly a performative function is suggested not only by the low number of deportations related to the considerable means deployed in terms of human and financial resources, but also by the modest number of arrests, decisions, and detentions compared to the population of undocumented migrants. Although this figure is, almost by definition, unknown, its most conservative assessment can be made via the statistics of people benefiting from State Medical Assistance, which is provided to those irregularly present in French territory: 320,000 persons. Nevertheless, this figure gives a very partial view of the actual demographic reality, as many people entitled to this health insurance do not request it, and it is more reasonable to think that the actual number could be at least twice as high (Lebourcq 2019).

In other words, in metropolitan France, less than 5 percent of the undocumented migrants are detained each year and hardly more than 1 percent are deported. Given such poor performance, the social performativity of these policies has two objectives and two targets. On the one hand, it is meant to show to the general public the determination of the government to combat illegal immigration, even if many of those arrested and detained actually have close family ties or seek refugee status. On the other hand, it is directed toward undocumented migrants themselves in order to inculcate in them a sense of their illegitimacy and, if one considers the indignity of the vexing conditions of their arrest and detention, of their unworthiness.

The attitude of governments toward the most vulnerable segments of their population—in particular, their degree of care or, on the contrary, indifference—is an indicator of their ultimate ethical values. The range of these attitudes has been studied for health systems in general (Dauvrin, Lorant, Sandu, Devillé, Dia, Dias, Gaddini, Ioannidis, Jensen, Kluge, Mertaniemi, Puigpinos i Riera, Sarvary, Strabmayr, Stankunas, Soarea, Weibel, Priebe 2012) and more recently for responses to the coronavirus infection (Boinnard 2020).

When the pandemic started, Spain closed all its detention centers, considering that preventative measures could not discriminate against undocumented migrants and moreover that their confinement in these facilities had no remaining legal basis as they could not be deported. Portugal decided to grant a temporary residence permit to all migrants and asylum seekers who had pending applications in order to ensure their access to public services, including health facilities. By contrast, the United States has had approximately 60,000 undocumented migrants in its overcrowded detention centers since the beginning of the pandemic, with an estimated 20 percent infection rate among the 19,000 tested by the Immigration and Customs Enforcement agency; nevertheless, the country has continued to organize deportations to Mexico and the Northern Triangle via 180 flights, at the risk of spreading of the virus.[23]

In between these extremes, France has chosen to reduce its detained population but not to close its detention centers, despite their insalubrious conditions. Most European countries have done the same. Their policies in that regard are not significantly different from those they already carry out in the Mediterranean and at their internal borders, particularly in the Alps, where European countries have considerably increased the risks of migrants' journeys by intensifying state repression against those who try these dangerous crossings and preventing those who attempt to assist them from doing so.[24] Such policies reflect a profound indifference toward what the life of these exiles is worth.

Notes

1. Their letter was published by the website infoLibertaire.net dedicated to the dissemination of news obtained from more than 150 sources in the activist media so as to serve as a repertoire of alternative media (see Infolibertaire 2020).
2. The statement was published by the website of the Assembly Against Administrative Detention Centers, an organization created in January 2019 in support of the collective struggles led by migrants in these centers (see A bas les CRA 2020).
3. The decree of March 16 prohibits all movements outside except under very specific circumstances with adequate permission (see https://www.legifrance.gouv.fr/eli/decret/2020/3/16/PRMX2007858D/jo/texte).
4. The language of the law 2020-290 is particularly dramatic in speaking of "health disaster" (*catastrophe sanitaire*; see https://www.legifrance.gouv.fr/affichTexte.do?cidTexte=JORFTEXT000041746313&categorieLien=id).
5. These fines amount to $175 million. For details, see La Gazette des Communes (2020).
6. On January 1, there were 70,651 persons incarcerated. Short-stay prisons housed 48,288 prisoners, among whom 44 percent were awaiting trial. They had an average density of 138 percent per cell, with four facilities exceeding 200 percent (see Republic of France, Ministry of Justice 2020).
7. In 2019, there were 1,814 places in the administrative detention centers. There were 18,906 actual deportations that year, representing only 40 percent of those housed (see Republic of France, Cour de Comptes 2020).
8. A detailed and useful chronicle of this mobilization, of the authorities' response, and of the reactions of the inmates and detainees has been produced by the French section of the International Prison Observatory (OIP 2020), for correctional facilities and by Gisti, the Group of Information and Support of Migrants, for detention centers (see Gisti 2020a) .
9. The Controller General of Facilities of Deprivation of Liberty is an independent public body created in 2007 that controls all institutions where people are deprived of their liberty. See the statement and the letters to the ministers (Controleur General des Lieux de Privation de Liberte 2020a).
10. The Defensor of Rights is an independent public body in charge of guaranteeing the respect of human rights. See his statement to the government (Defenseur de Droits 2020).
11. The letter was published on May 3, three days after the most recent condemnation of the French state by the European Court of Human Rights for its inhumane treatment of prisoners. It is available through the Observatoire International des Prisons (2020).
12. The concern regarding the danger incurred by prisoners and detainees was not specific to France. On March 25, the UN High Commissioner for Human Rights, Michelle Bachelet, called on governments to protect the health and safety of people in detention and other closed facilities, including their staff (UN Office of the UN High Commissioner for Human Rights 2020).
13. These statistics were provided by the special advisor for prison of the minister of justice (interview by the author, June 15, 2020).
14. A detailed presentation of the situation of each detention center was produced on March 20 by Cimade (2020a).
15. These figures were obtained from the Observatory of the Detention of Foreigners (emails on file with the author, of March 16, 2020, and March 26, 2020).
16. See the full text of the decision of the Council of State in Conseil d'Etat (2020) and the response of the organizations in Gisti (2020b).
17. Members of Parliament and observers of the Controller General of Facilities of Deprivation of Liberty can visit detention centers. See, for example, the statement by European Parliament member Manuel Bompard (2020) and Controleur General des Lieux de Privation de Liberte (2020b).
18. The history of detention centers has been recounted by Nicolas Fischer (2017), who has also conducted an ethnographic research in one of the largest of them, focusing his attention on the role of the NGO present to assist in legal cases and confront difficult dilemmas.
19. At the time, the government changed the rules of the legislative elections from majority voting to proportional representation, which allowed, for the first time under the Fifth Republic, the presence of the far right in the French Parliament. Archival footage is available via the French National Audiovisual Institute (INA 1984).

20. This "politics of number," as it was coined, concerned also the statistics of crime. For the detention centers, the figure that was never publicized was that of the cost (Blic 2009).
21. A yearly report has been produced by Cimade since 2006, providing precious quantitative and qualitative information about detention centers (see Cimade 2020b).
22. An overview of both the statistical data and individual situations is presented in the *2018 Report on Administrative Detention* Centers written by the NGOs present in these centers (see Cimade 2018).
23. On the closure of detention centers in Spain, see Majkowska-Tomkin (2020); on immigration regularization in Portugal, see Waldersee (2020); on practices of the US Immigration and Customs Enforcement agency, see reporting by the International Rescue Committee (2020).
24. According to the Missing Migrant Project conducted by the UN International Organization for Migration (IOM), 10,958 migrants have died crossing the Mediterranean in the past five years; in the first seven months of 2020, there were 497 deaths. These figures are necessarily conservative, as an unknown number of fatalities are not registered. For details, see IOM (2020). As the repression of immigration by European authorities increased and as the humanitarian efforts to rescue people in sinking boats have been hindered, the mortality rate—that is, the number of deaths related to the number of arrivals—has climbed from 2 percent to 8 percent, meaning that for 12 persons reaching the European coast at least one has died in the crossing, making this border the most dangerous in the world (see IOM-Global Migration Data Analysis Centre 2020).

Acknowledgments

This article is based on research conducted as part of a program on crises supported by the Nomis Foundation. This study was carried out exempted from the Institutional Review Board, and the people mentioned in the article are anonymized. I am grateful to Luc Ginot, public health director at the Ile-de-France Regional Health Agency, and Isabelle Grémy, director of the Ile-de-France Regional Health Observatory, for having facilitated my access to information and my understanding of the coronavirus crisis. I am indebted to the Observatory of the Detention of Foreigners and the organizations composing it, who serve as a watchdog for human rights issues and a legal activist to redress legal violations by the state in places where undocumented migrants are locked down, for the wealth of information contained in their daily exchanges about the situations in the detention centers, which are impenetrable institutions for researchers. I also thank all those in the prison and shelter systems—officials, managers, workers, inmates, and migrants—who have shared their knowledge and experience. As a disclosure, I must add that I am the president of Comede, the Committee for the Health of Exiles, a French nongovernmental organization that assists undocumented foreigners and asylum seekers in addressing their medical, social, and legal issues; Comede is a member of the Observatory of the Detention of Foreigners.

References

A BAS LES CRA. (2020) *On Demande Notre Libération Immédiate et la Fermeture Du Centre. Communiqué du Mesnil-Amelot.* [Online]. Available: https://abaslescra.noblogs.org/on-demande-notre-liberation-immediate-et-la-fermeture-du-centre-communique-du-mesnil-amelot/ [24 August 2020].

BLIC, Damien. (2009) Sans-Papiers: L'autre 'Chiffre' de la Politique D'expulsion. *Mouvements*, 2 July. [Online]. Available: https://mouvements.info/sans-papiers-lautre-chiffre-de-la-politique-dexpulsion/ [24 August 2020].

BOINNARD, Léa. (2020) Étrangers en situation irrégulière et crise sanitaire: sélection de réponses étatiques à la vulnérabilité de cette population. *Revue Des Droits Et Des Libertés Fondamentales,* Chronicle 45.

BOMPARD, Manuel. (2020) *Il Faut Fermer Les Centres de Retention.* [Online]. Available: https://m.facebook.com/story.php?story_fbid=1626996864123358&id=837898283033224 [24 August 2020].

BUFFET, François-Noël. (2017) *Asile, Immigration, Intégration Et Nationalité.* [Online]. Available: https://www.senat.fr/rap/a17-114-2/a17-114-21.pdf [24 August 2020].

CIMADE. (2018) *Centres Et Locaux de Retention Administrative, 2018 Rapport.* [Online]. Available: https://www.lacimade.org/wp-content/uploads/2019/06/La_Cimade_Rapport_Retention_2018.pdf [24 August 2020].

CIMADE. (2020a) *Retention Corona Etat Des Lieux.* [Online]. Available: https://docs.google.com/spreadsheets/d/1FC68z_pGVOPvaenFw6BPX2n-epOu-gT5rZLQGfVQ2m8/edit#gid=0 [24 August 2020].

CIMADE. (2020b) *Publications Et Ressources/Reports Sur la Retention Administrative.* [Online]. Available: https://www.lacimade.org/publication/?type-publication=rapports-sur-la-retention-administrative&numpage=2&num-page=1 [24 August 2020].

CONSEIL D'ETAT. (2020) *Decision 27 March 2020 no.* 439720. [Online]. Available: https://www.conseil-etat.fr/ressources/decisions-contentieuses/dernieres-decisions-importantes/conseil-d-etat-27-mars-2020-demande-de-fer-meture-temporaire-des-centres-de-retention-administrative-cra [24 August 2020].

CONTRÔLEUR GÉNÉRAL DES LIEUX DE PRIVATION DE LIBERTE. (2020a) *Situation Sanitaire Des Prisons Et Centres de Rétention Administrative: le CGLPL Demande la Prise de Mesures Pour la Protection Des Personnes Privées de Liberté.* [Online]. Available: https://www.cglpl.fr/2020/situation-sanitaire-des-prisons-et-centres-de-retention-administrative-le-cglpl-demande-la-prise-de-mesures-pour-la-protection-des-personnes-privees-de-liberte/ [24 August 2020].

CONTRÔLEUR GÉNÉRAL DES LIEUX DE PRIVATION DE LIBERTE. (2020b) *COVID-19: Ie CGLPL s'est Rendu Dans Les Centres de Rétention Administrative de Paris-vincennes Et Du Mesnil-Amelot.* [Online]. Available: https://www.cglpl.fr/wp-content/uploads/2020/04/Communiqu%C3%A9-Coronavirus-CRA-Vincennes-et-Mesnil.pdf [24 August 2020].

DAUVRIN, Marie, LORANT, Vincent, SANDU, Sima, DEVILLÉ, Walter, DIA, Hamidou, DIAS, Sonia, GADDINI, Andras, IOANNIDIS, Elisabeth, JENSEN, Natasja, KLUGE, Ulrike, MERTANIEMI, Ritva, PUIGPINOS I RIERA, Rosa, SARVARY, Attila, STRABMAYR, Christa, STANKUNAS, Mindaugas, SOAREA, Joachin, WEIBEL, Maria, and PRIEBE, Stefan. (2012) Health care for irregular migrants: Pragmatism across Europe. A qualitative study. *BMC Research Notes*, 5, 99.

DEFENSEUR DES DROITS. (2020) *Covid-19: Face Aux Risques de Contamination, Ie Défenseur Des Droits Demande la Fermeture Des Centres de Rétention Administrative.* [Online]. Available: https://www.defenseurdes-droits.fr/actualites/2020/03/covid-19-face-aux-risques-de-contamination-le-defenseur-des-droits-demande-la [24 August 2020].

DE GENOVA, Nicholas, and PEUTZ, Nathalie. (2010) *The Deportation Regime: Sovereignty, Space and the Freedom of Movement* (Durham, NC: Duke University Press).

FASSIN, Didier. (2019) *Life: A Critical User's Manual* (Cambridge, UK: Polity Press).

FASSIN, Didier. (2020) L'inégalité des vies en temps d'épidémie. *Libération,* March 18. [Online]. Available: https://www.liberation.fr/debats/2020/03/18/l-inegalite-des-vies-en-temps-d-epidemie_1782169 [24 August 2020].

FISCHER, Nicolas. (2017) *Le Territoire de L'expulsion. La Rétention Administrative Des Étrangers et L'État de Droit en France* (Lyon, France: ENS éditions).

GISTI. (2020a) *Enfermement en Periode de COVID-19: Fil d'infos 17 Mars–15 Mai 2020.* [Online]. Available: https://www.gisti.org/spip.php?article6362 [24 August 2020].

GISTI. (2020b) *Le Conseil D'état Refuse la Fermeture Des Centres de rétentio: Une Protection au Rabais Pour Les Étrangers.* [Online]. Available: https://www.gisti.org/spip.php?article6346 [24 August 2020].

HERZFELD, Michael. (1993) *The Social Production of Indifference. Exploring the Symbolic Roots of Western Bureaucracy* (Chicago, IL: University of Chicago Press).

INA (French National Audiovisual Institute). (1984) *Laurent Fabius: 'L'extrême Droite ce Sont de Fausses Réponses à de Vraies Questions.* [Online]. Available: https://www.ina.fr/video/I09082524 [24 August 2020].

INFOLIBERTAIRE. (2020) *[CRA] On Préfere Mourir de Faim Que de Cette Merde! Infos du CRA de Lesquin.* [Online]. Available: https://www.infolibertaire.net/cra-on-prefere-mourir-de-faim-que-de-cette-merde-infos-du-cra-de-lesquin/ [24 August 2020].

INTERNATIONAL RESCUE COMMITTEE. (2020) *COVID-19 Escalating in ICE Detention Centers as States Hit Highest Daily Records and ICE Deportation Flights Into Northern Triangle Continue.* [Online]. Available: https://www.rescue.org/press-release/covid-19-escalating-ice-detention-centers-states-hit-highest-daily-records-and-ice [24 August 2020].

JANUEL, Pierre. (2019) *La Coûteuse Machine à Expulser Les Étrangers.* [Online]. Available: https://www.dalloz-actualite.fr/flash/couteuse-machine-expulser-etrangers#.Xz8-jS2z26v [24 August 2020].

LA GAZETTE DES COMMUNES. (2020) *Plus D'un Million D'amendes Pendant le Confinement.* [Online]. Available: https://www.lagazettedescommunes.com/678602/coronavirus-plus-dun-million-damendes-pendant-le-confinement/ [24 August 2020].

LEBOURCQ, Fabien. (2019) *Est-il Vrai Que Les 320,000 Bénéficiaires de l'AME ne Représentent Que 12% Des Sans-Papiers?* [Online]. Available: https://www.liberation.fr/checknews/2019/10/09/est-il-vrai-que-les-320-000-benefici-aires-de-l-ame-ne-representent-que-12-des-sans-papiers_1756219 [24 August 2020].

MAJKOWSKA-TOMKIN, Magda. (2020) *Countries are Suspending Immigration Detention Due to Coronavirus: Let's Keep it that Way.* [Online]. Available: https://www.euronews.com/2020/04/29/countries-suspending-immi-gration-detention-due-to-coronavirus-let-s-keep-it-that-way-view [24 August 2020].

MUCHIELLI, Julien. (2020) *Centres de Rétention: Étrangers et Policiers Face au Coronavirus*. [Online]. Available: https://www.dalloz-actualite.fr/flash/centres-de-retention-etrangers-et-policiers-face-au-coronavirus#.Xz8p9y2z26t [24 August 2020].

OBSERVATOIRE INTERNATIONAL DES PRISONS (OIP). (2020) *En Finir avec la Surpopulation Carcérale: 'Monsieur le Président, L'occasion Est la ne la Manquez Pas*. [Online]. Available: https://oip.org/communique/en-finir-avec-la-surpopulation-carcerale-monsieur-le-president-loccasion-est-la-ne-la-manquez-pas/ [24 August 2020].

REPUBLIC OF FRANCE. (2020a) *Decree no. 2020-260 of 16 March*. [Online]. Available: https://www.legifrance.gouv.fr/eli/decret/2020/3/16/PRMX2007858D/jo/texte [24 August 2020].

REPUBLIC OF FRANCE. (2020b) *Law no. 2020-290 of 23 March*. [Online]. Available: https://www.legifrance.gouv.fr/affichTexte.do?cidTexte=JORFTEXT000041746313&categorieLien=id [24 August 2020].

REPUBLIC OF FRANCE, MINISTRY OF JUSTICE. (2020) *Statistique Des Établissements Des Personnes Écrouées en France*. [Online]. Available: http://www.justice.gouv.fr/art_pix/Stat_etablissements_janvier_2020.pdf [24 August 2020].

TOUBON, Jacques, HAZAN, Adeline, and BURGUBURU, Jean-Marie. (2020) Sauvegardons les droits fondamentaux pendant la crise sanitaire. *Le Monde*, March 21. [Online]. Available: https://www.lemonde.fr/idees/article/2020/03/20/coronavirus-sauvegardons-les-droits-fondamentaux-pendant-la-crise-sanitaire_6033892_3232.html [24 August 2020].

UN INTERNATIONAL ORGANIZATION FOR MIGRATION (IOM). (2020) *Missing Migrant Project*. [Online]. Available: https://missingmigrants.iom.int/region/mediterranean [24 August 2020].

UN IOM GLOBAL MIGRATION DATA ANALYSIS CENTRE. (2020) *Calculating 'Death Rates' in the Context of Migration Journeys: Focus on the Central Mediterranean*. [Online]. Available: https://publications.iom.int/system/files/pdf/mortality-rates.pdf [24 August 2020].

UN OFFICE OF THE UN HIGH COMMISSIONER FOR HUMAN RIGHTS. (2020) *Urgent Action Needed to Prevent COVID-19 'Rampaging Through Places of Detention'—Bachelet*. [Online]. Available: https://www.ohchr.org/EN/NewsEvents/Pages/DisplayNews.aspx?NewsID=25745&LangID=E [24 August 2020].

WALDERSEE, Victoria. (2020) *Portugal to Treat Migrants as Residents During Coronavirus Crisis*. [Online]. Available: https://www.reuters.com/article/us-health-coronavirus-portugal/portugal-to-treat-migrants-as-residents-during-coronavirus-crisis-idUSKBN21F0N7 [24 August 2020].

Postscript

"I consider myself a journalist, since what interests me is current events, what is occurring around me, what is happening in the world", answered Michel Foucault (2001: 1302) to the Brazilian scholar who was interviewing him, and he went on, evoking Nietzsche who "had been the first philosopher-journalist". There is definitely some provocation in this statement coming from someone who had carefully avoided anything contemporaneous in his academic work, both books and lectures, and had reserved his interventions on what was going on in his time to his intellectual activism. But in this clear separation he draws, there is precisely an indication of the potential issues faced by scholars who work on current events as they are an unstable material. Facts can be refuted and analyses disproved as situations change.

This is – in part – what I experienced with this essay. It was written in the summer of 2020, less than six months into the literally extraordinary response to the pandemic, with a generalized lockdown in numerous countries, including France. As I then mentioned, the situation of inmates and migrants was paradoxical since they were facing an increased risk despite their confinement. But regarding the former, there was a remarkable effort facilitated by circumstances (the activity of courts being almost interrupted) to reduce the overcrowding of prisons and protect the inmates, whereas for the latter, there was a constant refusal by the government to close detention centers which had become useless due to the context (absence of flights and closure of borders) and whose unsanitary conditions exposed their occupants to the virus generating fear and even panic among them. The contrast between the two institutions showed the state's unequal concern towards these populations and an implicit hierarchy in the values of their lives.

However, with time, this difference of treatment progressively waned, or better said, policies returned to "business as usual". Using the 1st of July as reference, the number of people with prison sentences immediately executed, which had spectacularly declined from 84,218 to 68,168 between 2019 and 2020, increased at a fast pace to reach 83,511 in 2021, whereas the number of those effectively detained, which had gone from 71,710 to 58,621, swelled to 67,971 (Administration Pénitentiaire, 2019, 2020, and 2021). In one year, the initial efforts to protect the inmates were largely abandoned despite two new waves of the pandemic which had provoked two lockdowns of the general population and despite a vaccination rate of barely 10 percent among inmates who were often crammed in individual cells occupied by two or three people. The concern for prisoners was thus short-lived. Conversely, the indifference towards migrants remained mostly unchanged, and their condition even worsened with the overcrowding of detention centers and the reduction of the housing programs for those living in public spaces. Notwithstanding the lack of hygiene and the impossibility of isolating themselves in the detention centers, 28,000 people were confined in these facilities, causing numerous clusters to be detected (Cimade, 2021). Still, in most cases, those locked up in these centers could not be sent back to their countries and ended up being released after 90 days. For example, out of 1,000 Algerians detained during the year, only 4 were actually deported. In parallel, the repression against migrants, sometimes families, often asylum seekers, who, for lack of state housing, were present in public spaces, be they streets, parks, forests, or beaches, intensified under the successive ministers of the interior's motto "no fixation point": tents were torn up, occupants teargassed, and belongings destroyed. This led exiles to seek out more remote places where they had no access to medical support and vaccination programs.

Thus, in a context of law-and-order policies, the benign attitude of the government towards prisoners at the height of the first wave of the pandemic was a mere parenthesis, in a brief moment of general stupor when priority was given to health over security or retribution. Noticeably, however, even in this ephemeral form, it had no equivalent towards asylum seekers and undocumented migrants, whose health was taken into account neither in their detention centers nor outside. To understand this relentless attitude of the authorities at a time when multiple measures were adopted to contain the pandemic in the general population, one has to take into account what Stuart Hall (1979) famously called "the great moving right show" in Britain in the 1970s, which has equivalents in the 2010s in various European countries. In France, as the presidential election approached, most political leaders thought that the outcome would be decided on the right of the political spectrum: indeed, six months before the election, opinion polls showed that the four candidates with the highest popularity were situated from the center right to the far right. Demonstrating signs of toughness, especially with respect to crime and immigration, which are the two major concerns of the population, was the choice made by the head of state to gain votes among the most conservative segment of the electorate.

During the first lockdown, the pandemic had generated uncertainty in what was supposed to be known and instability in what was supposed to be done. But the so-called "return to normal", with its consequences for prisoners and exiles, is a cautionary tale for social scientists working on current events since initial trends were reversed in the case of the former and worsened in the case of the latter. Far from generating more solidarity, at least towards these populations, the health crisis accentuated the inequalities and made life more difficult for the most vulnerable in a context of political shift of French society to the right with preoccupying consequences for fundamental liberties and human rights.

References

Administration Pénitentiaire. (2019-2020-2021). *Statistique Trimestrielle des Personnes Écrouées en France, Situation au 1er juillet 2019, 2020, et 2021.* Ministère de la Justice. http://www.justice.gouv.fr/art_pix/Trim_1907_VF.pdf.

Cimade. (2021). *Rapport 2020 sur les Centres de Rétention Administrative* (6 July). https://www.lacimade.org/publication/rapport-2020-sur-les-centres-et-locaux-de-retention-administrative/.

Foucault, M. (2001). Le Monde Est un Grand Asile. In *Dits et Écrits. Volume I* (pp. 1301–1302). *1954–1975.* Gallimard.

Hall, S. (1979). The Great Moving Right Show. *Marxism Today*, January, 14–20.

Part II: Ongoing debates

Introduction – Beyond complacency and acrimony: Studying human rights in a post-COVID-19 world

Giacomo Chiozza and Jeffrey King

Much has been written on the impact of COVID-19 on human rights since it first emerged in early spring 2020. This literature demonstrated that the pandemic has had a profoundly negative effect on human rights for people across the globe in many varied contexts. Studies written at the beginning of the pandemic consistently showed that governments' efforts to mitigate the spread of COVID-19, regardless of intent, often worsened human rights conditions for millions of people globally in both expected and unexpected ways.

We have witnessed the inadequate efforts of governments to mitigate the spread of the pandemic, along with the new normal of lockdowns, border closures, mask wearing, the vast inequalities laid bare by the pandemic, and we have felt the absence of millions of humans who lost their lives to COVID-19. We have also witnessed governments becoming more effective at responding to the pandemic based on lessons of the past, the inevitable social movements in reaction to government limitations on human rights, the consolidation of authoritarianism in many states, and the swift development of vaccines.

We now reside at a critical juncture within the ongoing pandemic. It has been more than two years (as of publication) since the pandemic began. Enough time has passed to allow us to assess the state of human rights under COVID-19 in a longer period than did the early literature on COVID-19 and human rights. We are also at a point in the pandemic where we can provide more holistic assessments and predictions of the state of human rights in a post-COVID-19 world, although we must acknowledge that new strains of COVID-19, the rise of vaccine nationalism, and continued resistance to mitigation efforts in various places make our assessments difficult.

The seven articles integral to this special issue represent the most up-to-date studies on a variety of topics, allowing us to assess the state of human rights under COVID-19 in the short and long terms. We recognize that our special issue can only cover a limited number of topics. More work needs to be done on a variety of topics, including on the experiences of the Global South. Our hope is that this special issue will pave the way toward more holistic, cohesive, and realistic assessments of the impact of COVID-19 on human rights for the past, present, and future.

ORCID

Giacomo Chiozza http://orcid.org/0000-0002-6046-0901
Jeffrey King http://orcid.org/0000-0002-9666-931X

OPEN ACCESS

The state of human rights in a (post) COVID-19 world

Giacomo Chiozza and Jeffrey King

ABSTRACT

As the pandemic spread globally, there was an explosion of scholarship written on the effects the pandemic had in numerous fields. Human rights scholars were no exception to this trend and sought to identify the effects of the pandemic on many related factors, including on gender violence, freedom of movement, protests, health care, and repression. Scholarship of this type, written in real time and responsive to the rapidly changing circumstances of the pandemic, was necessary for making sense of what was taking place, but provided little consideration for the long-term effects of the pandemic on human rights. Although the pandemic is not over, we believe that sufficient time has passed to allow us to think on the impact of the pandemic in a longer-term context. First, we provide a review of the existing literature on the effects of the pandemic on human rights, categorizing the literature as descriptive or prescriptive. Second, we introduce six articles contained in this special issue entitled "Beyond Complacency and Acrimony: Studying Human Rights in a Post-COVID-19 World" that in some ways address the shortcomings of the previous human rights literature. Finally, we provide concluding remarks we hope can act as inspiration for future scholarship.

Introduction

Since early 2020, the world has been gripped by an exceptional crisis: a worldwide pandemic that has killed approximately 4.5 million people as of this writing (Worldometers.info), caused a major global economic downturn, and upended all patterns of normal life. We now practice social distancing and wear face masks; we have endured quarantines, lockdowns, travel restrictions, school closings, and compulsory online work; we will undergo more testing, monitoring, and (we hope) widespread vaccination programs globally, although vaccinations have become an increasingly controversial issue. These elements count as momentous changes in the frame of everyday life for most people, without even considering the political, economic, and societal effects of the pandemic.

At the international level, the crisis has generated more acrimony than cooperation, as countries and international organizations have struggled to respond to the crisis. At the domestic level, the crisis has highlighted the relevance of leadership, state capacity, and information to devise an effective response. Looking at the typical government response, we can find elements of both coercion and tradeoff between the human rights in the Universal Declaration of Human Rights (UDHR). Governments have limited some rights (the right to movement, for example) to protect other types of rights (the right to health, most notably; Forman & Kohler, 2020; Lebret, 2020; Sekalala et al., 2020; Spadaro, 2020; Wong & Wong, 2020). The detrimental effects of the pandemic have also laid bare the vast inequalities within and across states during the pandemic, highlighting the fragility of human rights for large portions of the global population.

It is no wonder that the events of the pandemic and the responses of states to it have generated an extensive debate within the human rights literature. This debate comes in the wake of an acrimonious stand-off in the international human rights community between those who have been cautiously celebrating the worldwide improvement in human rights conditions, on one hand, and those who view the campaigns for the spreading of human rights as a bourgeois (or neoliberal) project that is both detrimental to equality and disrespectful of other cultures, on the other (Moyn, 2018; Sikkink, 2017).

The new debate triggered by the COVID-19 pandemic calls for a renewed effort in the study of human rights, one that seeks to be holistic in its theoretical approaches and comprehensive in its empirical assessments. The pandemic has highlighted the need for a theoretical framework to protect and promote human rights when the goal of preserving public health may clash with the goal of preserving human freedom, dignity, and equality. This article, and the special issue (Chiozza & King, 2022) of which it is part, contributes to this renewed effort for a novel theoretical framework in two ways.

First, our article reviews much of the extensive literature connecting COVID-19 to human rights. We organize this literature in two categories: descriptive, and prescriptive. The first category comprises literature that describes the main findings of COVID-19 on human rights. For example, studies on the impact of COVID-19 on domestic violence can be considered descriptive because these studies illustrate how incidents of domestic violence have increased because of lockdowns. Descriptive literature is important in helping scholars to understand the effects COVID-19 has had on various human rights conditions, but studies in this category often focus on the here and now rather than the long-term ramifications of COVID-19 on human rights.

A second category of literature that sometimes overlaps with the descriptive category is prescriptive literature. This strand of literature comprises studies that extend COVID-19 into existing debates in the human rights literature and seek to explain what states should, or should not, do to address the crisis. An example would be placing COVID-19 into debates regarding the legal rights of migrants (Kysel, 2021) or the impact of state policies on privacy (Eck & Hatz, 2020). This type of literature seeks to place the pandemic within the legal, ethical, and political parameters of the international human rights regime: It explains what kinds of human rights obligations states owe not only to their citizens and residents but also to people residing beyond their borders, it analyzes how specific state responses may harm human rights, and it raises alarm bells about potential abuses that may occur in the exceptional circumstances of a global pandemic.

The strength of this literature is to bring a degree of clarity to the human rights implications of state responses to the pandemic. The limit of this literature is its tendency to follow in the footsteps of each state response: border closures first, then lockdowns, then social distancing and mask wearing, and now vaccine mandates and vaccine passports. The prescriptive gaze is understandable, considering the context within which that literature was written, but nonetheless it remains a gaze that may close off the chance to detect any potential transformative effects of the pandemic on the fabric of the human rights regime.

The second purpose of this article is to introduce the six manuscripts, minus our own, contained in this special issue (Chiozza & King, 2022). We have been living with the pandemic for nearly two years. We are now at a point at which we can assess the impact of COVID-19 on human rights in a more long-term and holistic manner than the existing literature has done to date. Within the six articles of our special issue, our contributors are able to address many of the issues we highlight here. But while acknowledging that the pandemic is far from over, they also take a step forward and lay out an agenda for a new phase of scholarship on human rights.

Responses to the pandemic: The descriptive perspective

Tens of millions of words have been written on the topic of COVID-19 and human rights. Much of the literature on COVID-19 and human rights can best be described as *descriptive* in nature. This literature is extremely diverse but holds in common a focus on describing the deleterious effects COVID-19 has had on a variety of human rights conditions. This type of literature is undoubtedly important for our understanding of the effects that the pandemic has had on human rights conditions. However, much of this literature is limited in its scope, in many cases simply describing the effects of the pandemic on various human rights. In the following section, we provide a review of a selection of this descriptive literature, organized by topic.

COVID-19 and migrants/refugees

As COVID-19 cases emerged globally, governments struggled to stop the disease from spreading in their populations. One common policy response was the closure of international borders. This policy was intended to prevent COVID-19 from entering the country through international travelers. Measures of this type have had mixed success, but these border closure policies have had a consistently negative effect on migrants and refugees both within and without countries employing border closures.

At the beginning of the pandemic, more than 167 countries closed or partially closed their borders. Even in relatively open places such as the European Union, restrictions were put in place to prevent movement between member states (Ramji-Nogales & Goldner Lang, 2020). These types of border closures were intended to stop the spread of COVID-19 but had a devastating impact on migrants and refugees globally. Ramji-Nogales and Goldner Lang (2020), for example, pointed out that when borders were closed to all noncitizen travelers in the European Union in March of 2020, many migrants and asylum seekers from Africa became stuck in nonnative and unsafe states enroute. Even when refugees reached the borders of destination states, they were sometimes refused entry and were forced to return to their unsafe ports of origins (Crawley, 2021). The cumulative effect of border closures has forced refugees and migrants into increasingly precarious positions throughout the pandemic.

In other instances, refugees and migrants living within host states faced worsening conditions from lockdowns. Dempster et al. (2020), for instance, found that refugees were 60 percent more likely to work in industries that were most impacted by COVID-19 measures. As a result, migrants were more likely to lose their jobs, leading to increasing homelessness and food insecurity, all while being denied access to health care (Hill et al., 2021). Coupled with this, migrants have been subject to increasing amounts of vitriol and violence in many host countries, as they have been blamed for bringing COVID-19 into the states (Wang, 2020). To make matters worse, many governments have used migrants to implement policies that limit or suspend legal immigration and asylum procedures, in many cases in direct violation of the rights of migrants and refugees (Crawley, 2021; Garrett, 2020; Roksandić et al., 2021).

COVID-19 and lockdowns

To reduce the transmissibility of COVID-19, governments have commonly used lockdowns that required their populations to shelter-in-place for extended periods. In general, during lockdowns people are only allowed to leave their shelters under limited circumstances, such as for grocery store trips and medical appointments. In limiting the movements of their populations, lockdown orders were designed to prevent COVID-19 from spreading into the general population. However, as the literature shows, lockdowns have had tragic effects for a variety of populations, including for essential workers, detainees, children, the elderly, and the disabled (Openshaw & Travassos, 2020).

In particular, lockdowns have had significant negative consequences for the well-being of women in many countries (Aziz & Moussa, 2021). During the pandemic, reports of domestic violence increased in India by 94 percent (Nigam, 2020), in Brazil by 40 percent (Telles et al., 2021), in Hubei Province China by 90 percent, and in the United States by estimates ranging from 10 percent to 48 percent (Boserup et al., 2020; Agüero 2021). Unfortunately, findings of this sort are to be expected because of a well-known finding within the violence-against-women literature, that most acts of violence against women are perpetrated by family members. During lockdowns, women, many of whom can be described as vulnerable, are required to shelter-in-place with abusers. Coupled with this, during the pandemic victims have had less access to the justice system and police and social worker intervention. This effectively has disempowered women in favor of their potential abusers.

Other populations have also been shown to be highly vulnerable to lockdown measures, although this literature is much less robust in comparison to that on gender. Older adults, for example, are more likely to live alone or in nursing homes, and as a result are marginalized by lockdown measures, making them vulnerable to potential abuse (D'cruz & Banerjee, 2020). In a similar manner, the disabled have also become increasingly vulnerable to abuse during the pandemic (Quinn, 2021), with reports of increasing numbers of "do not resuscitate" orders being imposed on disabled individuals in the event of medical emergencies as an example. Prisoners have also become increasingly vulnerable, as countries have limited prison visits and oversight during lockdown (Metcalf, 2021; Muntingh, 2020).

COVID-19 and inequalities

When the pandemic was in its initial phases, some argued that it represented the "great equalizer": Everyone—regardless of class, gender, race, ethnicity, education, or sexual orientation—was expected to be equally vulnerable to getting (and dying from) COVID-19. That prediction did not materialize. Many of the inequalities that were present prior to the pandemic led to worse outcomes for vulnerable populations, such as racial minorities, women, and immigrants, who were subject to the effects of COVID-19 to a greater degree than more privileged populations.

Several studies have demonstrated that minority and migrant populations were more likely to die from COVID-19 in comparison to white populations in Western countries. According to Wilder (2021), minorities were five times more likely than non-Hispanic white people to be hospitalized during the early period of the pandemic in the United States and were much more likely to die from COVID-19, as well.

The reasons cited for this inequality are complex: Some scholars have blamed the greater presence of comorbidities in minority populations, others have pointed out the socioeconomic determinants of healthcare. Tai et al. (2021) found, for example, that minorities in the United States were in more vulnerable positions at the start of the pandemic, with significantly higher unemployment rates than white people. Minorities were also much more likely to work in sectors of the economy that did not allow them to work from home or to quarantine (Kantamneni, 2020). Although unemployment for African Americans did not rise as high as many had predicted (Couch et al., 2020), the types of jobs African Americans worked increased their risk of catching COVID-19.

Other scholars have argued that the adverse impact of COVID-19 on minorities compared to the white population in the United States has been further compounded by minorities generally having less access to preventive healthcare services. This has meant that minority populations are especially vulnerable to either receiving subpar health care or to receiving no health care if they contract COVID-19 (Okonkwo et al., 2021). In fact, many minorities in the United States actively avoid or distrust health-care systems to such an extent that they have avoided receiving increasingly common vaccines, leading to higher rates of mortality.

Another type of inequity that has gained significant attention is the digital divide: as governments all over the world locked down, the importance of a reliable internet connection became clearer. Regardless of their location in developed or developing countries, more privileged workers were better able to adjust to lockdown orders by simply shifting from working in-person to working remotely (Wang, 2021). In contrast, workers who lack access to a stable internet connection or who work in industries that could not shift online found themselves at a greater risk of contracting the virus or losing their jobs.

The digital divide is also present in the shift toward online education. Prior to the pandemic, hundreds of millions of children attended classes in person every day, with education seen as the best chance of raising millions of children out of poverty. With the emergence of the pandemic, the world has seen an unprecedented shift toward online learning, increasing the inequities between the haves and have-nots throughout the world. In wealthier countries and regions of the world with access to stable internet connections, the shift to online learning has been relatively seamless (Davis 2021).

However, millions of children lack access to internet, preventing them from taking part in remote learning. This has placed less-privileged students at a severe disadvantage once schools shifted online. In some countries, poorer students lost access to education entirely during lockdowns, creating what is termed a "learning loss" (Donnelly & Patrinos, 2020). A particularly troubling example comes from a recent report on India, which found that tens of thousands of children lost the ability to read due to the shuttering of in-person schools (Arya, 2021).

COVID-19 and regime type

The literature on regime type and COVID-19 falls into two broad categories. One focuses on estimating the effectiveness of regime types in responding to the pandemic, often comparing autocracies and democracies. The second category focuses on the threat the pandemic represents to democracy globally, whether by focusing on the erosion of democratic principles in democracies as a result of government responses or by focusing on the use of the pandemic by authoritarian states as a window of opportunity to consolidate their repressive capacities.

When the pandemic first emerged, there was a great deal of variation in government responses. Some countries reacted almost immediately, shutting borders, canceling flights, and placing large proportions of their populations into strict lockdowns. Subsequent studies have shown that this quick response decreased the number of daily deaths attributed to the initial emergence of the pandemic. One factor explaining how quickly states responded to the pandemic was regime type, with scholars arguing that autocracies reacted faster than democracies (Alon et al., 2020).

Cepaluni et al. (2021), for example, looked at political institutions and found that states with more democratic institutions experienced more deaths than states with less democratic institutions. Cheibub et al. (2020) argued that one reason why democracies reacted slower is because some entrenched democratic features hindered government responses initially, although democratic governments were later able to enact typical lockdown measures. Likewise, Yao et al. (2022) argued that democracies had more deaths initially not because of an unwillingness to restrict democratic rights but, instead, because democracies were incapable of doing so in a timely manner. In contrast, Edgell et al. (2021) categorized how states have violated democratic standards during the pandemic and found no connection between democracies violating democratic standards and COVID-19 deaths.

Other studies have looked beyond aggregate regime type when looking for the so-called "autocratic advantage." Frey et al. (2020), for example, noted that autocracies implemented more stringent lockdowns and were more pervasive with contract tracing. Conversely, democracies implemented less stringent lockdowns but were actually able to reduce geographic mobility more effectively. Given these somewhat contradictory and inconclusive findings on regime type, we do not have an accurate understanding of any autocratic advantage yet.

Another strand of literature has focused on the growing presence of authoritarian tactics in many democratic states. Initial efforts to combat the pandemic leaned toward the typical authoritarian toolbox: lockdowns, border closures, and state surveillance. In many countries, some form of surveillance was used initially for contract tracing (Liu & Zhao, 2021). In fact, 34 states immediately adopted digital surveillance programs after the pandemic began, with 22 of these being democracies (Eck & Hatz, 2020). For many states, including democracies, this type of surveillance has become the normal response, with domestic populations accepting this as the price to pay for response to the pandemic. This acceptance by democratic populations suggests that use of these tools represents a slippery slope toward authoritarianism in some instances.

Developments of this type have been particularly concerning for many scholars. Maerz et al. (2020) categorized the democratic principles most commonly violated by democracies during the initial stage of the pandemic and found that, although democracies were derogating on democratic principles in their responses to the pandemic, they did not experience any improvement in effectiveness at combating the pandemic. Thus, democracies were violating their democratic obligations, using more authoritarian methodologies, and receiving no increase in effectiveness.

Given this, some scholars have suggested that one of the chief effects of the pandemic is the rise of authoritarianism in many states. In repressive authoritarian states such as China, governments have used the pandemic to further consolidate their powers through such measures as greater and more pervasive surveillance capabilities (Liu & Zhao, 2021). In many authoritarian states, domestic surveillance systems were dramatically expanded, and they appear to be here to stay. In addition to this, the methods many authoritarian states used to combat the pandemic initially, such as lockdowns, are similar to normal repressive policies like a declaration of martial law and curfews. However, responding to a health crisis has allowed many authoritarian governments to bypass domestic complaints or international scrutiny in the name of public health. Thus, authoritarian states have actually used the pandemic as an opportunity to consolidate and, in certain instances, further repress their populations (Barceló et al., 2020).

COVID-19 and protests

According to Metternich (2020), 2019 was the year of protest. In contrast, 2020 was the year of the pandemic, with many fearing for the future of civil disobedience in the face of lockdowns, social-distancing rules, and other limitations put in place by governments to prevent the spread of COVID-19. Initial studies suggested that scholars were right to be fearful. Metternich (2020) found a severe decline in protest activities globally at the beginning of the pandemic. The effect of the pandemic, however, has been much more complex than simply concluding that protest activities are in decline.

If we look at protest activities from a country perspective, the answer is different than Metternich's (2020). Ferrero and Natalucci (2020) found that incidents of engagement in protests remained high in Argentina during the beginning of the pandemic. Similarly, many countries experienced large protests in support of the Black Lives Matter movement or in protest of George Floyd's murder (Van Dijcke & Wright, 2020). In other instances, some countries experienced widespread protests against various government measures, such as lockdowns, mask mandates, and vaccine mandates. Although initially it seemed that the future of protest activity was under threat, we now know that COVID-19 sparked further protest activity, especially among groups of people who previously were disengaged (Avetian et al., 2021). But more scholarship is needed to further explicate the effects of COVID-19 on protest activities (Clay et al., 2022).

Other scholarship has looked at the effects of protests on COVID-19 instead, asking if large-scale protests acted as "superspreader" events. Lange and Monscheuer (2021) provided an analysis of two large-scale COVID-denier protests that took place in Germany in 2020 and found that there was a significant increase in positive cases as a result. However, Dave et al. (2020) found the exact opposite for Black Lives Matter protests in the United States. This result is not surprising, as social justice protests tended to have greater mask wearing and social distancing. Thus, protest activity has been robust during the pandemic, with an increasing array of new protest tactics (Pleyers, 2020). Given this, fears of protests being severely constrained or eliminated in many parts of the world appear somewhat unfounded, but significant questions remain on protest activities in both the pandemic and postpandemic contexts (Chenoweth, 2022).

Responses to the pandemic: The prescriptive perspective

A second strand in the human rights literature also emerged at the beginning of the pandemic that we define as prescriptive. Prescriptive literature comprises studies that place the context of COVID-19 into preexisting debates within the field of human rights on such diverse topics as the right to privacy (Eck & Hatz, 2020), the right of assembly (Chenoweth, 2022), the right of movement (Ramji-Nogales & Goldner Lang, 2020), and the right to health (Forman & Kohler, 2020). Much of this literature highlights how states systematically fell short (or were in danger of doing so) of the norms, standards, and legal obligations of the international human rights regime when implementing policies in response to the pandemic. When looked at in retrospect, it appears that this literature sounded the "alarm bells" regarding state power encroaching into the realms of individual human rights across many global contexts.

The prescriptive literature also highlights several tensions that appear between government provision of different types of rights. In particular, the prescriptive literature has brought into sharp relief the challenges of providing a right to health during a pandemic—a right that is "individually held and collectively shared" (Wong & Wong, 2020)—while continuing to meet obligations for other types of rights that are directly and negatively impacted by government efforts to protect their populations from the pandemic (Toebes, 2015). This type of literature argues that "the authorities should at all times attempt to promote one hundred percent of all rights involved, and not establish a hierarchy of rights" (Du Plessis, 2021, p. 28). However, this literature also focuses on the practical realities of competing imperatives to protect populations from a global health crisis while maintaining individual autonomy, reflecting the fact that many countries have traded off certain rights in favor of a right to health. Given this, much of this literature also includes a normative element, loudly declaring state obligations to protect rights while also providing prescriptions for how to do so. In the following section, we provide a review of a selection of this literature.

COVID-19 and the dilemma of rights

When the government of China imposed draconic measures to lock down the province of Hubei in January 2020, it took steps that, according to Wang (2021), led to "China's Covid success story" but also to "a human rights tragedy." Wang (2021) contends that China had been able to tame, albeit not defeat, the virus at a high price—namely, the curtailment of the fundamental rights of millions of people who endured disproportionate, and possibly unnecessary, hardships amid censorship and surveillance.

Wang's (2021) assessment encapsulated one of the central concerns of the early prescriptive literature: In the name of public health, governments would both curtail certain individual rights and expand their coercive capacity, thus inflicting long-term harm to individual freedom and autonomy. In particular, the prescriptive literature reflects concerns that any curtailment of individual rights would trigger a cascading effect of adverse consequences on the entire array of human rights, including the loss of appetite for freedom among frightened citizens (Nay, 2020). Goodhart (2020) called this dynamic "negative interdependence."

Various studies have explicated the reasons why states would seek to expand their power during the pandemic. In some cases, government responses might be driven by inadequate or antiquated standard operating procedures endorsed by international organizations (Wong & Wong, 2020); in other cases, the decisions may be driven by the goal to avoid panic or to prevent the entire collapse of the health-care system of a country (Nacoti et al., 2020); but in some cases, the policies to combat COVID-19 may be no more than cynical attempts to consolidate power behind the veil of a national emergency (Guasti, 2020).

Regardless of the motivation, many scholars sought to remind those in positions of power that civil and political rights can be limited, but only in specific, strict, and temporary conditions (Hathaway et al., 2021; Joseph, 2020; Lebret, 2020). Spadaro (2020), for instance, delineated the terms of the debate by highlighting the rights potentially at risk from the measures to combat the pandemic: Lockdowns, masks, and quarantines would endanger the freedom of movement, the freedoms of assembly and association, the right to a private life, the freedom to manifest one's beliefs and religion, the right to work, and the right to education.

From that, Spadaro (2020) articulated a policy recommendation that is shared across several studies (Lebret, 2020; Ó Cathaoir, 2021; Santoro & Shanklin, 2020): While international human rights law would grant limitations and derogations to states' legal obligations in case of emergencies, citizens, activists, and scholars would need to exercise heightened scrutiny to ensure that all measures taken would be no more than strictly necessary, nondiscriminatory, and temporary.

COVID-19 and the dilemma of social rights

Other scholars have come to similar conclusions about the necessity of greater government scrutiny regarding social rights—that is, the right to health, the right to work, and the right to education. Much of this literature has highlighted the special challenges that the fulfillment of social rights entails. In particular, scholars pointed out how state responses not only revealed but also magnified several structural inequalities and patterns of discrimination across gender, race, age, and sexual orientation (Davis, 2021; Jimenez, 2021; Šehović & Govender, 2021; Theidon, 2020).

Given this, significant attention has been paid to how to determine whether government policies balance obligations toward social rights while addressing the pandemic. Article 12 of the ICESCR provided some guidance on this, stating that governments have "the burden of justifying such serious measures"[1] when derogating from social rights. To achieve this best outcome, Sekalala et al. (2020, 14), argued that "evidence-based decision-making," which should entail "rigorous pilot studies and risk assessments," should be carried out prior to implementing public health measures to combat the COVID-19 pandemic more widely.

Meanwhile, Flood et al. (2021) highlighted the trade-off dilemma from a human rights perspective more explicitly, arguing that government policies should comply with the precautionary principle, but from a civil rights perspective, and government policies should also comply with the proportionality principle—a difficult task for any state, as these two principles may lead to different contradictory conclusions about whether a policy—public health surveillance tools, for example—is respectful of human rights or not.

Using the Rio Declaration to articulate the precautionary principle, it maintained that, "Where there are threats of serious or irreversible damage, lack of full scientific certainty shall not be used as a reason for postponing cost-effective measures to prevent environmental degradation."[2] Although these words are for environmental policy, the standard for derogation of civil rights obligations is similar, but with scholars arguing that the standard of proof should be much higher: civil rights should be curtailed only if the policy is in a position to pass a much stricter test, a test that places the burden of proof on the decision maker who seeks to curtail civil and political freedoms. In one case, a policy may be adopted so long as it is not patently detrimental; in the other case, a policy may be adopted if there is positive evidence that it is beneficial (Flood et al., 2021).

For some scholars hailing from the Global South, the emphasis on the harm inflicted on civil and political rights within this debate reflects a specific Western, neoliberal bias, one that privileges the individual over the community (Bennoune, 2020; Gurmendi, 2020). Bennoune (2020, pp. 666, 675), for example, urged human rights scholars to go beyond a discourse that turns human rights into "a litany of prohibitions" and to start devising a language and an analysis that, although mindful of the reality of pervasive human rights abuses, also empowers states "to take positive action to guarantee human rights—to act in accordance with science to protect life and health, to guarantee provision of PPE, and to take effective steps to defeat the virus." In practical terms from this perspective, that would entail limiting, if not prohibiting, large gatherings, protests, and so on that are perceived as violations of individual rights.

Scholars addressing the dilemma of public health from the utilitarian perspective were even blunter in their recommendations. Savulescu et al. (2020, p. 628), for example, wrote, "Liberty and rights are only important insofar as they secure well-being. Thus, a utilitarian approach to the lockdown question may be prepared to override the right to privacy or liberty to protect well-being." In their view, it is a value choice: although societies may privilege freedoms over health, they need to reach a clear understanding of what price they are willing to pay for their preferences.

From the perspective of the human rights literature, therefore, the dilemma of protecting public health while maximizing individual rights remains an outstanding issue. The emerging literature on COVID-19 vaccines provides further illustration of these competing priorities that underlie the analysis of rights and obligations during a pandemic.

Vaccine policies: The new battleground

While people were facing the hardships of lockdowns and quarantines at the height of the first wave in 2020, vaccines were seen as a savior on a distant horizon. The development of safe and effective vaccines were truly the highlight of the pandemic when they were first rolled out in late 2020, as never before had humanity come together to develop an urgent preventative treatment so quickly. In fact, Santoro (2021, p. 327) argued that the pharmaceutical companies behind the development of these vaccines in record time should be praised as the unsung heroes of the pandemic: they "produced miracles and delivered us from our basements and attics" once their vaccines were approved. However, significant debate exists on the use of these vaccines: on the one hand, vaccines are seen as public goods that are humanity's best chance of ending the pandemic and, on the other, the reality is that these vaccines have fallen victim to the realpolitik of international politics.

When it comes to vaccine policies, the primary concerns in much of the literature are (1) "vaccine nationalism"—that is, the hoarding of a life-saving preventive remedy in the hands of a few wealthy governments for the exclusive benefit of their people; (2) the potential constraints that intellectual property (IP) rights pose for the production and affordability of the COVID-19 vaccines; and (3) the criteria to allocate scarce supplies of vaccines among the eligible populations in many parts of the world (Jecker et al., 2021; Khosla & Gruskin, 2021; Santoro & Shanklin, 2020; Šehović & Govender, 2021; Sekalala et al., 2020).

According to Forman and Kohler (2020), these concerns have been shaped by the experiences of past pandemics. They highlighted that one of the lessons learned from combating smallpox in the 1970s was the necessity to tackle the crisis on a global scale: "[S]mallpox anywhere means smallpox everywhere" (International AIDS Society–Lancet Commission 2021, p. 1525). The case of HIV/AIDS is another example where the callousness of the pharmaceutical industry response provided lessons and expectations that things would be better this time around (Santoro, 2021, p. 328). In that regard, initiatives such as the COVAX program arranged under the aegis of the WHO are seen as a step in the right direction, albeit with serious concerns about effectiveness (Sekalala et al., 2020).

The appeal to an enlightened self-interest whereby no one is safe unless everybody is safe, however, has remained largely unrealized. According to a study by Oxfam (2020), "Wealthy nations representing just 13 percent of the world's population have already cornered more than half (51 percent) of the promised doses of leading COVID-19 vaccine candidates." About five months later, in February 2021, things were no better: According to UN Secretary General Antonio Guterres (2021), "Just ten countries have administered 75 percent of all COVID-19 vaccines. Meanwhile, more than 130 countries have not received a single dose."

But if the current situation points to a failure of cooperation on an equitable distribution of COVID-19 vaccines worldwide, the extent to which such a failure would count as a failure to respect for international legal obligations for the fulfillment of the right to health and the right to enjoy the fruits of scientific discoveries remains a contested matter (Hathaway et al., 2021, p. 35). The extra-territorial application of international legal provisions requires a jurisdictional nexus: To that effect, Joseph and Dore (2021, p. 8) argued, "It is difficult at present to extrapolate a general duty under the ICCPR for a state to equitably share vaccines with other states, though such obligations could be evolving."

The early analysis of the human rights implications of COVID-19 vaccines highlights a number of salient issues and provides a point of reference for assessing the extent to which those policies were compliant with human rights standards. Surprisingly, however, the early reflections on vaccine policies have remained silent on an issue that has become a contentious battleground in the politics of many countries: the refusal of people who are eligible to receive a free vaccine to get vaccinated. Such refusals may be spurred by genuine anxiety, a sense of uncertainty, and a person's level of trust of authority and medical expertise, but they may also be fostered by the poison of conspiracy theories and fake news (Kerr et al., 2021; Loomba et al., 2021). Whatever the reasons, the people who decide not to be vaccinated often make a principled argument: my body, my choice. The corollary from that position is that vaccine mandates (i.e., policies that make it compulsory to be vaccinated) would constitute a serious breach of human rights obligations.

In what manner can the extensive literature on human rights help guide policy and help heal a serious cleavage in many societies? For a literature that had developed in a prescriptive manner—that is, by incorporating the current challenges of the pandemic into existing debates—there would be several angles for elaborating clearer positions in a contested field. Prior to the COVID-19 pandemic, the libertarian position on vaccine mandates was that mandates were consistent with the principles of freedom and autonomy as long as they were not implemented in a discriminatory manner. For example, Flanigan (2014) relied on the analogy of random gunfire in a crowded place—a prohibited act that is usually prosecuted as a felony or a misdemeanor—to conclude that "Citizens do not have the right to turn themselves into biological weapons that expose innocent bystanders to undue risks of harm." (p. 23)

Scholars who subscribe to utilitarian ethics have reached similar conclusions through different reasoning. Giubilini and Savulescu (2019, p. 237), for example, took the risks of vaccine side effects as the starting point of their analysis and concluded that, as has been the case for seatbelt legislation in many countries worldwide, "the risks of vaccines do not constitute strong enough reasons against coercive vaccination policies and that the same reasons that justify compulsory seat belt use—a measure now widely accepted and endorsed—also justify coercive vaccination policies." If taken into the context of COVID-19 vaccines, this argument would entail a careful assessment of the specific risks of all the different COVID-19 vaccines that have become available.

Although a comprehensive assessment of the place of COVID-19 vaccines within a human rights framework remains to be fully developed, the question of balancing different rights and navigating competing imperatives yet again emerges as a focal point for future scholarship (Murdie, 2022). Human rights scholars have long noted the issues highlighted above, but as with inequalities being laid bare, the pandemic has shown that this debate is far from over.

Human rights in a (post) COVID-19 world

At the end of an extensive overview of the status of human rights during the COVID-19 pandemic, Kjaerum (2021, p. 295) asked, "[T]o what extent will human rights play a role in the building back of societies after the COVID-19 crisis?" Underpinning that question is the concern that human rights may risk being overwhelmed by the real or imagined exigencies of post-COVID-19 societies unless scholars directly tackle the challenges raised by the pandemic. In this special issue, we take heed of Kjaerum's exhortation. We build on the rich work we have reviewed in the previous sections and contribute to a new phase in the debate on the status of human rights for a post-COVID-19 world, with a specific focus on how to protect human rights when the imperatives of public health and the imperatives of preserving human freedom, dignity, and equality may be at cross-purposes.

Emergencies and states of exceptions create windows of opportunity to restructure the power of the state *vis-à-vis* society to the advantage of the state. This is the specific focus of the first section of this special issue, in which Chenoweth (2022) and Badran and Turnbull (2022) analyze how processes of authoritarianism in democracies and autocracies seek to neutralize one of the most effective tools to tame the Leviathan: the right to civil and peaceful resistance. These two contributions operate at different levels of granularity: a macro-perspective in the case of Chenoweth and a micro-perspective of case studies of Egypt and Morocco for Badran and Turnbull.

From different perspectives, both illustrate interactive processes of learning and innovation by the state as well as by civil society movements. Greater restrictions on the ability to organize civil protests do not necessarily entail a reduction in civil protests or a surreptitious power grab, as shown by Chenoweth (2022), highlighting that although some movements may disband, other may become emboldened. However, pandemic restrictions on civil protests may lead to decreased chances of success for these emboldened movements. On the other hand, Badran and Turnbull (2022) show how "overshooting" WHO guidelines, along with a reputation as a moderate reformer in the case of Morocco, may serve as a yardstick to gauge whether the restrictive provisions most governments implemented during the pandemic reflect a genuine attempt at protecting public health or if these efforts reflect rising authoritarianism globally. The conundrum between screening and constraining so aptly analyzed by von Stein (2005) remains critical in addressing the potential consequences of government actions in a post-COVID-19 world.

The second section in this special issue directly tackles the challenges and tradeoffs of maintaining human rights while fighting the pandemic. Clay et al. (2022) rely on new and expanded data that track expert evaluations of the status of human rights to assess whether, and to what extent, the pandemic altered the enjoyment of human rights. The story they show is concerning. Clay et al. (2022) illustrate that human rights conditions worsened across the spectrum during 2020. The dynamic of "negative interdependence" feared by Goodhart (2020) leaves its footprints in the Clay et al. (2022) data. But Clay et al. (2022) also illustrate that dynamics of positive interdependence may also be at play, showing that, although human rights conditions may have been more fragile than expected in many countries, they appear to be more resilient in countries that demonstrated higher commitments to human rights.

If the Clay et al. (2022) analysis points to a sliver of hope in otherwise concerning scenarios, Koo (2022) demonstrates that levels of attention (or lack thereof) devoted to human rights conditions by domestic populations is an important pathway toward maintaining respect for human rights locally and potentially avoiding negative interdependence. In South Korea, people took to social media to comment on their government's policies; they also shared their reactions to the health crisis brought by the pandemic in other, especially Western, countries. People were less attuned to the human rights implications of the global pandemic at the local level. In the early phases of the pandemic, several scholars had urged that special attention should be given to the extent to which state responses were targeted, limited, and necessary. Koo's (2022) analysis confirms, with hard data, how important it is to maintain a sharp focus on the status of human rights, if human rights are to be preserved in times of crisis.

The weight of structural inequalities emerges in full force in the analysis of Brysk (2022): Women's rights found themselves under attack on several levels. The crisis has highlighted the deep reaches of patriarchy and gendered rights regimes amid rising violence against women, disproportional job losses and unequal risks of exposure to the COVID-19 virus for women, and regression in the recognition of reproductive rights. Brysk introduces a novel concept, "pandemic patriarchy," not only to illustrate the worsening of women's rights but also to highlight the structural conditions on which that worsening took place. Brysk (2022) makes a strong argument for a feminist ethic of care as the foundation for a novel theoretical approach that places the indivisibility, interdependence, and intersectionality of human rights as its core foundation. In so doing, Brysk (2022) sets the stage for the final section of the special issue, in which Murdie (2022) takes a bird's eye view of the lessons that could be derived from 20 months of scholarship on, and direct experience of, human rights during COVID-19.

Murdie (2022) identifies four specific lessons for future scholarship: the need to have a better grasp of public opinion on human rights; the need to embrace a more holistic analysis of human rights beyond the near exclusive focus on physical integrity rights by quantitative scholarship; the need to address the imperative of preserving transparency and information access while combatting the poison of conspiracy theory and fake news; and the need to assess whether, and under what conditions, human rights rhetoric is strategically used to mask surreptitious power grabs or to undermine some rights at the expense of others. The research agenda laid out by Murdie (2022) shows that ingrained assumptions in the study of human rights need to be revisited. From Murdie's (2022) analysis, we can conclude that this is not the time for either acrimony or complacency. It is a time for a new engagement for the human rights of a post-COVID-19 twenty-first century.

Conclusion

In this article, we have reviewed the extensive literature on COVID-19 and human rights and argued that much of it has been limited in scope, either by simply describing (descriptive) the effects of COVID-19 on human rights or by placing COVID-19 into existing and familiar debates about the obligation of states in times of crisis (prescriptive). We have numerous examples of studies that focus on a single human right or subset of rights, for instance. We also have numerous examples in which COVID-19 is placed within existing debates, as well. Much of this literature also lacks consideration for the long-term effects of COVID-19 in a post-COVID-19 context. As a result, we argue that not enough consideration is given to studying the effects of COVID-19 on human rights in a holistic and long-term manner. We describe the state of this literature as acrimonious and complacent as a result: acrimonious in the presence of COVID-19 in familiar and contentious debates; complacent in the lack of consideration for the long-term effects of COVID-19 on human rights in a late-pandemic and post-COVID-19 context.

However, given the all-encompassing effect COVID-19 has had on human rights, we believe that it is necessary to speculate on the effects of COVID-19 in a more holistic and long-term manner. The result of this belief is this special issue of *Journal of Human Rights*. Within this issue, six articles (excluding our own) cover a variety of topics, including on protests, regime type and authoritarian consolidation, public opinion and government responses, new human rights data on COVID-19, and considerations for the future.

In these articles, the authors address many of the weaknesses we have highlighted, providing some consideration for the long-term ramifications for human rights in a post-COVID context. Our special issue, unfortunately, cannot possibly address all areas of the literature on COVID-19 and human rights, however. Given this, a further objective of this special issue is to continue a conversation begun here. We hope this special issue will generate more research on the long-term and holistic effects of COVID-19 on human rights in a post-COVID context.

From our review of the literature, it is clear that significant work remains, including on topics that are largely unexplored in an academic sense. The literature on public opinion and COVID-19 is one example of this. We encountered significant numbers of articles (nonacademic) on public opinion. However, the academic literature is much sparser in comparison. One avenue we believe to be ripe for future exploration is the topic of changing attitudes toward the authoritarian toolset within many democracies and what implications this increased acceptance has for the long-term health of democracies globally.

We also encountered a significant imbalance within the academic literature on developed states and the Global South. Using the literature on domestic violence incidents as an example, hundreds of studies have gone under review on the topic from a Western perspective. However, far fewer studies have been carried out within the Global South context. Likewise, hundreds of studies have covered the derogation of certain rights in favor of public health measures from the Western perspective. However, in many cases this literature assumes there is a functioning health system present in the domestic environment that can be "traded off." However, a functioning health system in developing countries is not a given in many instances, making this debate largely moot. Given this, we believe much more needs to be done to explicate the experiences of the Global South during the pandemic.

Notes

1. These words are from General Comment No. 14 to the International Covenant on Economic, Social, and Cultural Rights (Committee on Economic, Social & Cultural Rights, 2000).
2. These words are from Principle 15 of the Rio Declaration on Environment and Development (United Nations, General Assembly, 1992).

Acknowledgments

We would like to thank Sammy Badran, Alison Brysk, José Antonio Cheibub, Erica Chenoweth, K. Chad Clay, Jeong-Woo Koo, Amanda Murdie, and Brian Turnbull for comments and suggestions throughout the course of this project. We extend special thanks to the Sir Easa Saleh Al-Gurg Professorship for providing the support to host two (online) roundtables at the American University of Sharjah where this article, as well as all the articles in this special issue, were presented. The work in this article was supported in part by the Open Access Program from the American University of Sharjah. The article represents the opinion of the authors and does not mean to represent the opinions or positions of the American University of Sharjah or the Sir Easa Saleh Al-Gurg Group. Mistakes, omissions, and other assorted infelicities are our own responsibility.

ORCID

Giacomo Chiozza http://orcid.org/0000-0002-6046-0901
Jeffrey King http://orcid.org/0000-0002-9666-931X

References

Agüero, J. M. (2021). COVID-19 and the rise of intimate partner violence. *World Development, 137*, 105217–105217. doi:10.1016/j.worlddev.2020.105217

Alon, I., Farrell, M., & Li, S. (2020). Regime type and COVID-19 response. *FIIB Business Review, 9*(3), 152–160. doi:10.1177/2319714520928884

Arya, D. (2021). *Covid-19: The Indian children who have forgotten how to read and write.* BBC. Retrieved November 29, 2021, from https://www.bbc.com/news/world-asia-india-58281442.

Avetian, V., Casanueva, A., Sardoschau, S., Saxena, K. (2021). *Social Protest in Times of Social Distancing: Black Lives Matter and COVID-19.* (April 22, 2021). Retrieved November 12, 2021, from https://ssrn.com/abstract=3831819 or 10.2139/ssrn.3831819

Aziz, Z. A., & Moussa, J. (2021). COVID-19 and violence against women: Unprecedented impacts and suggestions for mitigation. In M. Kjaerum, M. F. Davis, A. Lyons (Eds.), *COVID-19 and human rights* (pp. 100–115). Routledge.

Badran, S. & Turnbull, B. (2022). The COVID-19 pandemic and authoritarian consolidation in North Africa. *Journal of Human Rights, 21*(3), 263–282.

Barceló, J., Rahn, T. H., Cheng, C., Kubinec, R., Messerschmidt, L. (2020). Suppression and timing: Using COVID-19 policies against political dissidents? Retrieved November 12, 2021, from 10.31235/osf.io/yuqw2.

Bennoune, K. (2020). "Lest we should sleep": COVID-19 and human rights. *American Journal of International Law, 114*(4), 666–676. doi:10.1017/ajil.2020.68

Boserup, B., McKenney, M., & Elkbuli, A. (2020). Alarming trends in US domestic violence during the COVID-19 pandemic. *The American Journal of Emergency Medicine, 38*(12), 2753–2755.

Brysk, A. (2022). Pandemic patriarchy: The impact of a global health crisis on women's rights. *Journal of Human Rights, 21*(3), 283–302.

Cepaluni, G., Dorsch, M., & Branyiczki, R. (2021). Political regimes and deaths in the early stages of the COVID-19 pandemic. *Journal of Public Finance and Public Choice, 2021*, 724. doi:10.1332/251569121X16268740317724

Cheibub, J. A., Hong, J. Y. J., Przeworski, A. (2020). Rights and deaths: Government reactions to the pandemic. (July 7, 2020). Retrieved November 12, 2021, from https://ssrn.com/abstract=3645410 or 10.2139/ssrn.3645410

Chenoweth, E. (2022). Can nonviolent resistance survive COVID-19? *Journal of Human Rights, 21*(3), 304–316.

Chiozza, G., & King, J. (2022). Introduction to a special issue on beyond complacency and acrimony: Studying human rights in a post-COVID-19 world. *Journal of Human Rights, 21*(3), 245.

Clay, K. C., Abdelwahab, M., LaVelle, M., Parker, A., Rains, M., Bagwell, S., Barney, M., Burkle, E., Hawley, T., & Kehoe-Rowden, T. (2022). The effect of the COVID-19 pandemic on human rights practices: Findings from the Human Rights Measurement Initiative's 2021 Practitioner Survey. *Journal of Human Rights, 21*(3), 317–333.

Committee on Economic, Social and Cultural Rights. (2000). *General Comment 14, The Right to the Highest Attainable Standard of Health* (Twenty-second session, 2000), UN Doc. E/C.12/2000/4 (2000), Retrieved November 18, 2021, from http://hrlibrary.umn.edu/gencomm/escgencom14.htm.

Couch, K. A., Fairlie, R. W., & Xu, H. (2020). Early evidence of the impacts of COVID-19 on minority unemployment. *Journal of Public Economics, 192*(December), 104287.

Crawley, H. (2021). The politics of refugee protection in a post-covid-19 world. *Social Sciences, 10*(3), 81–95. doi: 10.3390/socsci10030081

"Coronavirus Cases." *Worldometer.* Retrieved September 1, 2021, from https://www.worldometers.info/coronavirus/?utm_campaign=homeAdvegas1?%22

Dave, D. M., Friedson, A. I., Matsuzawa, K., Sabia, J. J., Safford, S. (2020). Black lives matter protests, social distancing, and COVID-19. IZA Discussion Papers 13388, Institute of Labor Economics (IZA). Retrieved November 12, 2021, from https://ideas.repec.org/p/iza/izadps/dp13388.html.

Davis, M. F. (2021). The human (rights) costs of inequality: snapshots from a pandemic. In M. Kjaerum, M. F. Davis, A. Lyons (Eds.), *COVID-19 and human rights* (pp. 67–81). Routledge.

Dempster, H., Ginn, T., Graham, J., Ble, M. G., Jayasinghe, D., & Shorey, B. (2020). *Locked down and left behind: The impact of COVID-19 on refugees' economic inclusion. Policy Paper 179.* Center for Global Development and Refugees International. Retrieved November 20, 2021, from https://www.cgdev.org/publication/locked-down-and-left-behind-impact-covid-19-refugees-economic-inclusion.

D'cruz, M., & Banerjee, D. (2020). 'An invisible human rights crisis': The marginalization of older adults during the COVID-19 pandemic–An advocacy review. *Psychiatry Research, 292*, 113369. doi:10.1016/j.psychres.2020.113369

Donnelly, R., Patrinos, H. A. (2020). Is the COVID-19 slide in education real? *World Bank Blogs*, Retrieved November 19, 2021, from https://blogs.worldbank.org/education/covid-19-slide-education-real.

Du Plessis, G. A. (2021). COVID-19 and limitations to the international right to freedom of religion or belief. *Journal of Church and State, 63*(4), 619–647. doi:10.1093/jcs/csaa082

Eck, K., & Hatz, S. (2020). State surveillance and the COVID-19 crisis. *Journal of Human Rights, 19*(5), 603–612. doi:10.1080/14754835.2020.1816163

Edgell, A. B., Lachapelle, J., Lührmann, A., & Maerz, S. F. (2021). Pandemic backsliding: Violations of democratic standards during Covid-19. *Social Science & Medicine, 285*, 114244. doi:10.1016/j.socscimed.2021.114244

Ferrero, J. P., & Natalucci, A. (2020). COVID-19 pandemic and social unrest: The social protest by other means. Reflections on the argentinian case. *Bulletin of Latin American Research, 39*(S1), 67–70. doi:10.1111/blar.13211

Flanigan, J. A. (2014). A defense of compulsory vaccination. *HEC Forum, 26*(1), 5–25. doi:10.1007/s10730-013-9221-5

Flood, C. M., Thomas, B., & Wilson, K. (2021). Mandatory vaccination for health care workers: An analysis of law and policy., *193*(6), E217–E220.

Forman, L., & Kohler, J. C. (2020). Global health and human rights in the time of COVID-19: Response, restrictions, and legitimacy. *Journal of Human Rights, 19*(5), 547–556. doi:10.1080/14754835.2020.1818556

Frey, C. B., Chen, C., & Presidente, G. (2020). Democracy, culture, and contagion: Political regimes and countries responsiveness to Covid-19. *Covid Economics, 18*, 232–238.

Garrett, T. M. (2020). COVID-19, wall building, and the effects on migrant protection protocols by the Trump administration: The spectacle of the worsening human rights disaster on the Mexico-US border. *Administrative Theory & Praxis, 42*(2), 240–248. doi:10.1080/10841806.2020.1750212

Guasti, P. (2020). The impact of the COVID-19 pandemic in central and eastern Europe: The rise of autocracy and democratic resilience. *Democratic Theory, 7*(2), 47–60. doi:10.3167/dt.2020.070207

Giubilini, A., & Savulescu, J. (2019). Vaccination, risks, and freedom: The seat belt analogy. *Public Health Ethics, 12*(3), 237–249. doi:10.1093/phe/phz014

Goodhart, M. (2020). Revisiting interdependence in times and terms of crisis. *Journal of Human Rights, 19*(5), 520–527. doi:10.1080/14754835.2020.1814709

Gurmendi, A. (2020). COVID-19 symposium: COVID-19 and the 'Western Gaze.' *Opinio Juris*, 7 April 2020, Retrieved November 12, 2021, from http://opiniojuris.org/2020/04/07/covid-19-symposium-covid-19-and-the-western-gaze/.

Guterres, A. (2021). Remarks to the security council open meeting on ensuring equitable access to COVID-19 vaccines in contexts affected by conflict and insecurity. Speech transcript Retrieved October 1, 2021, from https://www.un.org/sg/en/content/sg/speeches/2021-02-17/ensuring-equitable-access-covid-19-vaccines-contexts-affected-conflict-and-insecurity-remarks-security-council.

Hathaway, O. A., Lim, P. J., Phillips-Robins, A., & Stevens, M. (2021). The COVID-19 pandemic and international law. *Cornell International Law Journal, 54*(2), 149–244.

Hill, J., Rodriguez, D. X., & McDaniel, P. N. (2021). Immigration status as a health care barrier in the USA during COVID-19. *Journal of Migration and Health, 4*, 100036.

International AIDS Society–Lancet Commission (2021). Human rights and fair access to COVID-19 vaccines: The International AIDS Society–Lancet Commission on Health and Human Rights. *The Lancet, 397*(10284), 1524–1527. doi:10.1016/S0140-6736(21)00708-X

Jecker, N. S., Wightman, A. G., & Diekema, D. S. (2021). Vaccine ethics: An ethical framework for global distribution of COVID-19 vaccines. *Journal of Medical Ethics, 47*(5), 308–317.

Jiménez, E. C. (2021). Racial justice to the forefront: Do black lives matter in international law? In M. Kjaerum, M. F. Davis, A. Lyons (Eds.), *COVID-19 and human rights* (pp. 82–99). Routledge.

Joseph, S. (2020). International human rights law and the response to the Covid-19 pandemic. *Journal of International Humanitarian Legal Studies, 11*(2), 249–269. doi:10.1163/18781527-bja10004

Joseph, S., & Dore, G. J. (2021). *Vaccine apartheid: A human rights analysis of COVID-19 vaccine inequity.* Retrieved November 12, 2021, from SSRN: https://ssrn.com/abstract=3876848 or http://dx.doi.org/10.2139/ssrn.3876848.

Kantamneni, N. (2020). The impact of the COVID-19 pandemic on marginalized populations in the United States: A research agenda. *Journal of Vocational Behavior, 119*(June), 103439. doi:10.1016/j.jvb.2020.103439

Kerr, J. R., Schneider, C. R., Recchia, G., Dryhurst, S., Sahlin, U., Dufouil, C., Arwidson, P., Freeman, A. L. J., & van der Linden, S. (2021). Correlates of intended COVID-19 vaccine acceptance across time and countries: Results from a series of cross-sectional surveys. *BMJ Open, 11*(8), e048025. doi:10.1136/bmjopen-2020-048025

Khosla, R., & Gruskin, S. (2021). Equity without human rights: A false COVID-19 narrative? *BMJ Global Health, 6*(7), e006720. doi:10.1136/bmjgh-2021-006720

Kjaerum, M. (2021). The post-crisis human rights Agenda. In M. Kjaerum, M. F. Davis, A. Lyons (Eds.), *COVID-19 and human rights* (pp. 293–307). Routledge.

Kjaerum, M., Davis, M. F., & Lyons, A. (Eds.). (2021). *COVID-19 and human rights.* Routledge.

Koo, J.-W. (2022). Global perceptions of South Korea's COVID-19 policy responses: Topic modeling with tweets. *Journal of Human Rights, 21*(3), 334–353.

Kysel, I. M. (2021). Seizing opportunities to promote the protection of rights of all migrants. In M. Kjaerum, M. F. Davis, A. Lyons (Eds.), *COVID-19 and human rights* (pp. 150–169). Routledge.

Lange, M., Monscheuer, O. (2021). Spreading the disease: Protest in times of pandemics. *ZEW-Centre for European Economic Research Discussion Paper,* (21-009), Retrieved November 20, 2021, from https://ssrn.com/abstract=3787921 or 10.2139/ssrn.3787921.

Lebret, A. (2020). COVID-19 pandemic and derogation to human rights. *Journal of Law and the Biosciences, 7*(1), lsaa015. doi:10.1093/jlb/lsaa015

Liu, J., & Zhao, H. (2021). Privacy lost: Appropriating surveillance technology in China's fight against COVID-19. *Business Horizons, 64*(6), 743–756.

Loomba, S., de Figueiredo, A., Piatek, S. J., de Graaf, K., & Larson, H. J. (2021). Measuring the Impact of COVID-19 vaccine misinformation on vaccination intent in the UK and USA. *Nature Human Behaviour, 5*(3), 337–348. doi:10.1038/s41562-021-01056-1

Maerz, S. F., Lührmann, A., Lachapelle, J., Edgell, A. B. (2020). Worth the sacrifice? Illiberal and authoritarian practices during Covid-19 (September 2020). V-Dem Working Paper 110, Retrieved November 12, 2021, from SSRN: https://ssrn.com/abstract=3701720 or http://dx.doi.org/10.2139/ssrn.3701720

Metcalf, H. (2021). Life and death in prisons. In M. Kjaerum, M. F. Davis, A. Lyons (eds.), *COVID-19 and human rights* (pp. 133–149). Routledge.

Metternich, N. W. (2020). Drawback before the wave?: Protest decline during the Covid-19 pandemic. (May 5, 2020), Retrieved November 12, 2021, from 10.31235/osf.io/3ej72.

Moyn, S. (2018). *Not enough: Human rights in an unequal world.* Harvard University Press.

Muntingh, L. M. (2020). Africa, prisons and COVID-19. *Journal of Human Rights Practice, 12*(2), 284–292. doi:10.1093/jhuman/huaa031

Murdie, A. (2022). Hindsight is 2020: Lessons from the COVID-19 pandemic for future human rights research. *Journal of Human Rights, 21*(3), 354–364.

Nacoti, M., Ciocca, A., Giupponi, A., Brambillasca, P., Lussana, F., Pisano, M., … Montaguti, C. (2020). At the epicenter of the Covid-19 pandemic and humanitarian crises in Italy: changing perspectives on preparation and mitigation. *NEJM Catalyst Innovations in Care Delivery, 1*(2), 1–5. doi:10.1056/CAT.20.0080

Nay, O. (2020). Can a virus undermine human rights? *The Lancet. Public Health, 5*(5), e238–e239. doi:10.1016/S2468-2667(20)30092-X

Nigam, S. (2020). COVID-19: India's response to domestic violence needs rethinking. *South Asia Journal* (May 12, 2020), Retrieved November 20, 2021, from https://ssrn.com/abstract=3598999 or http://dx.doi.org/10.2139/ssrn.3598999.

Ó Cathaoir, K. (2021). Human rights in times of pandemics: Necessity and proportionality. In M. Kjaerum, M. F. Davis, A. Lyons (Eds.), *COVID-19 and human rights* (pp. 35–51). Routledge.

Okonkwo, N. E., Aguwa, U. T., Jang, M., Barré, I. A., Page, K. R., Sullivan, P. S., Beyrer, C., & Baral, S. (2021). COVID-19 and the US response: accelerating health inequities. *BMJ Evidence-Based Medicine, 26*(4), 176–179. doi:10.1136/bmjebm-2020-111426

Openshaw, J. J., & Travassos, M. A. (2020). COVID-19, quarantines, sheltering-in-place, and human rights: The developing crisis. *The American Journal of Tropical Medicine and Hygiene, 103*(2), 578–580.

Oxfam. (2020). Small group of rich nations have bought up more than half the future supply of leading COVID-19 vaccine contenders. Press release. Retrieved October 1, 2021, from https://www.oxfam.org/en/press-releases/small-group-rich-nations-have-bought-more-half-future-supply-leading-covid-19.

Pleyers, G. (2020). The Pandemic is a battlefield. Social movements in the COVID-19 lockdown. *Journal of Civil Society, 16*(4), 295–312. doi:10.1080/17448689.2020.1794398

Quinn, G. (2021). Covid-19 and disability. In M. Kjaerum, M. F. Davis, A. Lyons (Eds.), *COVID-19 and human rights* (pp. 116–132). Routledge.

Ramji-Nogales, J., & Goldner Lang, I. (2020). Freedom of movement, migration, and borders. *Journal of Human Rights, 19*(5), 593–602. doi:10.1080/14754835.2020.1830045

Roksandić, S., Mamić, K., & Mikac, R. (2021). Migration in the time of COVID-19—Policy responses and practices in croatia concerning the Western Balkan Routes and readiness for the post-COVID-19 society in which the right to health care for the most vulnerable is guaranteed. *Frontiers in Human Dynamics, 3*, 595189. doi: 10. 3389/fhumd.2021.595189.

Santoro, M. A. (2021). Why the United Nations is not the ideal forum for business and human rights: The UNGPs and the right to COVID-19 vaccine access in the Global South. *Business and Human Rights Journal, 6*(2), 326–335. doi:10.1017/bhj.2021.27

Santoro, M., & Shanklin, R. (2020). Human rights obligations of drug companies. *Journal of Human Rights, 19*(5), 557–567. doi:10.1080/14754835.2020.1820315

Savulescu, J., Persson, I., & Wilkinson, D. (2020). Utilitarianism and the pandemic. *Bioethics, 34*(6), 620–632.

Šehović, A. B., & Govender, K. (2021). Addressing COVID-19 vulnerabilities: How do we achieve global health security in an inequitable world. *Global Public Health, 16*(8–9), 1198–1208. doi:10.1080/17441692.2021.1916056

Sekalala, S., Forman, L., Habibi, R., & Meier, B. M. (2020). Health and human rights are inextricably linked in the COVID-19 response. *BMJ Global Health, 5*(9), e003359. doi:10.1136/bmjgh-2020-003359

Sikkink, K. (2017). *Evidence for hope: Making human rights work in the 21st Century*. Princeton University Press.

Spadaro, A. (2020). COVID-19: Testing the limits of human rights. *European Journal of Risk Regulation, 11*(2), 317–325. doi:10.1017/err.2020.27

Tai, D. B. G., Shah, A., Doubeni, C. A., Sia, I. G., & Wieland, M. L. (2021). The disproportionate impact of COVID-19 on racial and ethnic minorities in the United States. *Clinical Infectious Diseases, 72*(4), 703–706. doi: 10.1093/cid/ciaa815

Telles, L. E. B., Valenca, A. M., Barros, A. J. S., & da Silva, A. G. (2021). Domestic violence in the COVID-19 pandemic: A forensic psychiatric perspective. *Revista Brasileira de Psiquiatria, 43*(3), 233–234. doi:10.1590/1516-4446-2020-1060

Theidon, K. (2020). A forecasted failure: Intersectionality, COVID-19, and the perfect storm. *Journal of Human Rights, 19*(5), 528–536. doi:10.1080/14754835.2020.1822156

Toebes, B. (2015). Human rights and public health: Towards a balanced relationship. *The International Journal of Human Rights, 19*(4), 488–504. doi:10.1080/13642987.2015.1044814

United Nations, General Assembly. (1992). *Report of the United Nations Conference on Environment and Development, Annex I, Rio Declaration on Environment and Development*, A/CONF.151/26 (Vol. I) (Rio de Janeiro, 3–14 June 1992), Retrieved November 18, 2021, from https://www.un.org/en/development/desa/population/migration/generalassembly/docs/globalcompact/A_CONF.151_26_Vol.I_Declaration.pdf.

Van Dijcke, D., Wright, A. L. (2020). Using mobile device traces to improve near-real time data collection during the George Floyd Protests. (June 7, 2020). Retrieved November 12, 2021, from SSRN: https://ssrn.com/abstract=3621731 or 10.2139/ssrn.3621731.

von Stein, J. (2005). Do treaties constrain or screen? Selection bias and treaty compliance. *American Political Science Review, 99*(4), 611–622.

Wang, R. Y. (2020). Is remote working a privilege? A spatial Durbin approach of digital infrastructure and workplace mobility change during the COVID-19 pandemic in the US. (August 3, 2021). Retrieved November 20, 2021, from SSRN: https://ssrn.com/abstract=3898272 or 10.2139/ssrn.3898272.

Wang, Y. (2021). China's Covid success story is also a human rights tragedy. *Human Rights Watch* (26 January 2021), Retrieved November 20, 2021, from https://www.hrw.org/news/2021/01/26/chinas-covid-success-story-also-human-rights-tragedy.

Wilder, J. M. (2021). The disproportionate impact of COVID-19 on racial and ethnic minorities in the United States. *Clinical Infectious Diseases, 72*(4), 707–709. doi:10.1093/cid/ciaa959

Wong, W. H., & Wong, E. A. (2020). What COVID-19 revealed about health, human rights, and the WHO. *Journal of Human Rights, 19*(5), 568–581. doi:10.1080/14754835.2020.1819778

Yao, L., Li, M., Wan, J. Y., Howard, S. C., Bailey, J. E., & Graff, J. C. (2022). Democracy and case fatality rate of COVID-19 at early stage of pandemic: A multicountry study. *Environmental Science and Pollution Research International, 29*(6), 8694–8704. doi:10.1007/s11356-021-16250-x

Windows of opportunity to worsen human rights

Can nonviolent resistance survive COVID-19?

Erica Chenoweth

ABSTRACT
When the COVID-19 pandemic arrived on the scene, the near-universal imposition of lockdowns and public health restrictions prompted many human rights advocates to sound the alarm regarding freedoms of assembly, expression, privacy, and movement. Even though they have not yet appeared to reduce the occurrence of protests in many countries, such restrictions may nevertheless diminish the ability of mass movements to effectively organize and win key concessions. In this article, I present new descriptive data on the outcomes of people-power movements, which suggest that, despite their heightened popularity, maximalist nonviolent campaigns are seeing their lowest success rates in more than a century. I describe how the diffusion of restrictions on peaceful assembly and expression accompanies a broader toolkit of authoritarian strategies that have become standardized over the past 15 years in response to people-power movements. I then turn to three tensions that present dilemmas for movements emerging from the pandemic and its associated lockdowns. I conclude by laying out key research questions that emerge from these trends and dilemmas that require sustained attention from scholars and practitioners of nonviolent resistance.

Introduction

One might expect that during a global pandemic and global lockdown, people would stay in their homes, protected from the virus and focusing on making ends meet during economic collapse. Instead, despite an initial decline in protest events around the world from January to April 2020 (Metternich, 2020), people all around the world have become more active in attempts to hold their governments accountable through people power. A recent study claims that the number of protest movements around the world tripled between 2006 and 2020; according to that study's authors, "the coronavirus has accentuated social unrest" (Ortiz et al., 2022: 19).

These mass mobilizations have included large-scale uprisings calling for the toppling of dictatorial regimes, national reckonings over racism in public life and accountability in policing, and more. For example, in Belarus, people rose up in late 2020 against the dictatorship of Alexander Lukashenko, a Russian-backed autocrat who rounded up or expelled his opposition and intimidated voters in the run-up to problematic national elections. In the United States, in response to the killings of George Floyd, Breonna Taylor, and Ahmaud Arbery—and on the heels of the multi-year Black Lives Matter movement that had brought issues of systemic racism and police brutality to the fore of the public agenda—Americans took to the streets to mobilize the largest and broadest mass protests in its history. Between 10 and 25 million people reportedly participated in the nationwide protests during the summer of 2020—the same period during which the country was experiencing thousands of deaths per day from COVID-19 (Buchanan et al., 2020). Several months later, people in Nigeria rose up demanding an end to police brutality, corruption, and extortion through the EndSARS movement, which galvanized hundreds of thousands of people to confront security forces in an unprecedented public mobilization in that country. Many other movements—from those opposing vaccinations and mask mandates in the United States to those demanding urgent action on climate change worldwide to those calling for the repeal of agricultural laws opposed by small farmers in India—were active during this period as well.

Yet when the COVID-19 pandemic arrived on the scene, the near-universal imposition of lockdowns and public health restrictions prompted many human rights advocates to sound the alarm regarding freedoms of assembly, expression, privacy, and movement (Roth, 2020). Even though the incidence of protest has persisted around the world, restrictions on assembly and expression may have nevertheless diminished the ability of mass movements to effectively organize and win key concessions.

In this article, I draw on the Nonviolent and Violent Campaign Outcomes (NAVCO) data to argue that, although mass mobilization has indeed persisted and even increased in quantity, the success rates of nonviolent resistance have plummeted. Many people-power movements against autocratization that emerged or were ongoing when COVID-19 arrived have been unable to sustain enough mass participation or build enough political pressure to lead to key breakthroughs. Paying attention not only to the incidence of protest but also to the outcomes of movements that use it can tell us a good deal about the ways in which governments are adapting to people power. The descriptive trends presented here are concerning for those interested in protecting peaceful assembly rights, as well as the ways in which people power can protect and expand human rights. Moreover, consistent with the analysis by Murdie (2022) in this issue, the pandemic has shown that the language of rights and the strategies of peaceful protest are not necessarily fostering freedom, equality, and respect of others.

In this article, I contribute to the special issue's overarching focus in several ways (Chiozza & King, 2022a). First, I present new descriptive data on the onset and outcomes of people-power movements. I focus on three key trends—including the troubling fact that, despite their heightened popularity, maximalist nonviolent campaigns are seeing their lowest success rates in over a century. I describe the global diffusion of restrictions on peaceful assembly and expression, which accompanies a broader toolkit of authoritarian strategies that have become standardized over the past 15 years in response to people-power movements. I then turn to three tensions that present dilemmas for movements emerging from the pandemic and its associated lockdowns. I conclude by laying out key research questions that emerge from these trends and dilemmas that require sustained attention from scholars and practitioners of nonviolent resistance.

Protest in the context of a global pandemic

When COVID-19 arrived on the world scene, an unprecedented number of mass movements had been mobilizing for democratic reforms and human rights in the midst of autocratic backsliding, from Hong Kong to Sudan to India and beyond (Chenoweth, 2021). The year 2020 itself saw record-shattering protest participation in some countries (Ortiz et al., 2022), including in the United States (Buchanan et al., 2020). Across multiple countries, surveys of activists indicated that renewed opportunities for digital activism and a unifying *esprit de corps* among organizers and activists led to a surprising wave of optimism about the future of resistance (Pinckney & Rivers, 2020a).

Tactical innovations during the pandemic have revised what it means to peaceably assemble. Car caravans, virtual rallies, and various forms of online organizing fueled by shared documents edited and stored in the cloud have provided important organizational capacity and stamina to many ongoing movements seeking to protect or expand their political power (Chenoweth et al.,

2020; Kowalewski, 2020; Pinckney & Rivers, 2020b; Pleyers, 2020; Pressman & Choi-Fitzpatrick, 2020; Sykes, 2020). These tactical innovations in many places quickly gained the attention of state authorities, which have responded with road blockades, internet shutdowns, and arrests of producers of online toolkits intended to suppress dissent (see, e.g., Daraghi, 2020).

Indeed, the persistence of popular protest during the pandemic prompted numerous optimistic assessments, including from this author, about the future of nonviolent resistance more generally (Chenoweth et al., 2020; Pinckney & Rivers, 2020a). Not only were there more tactical innovations on display—from stay-at-home protests to car caravans to the explosion of mutual aid organizations—there also was some much-needed time for many organizations and movements to regroup and strategize (Chenoweth, 2020; Kowalewski, 2020; Pressman & Choi-Fitzpatrick, 2020). Multinational surveys indicated that activists approached their work with a new sense of creativity and optimism (Pinckney & Rivers, 2020b), and that they perceived heightened public interest in their issues and concerns because of increased public attention to the inequalities laid bare by the pandemic (Murdie, 2022; Pinckney & Rivers, 2020b).

Yet there was always another danger, one signaled by concerned scholars, journalists, lawyers, and advocates of human rights. That was the danger that governments could use the pandemic as a pretext to usurp power, dealing a potentially irreversible blow to much of the progress that has been made in the development of human rights over the past 80 years (Bennoune, 2020; Brysk, 2022; Chiozza & King, 2022a; Clay, 2022; Hertel et al., 2020; Murdie, 2022; Roth, 2020; Theidon, 2020). These concerns were amplified by the fact that the pandemic also arrived during a period in which the world was already undergoing a global resurgence of autocracy—what some have called the "third wave of autocratization" (Lührmann & Lindberg, 2019; Maerz et al., 2020). Antidemocratic parties in Hungary, Poland, Brazil, Turkey, and the United States have attempted to usurp power in their countries, rolling back the degree to which governments respond to their publics (Burows & Stephan, 2014). In this special issue, Badran and Turnbull (2022) note numerous examples of authoritarian consolidation in North Africa as well.

The widespread continuation of mass mobilization—in spite of the global pandemic—reflects how economic crisis, the ongoing public health emergency, and creeping authoritarianism have motivated people to continue to rise up against corrupt, ineffective, and autocratic governments (Ortiz et al., 2022). Yet it is not clear the extent to which mass protests have produced meaningful change, especially compared to earlier eras of people-power movements. Ortiz et al. (2022: 67) reported that 42 percent of the protest movements they tallied achieved at least some concessions. Their sample included all protest movements expressing a range of grievances and demands in 101 countries between 2006 and 2020, when the pandemic was still in full swing. Examining NAVCO Data—which include a global sample of mass movements expressing maximalist claims such as the toppling of an incumbent national regime or territorial independence from 1900 to 2021—allows for a comparison between campaigns that emerged during the pandemic and those from prior decades.

The NAVCO data

The data I present below are drawn from the NAVCO Dataset, a global dataset I maintain on maximalist campaigns that rely primarily on nonviolent and violent resistance.[1]

Nonviolent resistance, or "people power," is the use of coordinated collective action by civilians who do not resort to violence (Carter, 2012; Randle, 1994). Nonviolent resistance is one of the most universally available techniques for people struggling for change, making it one of the most inclusive (Chenoweth, 2021). Protest is one of many methods of nonviolent resistance, which also includes strikes, boycotts, and other forms of noncooperation. Even during the height of the global pandemic, it remained available as an option to millions of people worldwide.

In this article, I use the terms "nonviolent resistance", "civil resistance", and "people power" interchangeably. Methods of nonviolent resistance include protests, strikes, sit-ins, boycotts, and other forms of noncooperation, as well as the development of alternative institutions like cooperative markets, mutual aid associations, and underground schools. When people engage in these techniques without directly harming other people, I classify them as engaging in nonviolent resistance. When people apply these techniques in a coordinated way over a concentrated period of time, I call this a nonviolent campaign, mobilization, or uprising. I treat the terms "campaign", "mobilization", and "uprising" synonymously for the purposes of this article, although in the broader literature the term "campaign" connotes a more organized and intentional collective activity than the terms "mobilization" and "uprising" which connote spontaneity, a lack of formal organization, and collective action that takes place during a particular time period. In reality, mass uprisings typically involve some combination of purposive organizing and spontaneous mobilization, so the lines between mass campaigns and mass uprisings can be blurred.

It is often the case that when people use nonviolent resistance, the authorities respond to them using coercion or violence, including lethal force. Moreover, at times, people who associate themselves with the broader mobilization engage in provocative actions, producing a violent flank. Thus, violence sometimes occurs in the context of a primarily nonviolent campaign. However, many maximalist campaigns feature vast majorities of people engaging in disciplined, intentional, nonviolent methods in ways that allow scholars to appropriately classify their overall campaigns as primarily nonviolent (or primarily nonviolent with a violent flank). This is particularly true when comparing them against armed campaigns, in which organized rebels and insurgents wage sustained guerrilla warfare or insurgency against their opponents.

Maximalist campaigns are those uprisings in which at least 1,000 people are actively participating and whose demands involve the removal of the incumbent national leader or territorial independence. These campaigns are chosen to increase data reliability, as large-scale maximalist campaigns are more likely to be reported on and are therefore easier to identify across time and space than smaller campaigns with less radical demands. Many, although not all, of the campaigns identified as primarily nonviolent involve an expressed commitment to peaceful, nonviolent resistance. Other nonviolent campaigns simply employ tactics of nonviolent resistance without necessarily making a doctrinal commitment to the technique. The data are collected from numerous source materials, including news reports, expert analyses or field reports, scholarly research, other datasets on protest and collective action, and eyewitness accounts; these techniques were discussed in Chenoweth & Shay (2019).

I follow prior research by classifying campaign outcomes according to the stated maximalist goal (Chenoweth & Stephan, 2011). If the campaign ousts the incumbent national leader (as in the ouster of Omar al-Bashir in Sudan in 2019) or achieves territorial independence (as occurred in East Timor in 1999) as a direct result of the collective action, the campaign is classified as a success. This classification scheme has many notable shortcomings, including that it does not include information about counterrevolutionary attempts, the duration or consolidation of the victory, or the long-term trajectory of the country in the aftermath of a successful people-power movement. Others have taken up these issues ably (e.g., Pinckney, 2020a). But this discrete and narrow conceptualization of success does allow for a systematic comparison across cases, if not a comprehensive one. Regardless, for the purposes of this article, I rely on this concept of success as a way to compare people-power movements over time.

The scope of the dataset is limited in several more ways. First, the dataset does not account for nonmaximalist goals, such as various reform or justice claims. As such, movements like Black Lives Matter, End SARS, the Farmers Movement in India, and others without a maximalist claim are not included in the dataset as distinct campaigns. Second, the dataset does not account for movements with nonmaximalist, transnational claims, such as the climate movement, antiwar movements, or the global feminist movement. Other studies have evaluated the rise and outcomes of many nonmaximalist movements such as these over the past 15 years (Ortiz et al., 2022).

Despite the limited scope of the type of campaigns evaluated in the NAVCO dataset, the dataset does provide a way to systematically assess the emergence and outcomes of a comparable set of cases over a significant time span. As such, it provides a useful metric for overall global trends in mass mobilization.

Key trends in maximalist people-power movements during COVID-19

This section notes three key trends that overlapped with the onset of the global pandemic in 2020: the primacy of people power, the plummeting of success rates of nonviolent resistance, and the diffusion of protest restrictions.

Trend #1: The primacy of people power

Setting aside COVID-19, the first two decades of the 21st century have seen more mass protest movements calling for the toppling of governments than there were during the entire 20th century. Since 2000, there have been nearly 200 such movements, including many that are ongoing (Figure 1). As of January 2020, people-power movements were responding to a global wave of autocratic backsliding in places as diverse as Poland, Hungary, Turkey, Brazil, the Philippines, India, and the United States.

Notwithstanding a short-term decline in protest events during the spring of 2020 (Metternich, 2020), many of these campaigns persisted once the pandemic set in, due to political emergencies that required immediate mass mobilization. For instance, oppositionists in Belarus organized a major attempt to dislodge Alexander Lukashenko from power there, in the aftermath of an unfair election. In February 2021, after a military *junta* seized power in Myanmar, a civil disobedience movement developed to restore democracy and initiate constitutional reforms that would curtail the military's power in the future; it has since largely given way to civil war. When protesters in Cuba poured into the streets in July 2021 to demand economic justice and an end to corruption, some said they had broken through a barrier of fear, leading people to revolt on a scale that few people in the country could recall in their lifetimes. At the same time, people from all walks of life in Eswatini rose up against the absolute monarchy there, calling for democratic reforms and demanding accountability for incidents of police brutality, torture, and arbitrary killings of civilians.

These and other mass movements reflect grassroots demands for well-being, accountability, representation, and government responsiveness—a primary way through which human rights practices have diffused across the world during the past century (Chenoweth & Stephan, 2011; Ortiz et al., 2022; Pinckney, 2020a).

Trend #2: Declining success rates

Given the global rise of people-power campaigns—and the unprecedented levels of involvement by ordinary people in hundreds of campaigns worldwide, the second trend is surprising and troubling. Over the past two decades, the success rates of people-power campaigns have been steadily declining (Chenoweth, 2020, 2021). But 2020 and 2021 have been the worst years on record for people power since the 1930s. In the same year that the Taliban insurgency toppled the Afghan government and drove out the US military intervention, people-power campaigns in Myanmar and Belarus were brutally crushed. For the first time since the 1940s—a decade dominated by state-backed partisan rebellions against Nazi occupations—nonviolent resistance does not have a statistically significant advantage over armed insurrection in terms of discrete

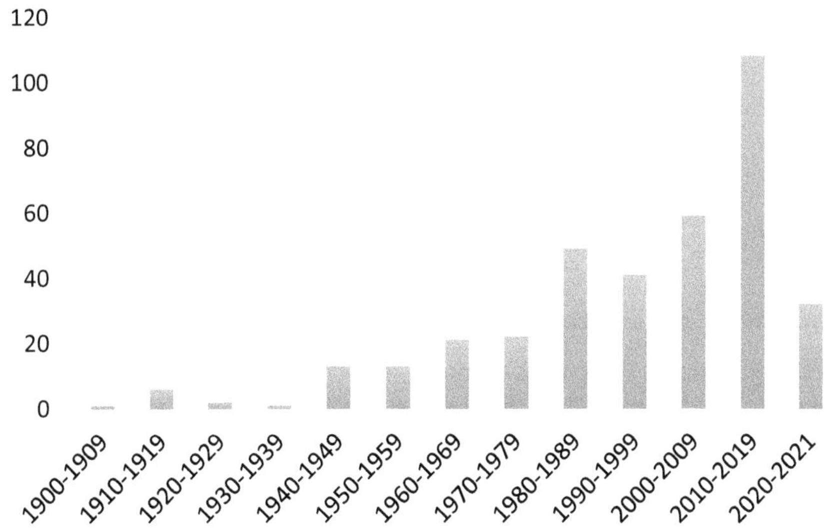

Figure 1. Onsets of maximalist nonviolent campaigns, 1900–2021 ($n = 368$). Source: NAVCO Database, v. 1.4.

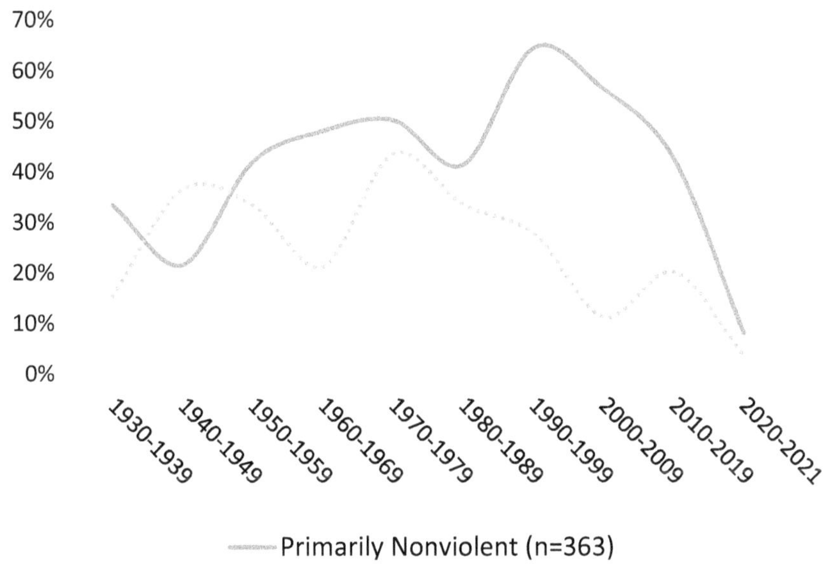

Figure 2. Success rates of maximalist campaigns, 1930–2021 ($n = 623$). Data for 2021 are through August. Source: NAVCO Database, v. 1.4.

success rates. In Figure 2, the success rates of armed resistance campaigns are included for reference.

There are multiple potential explanations for this decline in successes by people-power movements, which have been covered in depth elsewhere (Chenoweth, 2021). But one of the most important factors relates to the adaptive measures states have taken to prevent, deter, and suppress mass movements. These "smart repression" techniques involve a combination of divide and rule strategies, digital repression, propaganda and misinformation, and the declaration of emergency powers in the context of crises (Smithey & Kurtz, 2018). Crises like COVID-19 have provided the pretext for shutting down protests, in particular, on the basis of maintaining public health (Daraghi, 2020).

The use of techniques of smart repression goes beyond consolidated autocracies, and so does using the pandemic as a pretext for demobilizing movements. In India, for example, Roth (2020) noted that the Modi government's declaration of a three-week lockdown effectively demobilized massive protests in opposition to the Citizenship Amendment that was viewed as exclusionary and discriminatory toward Muslims, even as millions later participated in a nationwide strike related to the Farmer's Movement. Numerous countries declared public gatherings as unlawful. As Metternich showed, these measures did result in immediate declines in public protest (2020). That relates to the third key trend.

Trend #3: Diffusion of protest restrictions

During COVID-19, multiple observers have noted the ways in which restrictions on public gatherings can quickly overreach to limit freedom of assembly, expression, and protest (Libal & Kashwan, 2020). The International Center for Not-for-Profit Law (ICNL) noted that 153 countries around the world have adopted measures that restrict assembly; 59 have adopted measures that restrict expression; and 110 have made emergency declarations that expand the power and discretion of the executive branch (DeBlock & Ognenovska, 2022).

But these restrictions have emerged alongside a growing recognition of the political power of popular movements, which had led many governments—autocratic and otherwise—to broaden their crackdowns against human rights defenders, activists, organizers, and dissidents before the pandemic even began. When threatened by people power, today's autocrats and aspiring autocrats rely on the expansion of surveillance, adept use of social media to spread disinformation and mobilize their own supporters, jailing or terrorizing dissidents or their families, and purging or shoring up their inner entourage and security forces to ensure their loyalty in crucial moments (Smithey & Kurtz, 2018). Authoritarians often appeal to their supporters through rallies and other displays of popularity to try to challenge the opposition's claims to popular legitimacy. They also denounce protesters and dissidents as "terrorists," "criminals," and "traitors," declaring them threats to national security and inciting their supporters to attack them. Populist and polarized politics play to autocrats' advantage. Being able to divide and rule is a core survival strategy of most dictatorships, and the ability to mobilize loyalists in the streets inflames underlying tensions and divisions within society, sowing chaos among the opposition and popular doubts about democratic movements' claims. In recent years, the authoritarian toolkit has become increasingly widespread, in part because it has proved to be so effective in suppressing dissent (Chenoweth, 2021).

Public health crises simply exacerbate these trends. Historically, epidemics have often produced patterns of government coercion and resistance. In the name of the collective good, public officials have enforced strict physical distancing measures, such as quarantine, as a way to control the spread of deadly viruses. The term *quarantine* gets its name from the Italian *quaranta*, referring to the 40 days that Venetian officials held merchants in temporary housing before they were allowed to enter the city during the Black Plague (Snowden, 2019). To enforce such measures, Venetian officials consolidated means of coercion both by bolstering their armed forces and by developing narratives that justified these measures for the public good and thereby enhanced their legitimacy. Such measures produced resistance from peasants, who struggled to survive under the restrictions, and from competing elites, who worried that they would emerge from the pandemic with reduced status. Venetian proto-states used their powers to stamp out resistance of all kinds, often with horrific brutality. Snowden (2019) traced the origins of the modern state not to Westphalia but, rather, to the Venetian mini-states that assembled the trappings of statehood through the consolidation of coercion and the monopolization of violence. This episode demonstrates a particular lesson: When pandemics lift, the state often emerges much stronger. Of the contemporary emergency powers adopted by numerous states to control the COVID-19 pandemic, Kenneth Roth noted that it may be difficult to put the "genie back in the bottle once the crisis fades" (2020).

Of course, medieval Europe was a place of monarchs, warlords, and competing claims to autocratic rule. Today, the majority of the world's countries are still democracies, which is perhaps why there has been a more optimistic outlook about the fate of activism in the aftermath of this pandemic. Democratic states that emerge stronger should theoretically be accountable to their citizens at the ballot box if they overreach their authority to control the pandemic. But that assumes that people will be able to continue mobilizing to demand accountability among elected officials—and that such mobilization works.

Looking ahead: Three tensions for people power after COVID-19

Political protest is broadly recognized as a fundamental human right. Yet the global pandemic has crystallized numerous challenges to peaceful assembly that require urgent attention, renewal, and response. There are three key tensions relevant to the current time that complicate the renewal of these rights.

Tension #1: Health vs. assembly

Even where states have been pursuing lockdowns in good faith, these restrictions have put two important rights in tension: the right to personal health and safety, and the right to peaceably assemble. On the one hand, the emergence of the COVID-19 virus and the subsequent bans on public gatherings led to the rapid demobilization of various ongoing movements, such as the pro-democracy movement in Hong Kong. At the time, human rights advocates argued that these bans were being used cynically, as a convenient pretext to shut down ongoing dissent or to rob of their legitimacy those protestors who insisted on maintaining a street presence. It is clear that mask wearing and social distancing outdoors provided opportunities to accommodate the public health interests during the pandemic with the right of peaceful assembly. This is partly why so many of the tactical innovations developed during the pandemic involved socially distant protest, digital or online tactics, and outdoor protests that provided masks and hand sanitizer (Pinckney & Rivers, 2020a; Pressman & Choi-Fitzpatrick, 2020).

On the other hand, protections of peaceful assembly rights also meant that people protesting the lockdowns—including those participating in antilockdown protests and those participating in antimask or antivaccination demonstrations—have also made use of peaceful assembly and freedom of expression to promote misinformation and, in some cases, hate speech (Pet, 2021). Moreover, rallies and protests among those who have minimized or denied the pandemic and refused to take public health precautions (such as mandatory mask wearing and social distancing while indoors) while they exercised their rights to protest may have been responsible for spreading the virus to others. Hence the tensions between peaceful assembly and public health risks are tangible and real. As Koo notes in this special issue (2022), opinions vary about the legitimacy of restrictions on assembly given concerns about public health.

Tension #2: Digital activism vs. digital authoritarianism

The second tension emerging from the pandemic relates to the fact that so many activists turned to digital organizing and activism as a way to remain active during lockdowns—a celebrated move among some observers (Pinckney, 2020a; Pressman & Choi-Fitzpatrick, 2020). Yet as more activists have moved their planning, communication, and tactical innovations online, they have become more vulnerable to digital repression.

Indeed, we live in an age of digital authoritarianism—a form of authoritarianism that exploits the tools of digital technology to undermine, subvert, and suppress opposition groups, including activists. Such digital repression happens in multiple ways, from direct surveillance of activists' communications to online harassment and intimidation to the rapid diffusion of state propaganda to the infiltration of movements to selective censorship (Gohdes, 2015; Guntisky, 2015; Pinckney, 2020b; Roth, 2020). Human rights defenders have pointed to the enhanced surveillance capacities of states to monitor dissident activity online, as well as the long-term privacy risks of digitizing the public health response to the pandemic. For instance, the ICNL identified at least 61 countries that have passed laws that raise grave concerns about privacy (DeBlock & Ognenovska, 2022). These measures have also expanded the vulnerabilities for movements.

Tension #3: Reopening civic space in a time of right-wing populism

After World War II, people-power movements were among the key drivers leading to the global spread of democracy and human rights (Haggard & Kauffman, 2016). Between 1900 and 1999, more than 100 people-power movements demanded the toppling of the incumbent national regime (Chenoweth, 2021). About 60 percent of them succeeded in doing so, although other attempts were crushed. A vast majority of these breakthroughs led to democratic transitions and consolidation. Many of the successful movements of the past featured strikes, economic noncooperation, and underground organizing, often culminating in massive street demonstrations that brought orderly, daily life to a standstill. Remarkable levels of public pressure in the United States, Poland, the Czech Republic, Serbia, Chile, the Philippines, Zambia, Sudan, Brazil, and elsewhere encouraged political, economic, and security elites to throw their support behind democratic reforms. Historically, mass nonviolent resistance—which typically involves the active participation of women and men, children and elders, poor and middle-class people, urban and rural groups, people with varying physical abilities, and communities from all walks of life—has been a fundamentally inclusive technique of political change, which is partly why it was more likely than armed revolutions to lead to democratization (Chenoweth, 2021; Chenoweth & Stephan, 2011; Pinckney, 2020a).

Yet today, we are not seeing the same democratic dividends from civil resistance campaigns as we did during the twentieth century. Instead, over the past 15 years, democracy has continued to recede globally, as autocrats and aspiring authoritarians have become much more successful in defeating these movements.

Part of the reason for this change is that governments have successfully defeated many of these challenges, strengthening their political positions and consolidating authoritarian control. But another key trend is a surge of illiberal popular movements to rival those calling for democratic change. Some movements included in Figures 1 and 2 have made explicitly antidemocratic demands, such as the restoration of autocratic rule in Tunisia in August 2021, Egypt in 2013, and Thailand in 2014. The movement that brought al Sisi to power in Egypt in 2013, for instance, actively demanded that the military remove Mohammed Morsi from power, initiating a years-long dictatorship in which dissent has been mercilessly crushed.

Some other recent movements have used disruptive techniques to subvert democratic election results in places like Bolivia among opponents of Evo Morales in 2019, and in the United States among adherents to Trump's "big lie." In Germany, far-right groups have reportedly been reading Gene Sharp and other strategists of nonviolent resistance, hoping to use those theories to broaden their support and political leverage (Bennhold, 2018).

In other words, the techniques of people power—long associated with progressive aims and causes—have been cynically appropriated by those who would use these techniques to dispossess, disenfranchize, or subjugate others. Antidemocratic movements account for scores of recent popular campaigns. Although far-right groups have often used street protests and rallies to expand their bases, a self-conscious strategy of nonviolent resistance by far-right and antidemocratic groups is a relatively new phenomenon (Petz, 2021).

A crucial priority in the renewal and recommitment to rights of peaceful assembly will be to press for the equal protection of these rights. But it is also important to recognize that the ecosystem of groups and movements that are deploying tactics of nonviolent action is much more complex than it was prior to the pandemic. Various tactics of people power—large-scale protest, sit-ins, nonviolent occupations, public shaming and heckling, walk-outs, and other forms of non-cooperation—have been commandeered by groups and individuals associated with conservative and far-right causes, including those fighting against public health measures, as well as those groups with decidedly antidemocratic agendas. Such groups have been exercising the full range of their rights throughout the pandemic, building their bases of supporters, enhancing their messaging, obtaining tactical and organizational experience, and building resilience for what is to come.

Toward a post-COVID-19 research agenda on nonviolent resistance

People-power movements may have suffered serious setbacks as a result of the pandemic, and they may be emerging with a tricky set of tensions they must navigate. However, as the pandemic has run its course, the world's other urgent crises have not evaporated. Instead, arguably, most of them have deepened or accelerated. As before the pandemic, rising global inequality, climate volatility, a global economic crisis, the rise of far-right movements, a wave of populist authoritarian challenges to democracies worldwide, and declining trust in established institutions remain urgent challenges.

Grassroots movements often provide important resources for meeting such challenges by representing an array of civic attitudes, designing new policy proposals and solutions, helping to maintain key priorities at the top of the global political agenda, and holding politicians directly accountable for delivering on their promises. But many of the most skilled organizers around the world have been in survival mode during the pandemic, organizing communities for mutual aid and resilience rather than activating, mobilizing, and building political power. As a result, many of the ongoing and overlapping challenges we face require urgent attention and people-powered response that are difficult to summon.

What do these urgent trends, tensions, and challenges mean for the study of nonviolent resistance after the pandemic? Here I point to three fruitful avenues for future research by scholars of human rights and nonviolent resistance.

First, most research on nonviolent resistance has assumed that movements using these techniques have progressive, prodemocratic, or emancipatory aims. But far-right and antidemocratic groups have co-opted the techniques and rhetorical resources of nonviolent resistance (Bennhold, 2018; Petz, 2021), although they also express a violent and exclusionary rhetoric and often use violent means to pursue it. An enduring puzzle is therefore this: why are antidemocratic movements growing so broadly in popularity and power in so many countries around the world, including in the United States?

Second, the rapid decline of the success rates of nonviolent resistance campaigns all around the world raises questions about whether this is a truly global trend with a global cause. Because, as we have seen, the decline in success rates preceded the onset of the pandemic, it is unlikely that COVID-19 was the direct cause of this decline. However, the pandemic may have hastened the retreat of the postwar international order, and there is also an open question regarding the relationship between the postwar international order, the global spread of human rights norms, and the rise in the effectiveness of nonviolent resistance (Ritter, 2015). It may be that, in fact, the surprising success of nonviolent resistance in the late twentieth and early twenty-first centuries was an emblem of a bygone era rather than a pattern of human behavior that will persist in an age in which democracy is declining, human rights norms are under assault, and digital authoritarianism is on the march. This is a question that can only be answered with the passage of time.

Third, there is a real question about whether there are significant limits to nonviolent resistance during the disinformation age. Notably, the technique of nonviolent struggle was forged by practitioner-intellectuals who theorized that the primary power of nonviolent resistance emerged from the irresistibility of the truth. Gandhi called his autobiography *Experiments with Truth*. Some translate his technique—*satyagraha*—as "soul-force" or "truth-force." Vaclev Havel often commented on the fact that truth becomes much more appealing in the face of state lies, providing people with legitimacy and motivation to overcome corrupt power. Again, COVID-19 is not the direct cause of disinformation. However, it may be that lockdowns—and the reliance on social media for social connections—exacerbated the information silos that were already in place, further dividing polarized publics into more calcified views and identities. This emphasis raises questions about whether and how practitioners of nonviolent resistance can expand their bases of support and popular appeal when genuine understandings of truth are fundamentally contested depending on ones' partisan inclinations.

Conclusion and practical implications

Mass movements tend to win when they unsettle existing social relationships among those in power, gain allies, develop economic leverage by withholding their labor or their money, and develop the staying power and organizational base to withstand crackdowns (Schock, 2015). Those successes can strengthen chances for democracy when movements are genuinely inclusive, when the transition includes civil society groups at the negotiating table, and when the movement maintains its capacity to hold the new government accountable (Pinckney, 2020a). This requires far more than street protests improvised in the heat of the moment. Instead, the work of people power involves slow, painful coalition-building, public education about the movement's claims, and a plan to increase public pressure on people in positions of power and authority.

Movements share the common goals of building power, expanding their constituencies, and transforming their people power into institutional power even as their opponents continually try to demean, undermine, and suppress them. But even established democracies will continue to face mobilization from below, as protesters and counter-protesters mirror the deep levels of polarization present throughout most societies. As authoritarian movements gain ground, democratic movements worldwide are struggling to expand their constituencies among those who have grown frustrated with the systems of inequality and injustice that continue to plague democratic countries worldwide (Mampilly, 2021).

People power movements struggling for human rights and democracy today therefore need solidarity, skills, and support (Libal & Kashwan, 2020; Sikkink, 2020). Those movements that have succeeded in toppling long-standing dictatorships—such as in Sudan and Algeria in 2019—have faced difficult and fraught transitions that threaten human rights gains and often weaken popular coalitions. They struggle to hold the line with little recognition or assistance from the global community. Prodemocracy activists around the world—including in the United States—are confronting common challenges from a predictable authoritarian playbook. Opportunities for peer learning—through workshops, skills-shares, strategy sessions, and global summits for activists and organizers—may be critical to help to collect a thorough baseline of knowledge about how to navigate these challenges.

Note

1. Version 1.4; see the project's site at Harvard Dataverse: https://dataverse.harvard.edu/dataverse/navco.

Funding and acknowledgments

I thank Zesean Ali, Mayumi Cornejo, Michelle Poulin, and Hem Rizal for invaluable research assistance, and the Belfer Center for Science and International Affairs and the Carr Center for Human Rights Policy for supporting the data collection.

References

Badran, S. Z., & Turnbull, B. (2022). The COVID-19 pandemic and authoritarian consolidation in North Africa. *Journal of Human Rights, 21*(3), 263–282.

Bennhold, K. (2018). Germany's far right rebrands: Friendlier face, same doctrine. *The New York Times*, December 27. Web. https://www.nytimes.com/2018/12/27/world/europe/germany-far-right-generation-identity.html

Bennoune, K. (2020). Lest we should sleep: COVID-19 and human rights. *American Journal of International Law, 114*(4), 666–676. doi:10.1017/ajil.2020.68

Brysk, A. (2022). Pandemic Patriarchy: The impact of a global health crisis on women's rights. *Journal of Human Rights, 21*(3), 283–303. doi:10.1080/14754835.2022.2071105

Buchanan, L., Bui, Q., Patel, J. K. (2020). Black Lives Matter may be the largest movement in U.S. history. *The New York Times*, 3 July. Retrived August 13, 2020, from https://www.nytimes.com/interactive/2020/07/03/us/george-floyd-protests-crowd-size.html.

Burows, M., & Stephan, M. J. (2014). *Is authoritarianism staging a comeback?* Atlantic Council.

Carter, A. (2012). *People power and political change: Key issues and concepts.* Routledge.

Chenoweth, E. (2020). The future of nonviolent resistance. *Journal of Democracy, 31*(3), 69–84. doi:10.1353/jod.2020.0046

Chenoweth, E. (2021). *Civil resistance: What everyone needs to know.* Oxford University Press.

Chenoweth, E., Choi-Fitzpatrick, A., Pressman, J., Santos, F., Ulfelder, J. (2020). The global pandemic has spawned new forms of activism – and they're flourishing, *Guardian*, 20 April 2020, https://www.theguardian.com/commentisfree/2020/apr/20/the-global-pandemic-has-spawned-new-forms-of-activism-and-theyre-flourishing

Chenoweth, E., Shay, C. W. (2019). The NAVCO data project. Harvard Dataverse, https://dataverse.harvard.edu/dataverse/navco.

Chenoweth, E., & Stephan, M. J. (2011). *Why civil resistance works: The strategic logic of nonviolent conflict.* Columbia University Press.

Chiozza, G., & King, J. (2022a). Introduction to a special issue on beyond complacency and acrimony: Studying human rights in a post-COVID-19 world. *Journal of Human Rights, 21*(3), 245.

Chiozza, G., & King, J. (2022b). The state of human rights in a (post) COVID-19 world. *Journal of Human Rights, 21*(3), 246–262.

Clay, K. C. (2022). The effect of the COVID-19 pandemic on human rights practices: Findings from the Human Rights Measurement Initiative's 2021 Practitioner Survey. *Journal of Human Rights, 21*(3), 317–333.

Daraghi, B. (2020). How Algeria's regime used coronavirus to crush a revolution, *Independent*, 14 July 2020, https://www.independent.co.uk/independentpremium/world/algeriacoronavirus-protests-regime-government-a9618936.html.

DeBlock, A., & Ognenovska, S. (2022). COVID-19 Civic Freedom Tracker. Special Report, International Center for Not-for-Profit Law, Washington, DC.

Eligon, J. (2021). Racial double standard of Capitol Police draws outcry. *New York Times*, 7 January 2021, https://www.nytimes.com/2021/01/07/us/capitol-trump-mob-black-lives-matter.html.

Gerbaudo, P. (2020). The pandemic crowd: Protest in the time of Covid-19. *Journal of International Affairs, 73*(2), 61–76.

Gohdes, A. (2015). When Internet access becomes a weapon. *Washington Post*, February 25. https://www.washingtonpost.com/news/monkey-cage/wp/2015/02/24/internet-access-as-a-weapon/?utm_term=.b77fe28eb6fd

Guntisky, S. (2015). Corrupting the cyber-commons: Social media as a tool of autocratic resilience. *Perspectives on Politics, 13* (1), 42–45.

Haggard, S., & Kauffman, R. (2016). *Dictators and democrats: Masses, elites, and regime change.* Princeton University Press.

Hertel, S., Buerger, C., & Carbonetti, B. (2020). Introduction to a special issue on human rights in the time of COVID-19. *Journal of Human Rights, 19* (5), 519–519. doi:10.1080/14754835.2020.1830615

Koo, J.-W. (2022). Global perceptions of South Korea's COVID-19 policy responses: Topic modeling with tweets. *Journal of Human Rights, 21*(3), 334–353.

Kowalewski, M. (2020). Street protests in times of COVID-19: Adjusting tactics and marching "as usual." *Social Movement Studies.* 10.1080/14742837.2020.1843014?src=recsys

Libal, K., & Kashwan, P. (2020). Solidarity in times of crisis. *Journal of Human Rights, 19* (5), 537–546. doi:10.1080/14754835.2020.1830046

Lührmann, A., & Lindberg, S. (2019). A third wave of autocratization is here. *Democratization, 26*(7), 1095–1113. doi:10.1080/13510347.2019.1582029

Maerz, S. F., Lührmann, A., Hellmeier, S., Grahn, S., & Lindberg, S. I. (2020). State of the world 2019: Autocratization surges – Resistance grows. *Democratization, 27* (6), 909–927. doi:10.1080/13510347.2020.1758670

Mampilly, Z. (2021). Protests are taking over the world: What's driving them? *New York Times*, 3 October 2021, https://www.nytimes.com/2021/10/03/opinion/covid-protests-world-whats-driving-them.html

Metternich, N. (2020). Drawback before the wave? Protest decline during the Covid-19 pandemic. (SocArXiv, 2020), SocArXiv, https://files.osf.io/v1/resources/3ej72/providers/osfstorage/5eb1538962d4ab01396c7536?action=download&direct&version=2.

Murdie, A. (2022). Hindsight is 2020: Lessons from the COVID-19 pandemic for future human rights research. *Journal of Human Rights, 21*(3), 354–364.

Ortiz, I., Burke, S., Berrada, M., & Saenz Cortés, H. (2022). *World protests: A study of key protest issues in the 21st Century.* Routledge.

Petz, D. (2021). Why the far-right's use of nonviolent action should be questioned. *Waging Nonviolence,* 5 October 2021. https://wagingnonviolence.org/2021/10/why-far-right-use-nonviolent-action-should-be-questioned/

Pinckney, J. (2020a). *From dissent to democracy: The promise and perils of civil resistance transitions.* Oxford University Press.

Pinckney, J. (2020b). Amid coronavirus, online activism confronts digital authoritarianism, United States Institute of Peace, 28 April 2020, https://www.usip.org/publications/2020/04/amidcoronavirus-online-activism-confronts-digital-authoritarianism.

Pinckney, J., & Rivers, M. (2020a). Sickness or silence: Social movement adaptation to COVID-19. *Journal of International Affairs, 73* (2), 23–42.

Pinckney, J., Rivers, M. (2020b). Nonviolent action in the time of coronavirus. United States Institute of Peace, 25 March 2020, https://www.usip.org/publications/2020/03/nonviolent-actiontime-coronavirus.

Pleyers, G. (2020). The pandemic is a battlefield: Social movements in the COVID-19 lockdown. *Journal of Civil Society, 16* (4), 295–312. doi:10.1080/17448689.2020.1794398

Pressman, J., Choi-Fitzpatrick, A. (2020). Covid19 and protest repertoires in the United States: An initial description of limited change. *Social Movement Studies* 10.1080/14742837.2020.1860743.

Randle, M. (1994). *Civil resistance.* Fontana.

Ritter, D. (2015). *The iron cage of liberalism.* Oxford University Press.

Roth, K. (2020). How authoritarians are exploiting the Covid-19 crisis to grab power. *Human Rights Watch, 3*, 15.

Schock, K. (2015). *Civil resistance today.* Polity Press.

Sikkink, K. (2020). Solidarity key to post-COVID19 response. *Open Global Rights*, 28 April. [Online]. Retrieved August 13, 2020, from https://www.openglobalrights.org/solidarity-key-to-post-covid-19-response/?lang=English.

Smithey, L., & Kurtz, L. (2018). Smart repression. In Smithey and Kurtz , eds., *The Paradox of repression and social movements.* Syracuse University Press.

Snowden, F. (2019). *Epidemics and society: From the Black Plague to Ebola.* Yale University Press.

Sykes, E. (2020). How to protest in a pandemic [Online]. Retrieved August 13, 2020, from https://www.aclu.org/news/free-speech/how-to-protest-in-a-pandemic/.

Theidon, K. (2020). A forecasted failure: Intersectionality, COVID-19, and the perfect storm. *Journal of Human Rights, 19*(5), 528–536. doi:10.1080/14754835.2020.1822156

The COVID-19 pandemic and authoritarian consolidation in North Africa

Sammy Z. Badran and Brian Turnbull

ABSTRACT

Since the Arab Spring, North Africa has witnessed increased levels of authoritarianism and a general decline in human rights as authoritarian regimes have consolidated power. During the COVID-19 pandemic, regimes across the region have instituted greater restrictions on public gatherings in order to curb the spread of the virus, and some have used the pandemic to enhance powers and crush dissent. This article will investigate if these two phenomena are connected. Is the expansion of emergency powers and surveillance designed to primarily support public health, or is this emergency legislation designed to provide greater authoritarian power for regimes under the guise of fighting the pandemic? We find that considerable actions taken by these regimes were not solely designed to support public health, and instead have been exploited to curb dissent. The potential detrimental impact this expansion could have on human rights across the region could be severe. We compare emergency legislation in Morocco and Egypt since the beginning of the COVID-19 pandemic. Our analysis provides systematic insight into how authoritarian regimes respond to public health crises and details how these crises can be used by regimes facing contentious political action to quell dissent.

Introduction

On April 26, 2021, Deputy Interior Minister Noureddine Boutayeb addressed the Moroccan House of Representatives on the government's response to the COVID-19 pandemic over the past year. As a demonstration of the effectiveness of this response, he proudly noted that more than 5,700 people had been arrested per day for the violation of the "health emergency law." Over the course of a year, this amounted to an astonishing 1.5 million arrests (Odour, 2021). No small feat even for a well-consolidated autocracy, but Morocco had been continually praised internationally both before and during the pandemic for its notable achievements in the protection of human rights (Abouzzohour, 2020a).

However, this announcement would not have been a surprise to the many Moroccan social movements, whose demonstrators had been regularly harassed for defying social distancing and lockdown measures. Governments across the globe have instituted greater restrictions on public gatherings in the name of fighting the pandemic, and states have used these enhanced powers to restrict public demonstrations, consolidate power, and quell dissent. According to prodemocracy activists in Hong Kong, China used the COVID-19 crisis as a "golden opportunity" to justify its harsh crackdown on the prodemocracy movement in Hong Kong (Davidson, 2020). We see similar observations in North Africa. Since the end of the Arab Spring, Morocco and Egypt have witnessed increased levels of authoritarianism, a general decline in human rights, and the strengthening of autocratic power.

These cases raise important questions. Is the expansion of emergency powers and surveillance across North Africa primarily designed to support public health, or is it designed to provide greater authoritarian power for regimes under the cover of fighting the pandemic? As two very different authoritarian regimes, the cases of Morocco and Egypt help us answer these questions, as both have faced accusations of increased authoritarianism and curtailing of opposition since the beginning of the pandemic. Moreover, Morocco offers us a unique insight into how liberalizing authoritarian regimes use the pandemic to consolidate power, whereas Egypt serves as an example of an unpopular yet highly consolidated autocracy using the pandemic to normalize repressive measures domestically.

According to the EIU Democracy Index, Morocco currently ranks as the most democratic regime of North Africa with exception to Tunisia, the region's only liberal democracy (Economist Intelligence Unit, 2020). On the other hand, the EIU Democracy Index ranks Egypt as the least democratic regime, with the exception to Libya (which is mired in civil war).[1] Therefore, in order to better understand the effects of COVID-19 on authoritarian states in North Africa, we focus on Morocco and Egypt as the most stable authoritarian governments in the region, while also providing contrast on the democracy scales.

Overall, we find that Egypt and Morocco have been using the pandemic as a means to consolidate power. In both cases, the regime enacted and enforced recommendations provided by the World Health Organization (WHO) to protect their citizens during the pandemic. However, both regimes have also gone far beyond WHO recommendations in the expansion of surveillance and arrest powers. In the name of limiting the spread of the virus and combatting misinformation, both regimes have implemented powerful and intrusive surveillance structures alongside extensive arrest campaigns. Overall, pandemics of such a scale offer a significant window of opportunity for authoritarian regimes to consolidate power with a relatively lower risk of meaningful international and domestic pushback. This is not new, as scholars in this special issue have pointed out how the pandemic can be used to consolidate power or curtail human rights (Chiozza and King 2022). In the cases of Morocco and Egypt, despite a heavy rollback of personal freedom and civil protections, the international community has not unilaterally condemned these actions. The pandemic has also demonstrated to these regimes that, during health crises, they can act to consolidate power while also generally preserving their domestic approval, as long as those actions are perceived as supporting public health. We expect that these lessons not only will be internalized by the regimes examined in this analysis but will also be incorporated by fellow autocrats looking to upgrade their own authoritarian toolkits.

Authoritarian upgrading

Authoritarian regimes regularly seek out opportunities to upgrade and consolidate power. Heydemann and Leenders (2011) demonstrated that diffusion, or social learning, can occur among regimes and lead to "authoritarian resilience." During the Arab Spring, authoritarian regimes learned from each other, and often used these lessons to more effectively repress and demobilize protests. Regimes like those in Morocco or Algeria learned from preceding waves of protests in Tunisia and Egypt, and strategically responded to street protests using reforms and limited repression, such as early general elections and a partial devolution of power to the parliament in Morocco followed by limited bouts of repression (Badran, 2021). This diffusion of effective strategies led to authoritarian upgrading and consolidation.

A similar claim can be made for how authoritarian regimes, in the Middle East/North Africa (MENA) region and beyond, have learned from each other to consolidate power. Alrababa'h and Blaydes (2021) built on the well-established finding that authoritarian regimes engage in diversionary conflicts and "diversionary threat rhetoric" via regime-controlled media outlets to deflect attention away from domestic issues (like the economy). Chiozza and Goemans (2011) also found that leaders who anticipate being forcibly removed from office are more likely to engage in diversionary conflict. Even in Morocco, where civil society has been historically relatively free, the regime has regularly sought out opportunities to strengthen its power (Cavatorta, 2009; Zartman, 2015). Clay et al. (2022), Murdie (2022), and Brysk (2022) have all highlighted the interconnectedness and interdependence of human rights, and this implies that the curtailing of one human right affects others. Emergency measures enacted to limit freedom of movement directly curtail freedom of assembly. On a similar note, Chenoweth (2022), found that lockdowns following the pandemic led to an immediate recognition by nonviolent human rights advocates that freedom of assembly, press, expression, movement, and privacy would also be violated.

The literature has documented how regimes use crises (war or mass uprisings) and even liberalization (Morocco's vibrant civil society) as opportunities to consolidate power. We should view the COVID-19 pandemic in a similar light. We know that authoritarian governments globally have used pandemic responses to further consolidate their power via repression (Barceló et al. 2020). The pandemic has presented regimes, both democratic and authoritarian, with the ability to strengthen their surveillance capabilities via digital contact-tracing programs originally designed to restrict the spread of COVID-19 but also used to curtail dissent (Eck and Hatz 2020; Liu and Zhao 2021). The case of the 2019–2020 Hong Kong protests demonstrated how the state could use the pandemic to effectively crush dissent using disease control regulations to restrict political public gatherings (Ismangil and Lee 2021).

Chenoweth (2022) has argued that, although mobilization has continued throughout the pandemic, the success rates of the mass movements have declined. An example of this trend is the Algerian case, where the state has used the pandemic to accelerate prosecution of Hirak activists (Lahbib 2020). Similarly, Morocco has used the pandemic to control dissident voices online. Indeed, Chenoweth (2022) highlighted that mass movements are less successful in part due to "smart repression" techniques through digital repression and emergency measures the pandemic has encouraged.

Even democracies have been accused of democratic backsliding during the pandemic. The Hungarian Parliament was criticized by human rights organizations for passing the "COVID-19 Protection Act," an emergency law that allows for indefinite rule by decree (Hungarian Helsinki Committee 2020), and a historical analysis of past pandemics in the United States demonstrates that such crises have been used regularly to consolidate state power (Witt 2020).

The discussion on the appropriateness of pandemic control measures, given their dual-use function for regimes also seeking to repress political opposition, is further highlighted by the discussion over the ability of democracies to protect their citizens. Cepaluni et al. (2021) found that democratic states experienced a higher death rate during the pandemic than less democratic states. Alon et al. (2020) demonstrated that authoritarian regimes were more likely to initially cover up the emergence of the virus, although they agreed with Frey et al. (2020) that these same regimes tended to impose more effective lockdown and contact-tracing programs than democracies. Yao et al. (2021) revealed that democracies were not able to respond to the pandemic as quickly as autocrats and this led to higher initial death rates than nondemocracies. These slower responses were likely due to the effectiveness of democratic institutions in restricting the ability of the regimes to rapidly implement heavy-handed population control (Cheibub et al. 2020). These considerations should be kept in mind during our discussion on the violation of human rights by the Moroccan and Egyptian regimes. Spadaro (2020) has argued that effective pandemic control measures often require the temporary curtailment of freedoms, but they can be balanced with the protection of human rights if appropriate limitations are placed on regime action. Still, our discussion demonstrates the lack of a clear line and a general preference by the international community for pandemic control over the protection of human rights.

Methods

Across these examples, we see considerable evidence that regimes have used the outbreak of the COVID-19 pandemic to pass legislation that curtails human rights. These emergency powers have been justified as necessary for public health, but cursory examination indicates that significant portions of these laws do not support public health and are, instead, designed specifically to curb dissent. The potential detrimental impact this expansion could have on human rights across the region could be severe. Many authoritarian regimes across the region are likely looking at these cases as models on how to restrict public dissent without drawing criticism from human rights groups.

To investigate this dynamic, we conduct a comparative analysis of the emergency law packages passed in Egypt and Morocco from the beginning of the COVID-19 pandemic in March 2020 through the beginning of the international vaccine rollout in January 2021. This comparative analysis separates emergency legislation and regime actions into their core constituent parts, and then categorizes each part as either likely supportive of public health during a pandemic or likely not supportive. Our criteria for categorizing a part as supportive of public health was based on WHO guidelines. The WHO issued extensive advice throughout 2020 to governments on how best to curb the spread of COVID-19. As long as aspects of these emergency laws follow WHO guidelines, those parts are categorized as supportive. We then discuss in more detail why the parts were categorized as either supportive or not supportive of public health, and whether or not those parts also provided opportunity for authoritarian upgrading. Table 1 lists the guidelines used in this analysis.

We start the analysis with a chronological review of key events and legislation in each case, then progress into a comparative analysis on the design of these emergency laws in light of the guidelines. This is followed by a complementary discussion on how these laws have been enforced in practice with a focus on effective pandemic control along with regime overreach, and a critical review of divergent international responses, along with notable domestic support for both regimes. We conclude with a systematic comparison across the cases and discuss how regimes design emergency laws during times of crises with a focus on how they can use the immediate need to respond to a pandemic to also accomplish political repression goals.

Emergency law structure

Morocco

Since independence and prior to the pandemic Morocco had implemented an emergency law (state of exception—Article 35) only once. King Hassan II used the law to quell student protests

Table 1. COVID-19 guidelines.

1. Country-level coordination	Activation of a national public health emergency management system to coordinate key ministries.
2. Risk communication	Communicate with the public on what COVID-19 is, along with transparency on the rationale for restrictions on movement and actions to reduce COVID-19's spread.
3. Surveillance	Locating infections and points of high risk, alongside cataloging health resources and facilities. WHO recommends encouraging self-surveillance and reporting among the general population.
4. Points of entry	Regulating and surveilling points of entry by screening arriving and departing travelers, among other measures.
5. Infection prevention	Providing guidance on the need for protective measures, isolation, social distancing, minimizing crowds, and the targeted closing of schools, public transit, and workplaces when needed. These measures should be spread via key civil society and religious groups to encourage buy-in.
6. Maintain essential services	Health systems must be prioritized, but critical governmental, economic, and societal functions must be balanced and maintained alongside to ensure society can withstand the pandemic.

and an armed insurgency in 1965. Following five years of state violence against dissidents, known as the "Years of Lead," the king ended the state of exception, "because it was unpopular in the international community and damaged his prestige" (Tamburini 2021: 8). Tamburini (2021: 8) highlighted how King Hassan II skillfully lifted the state of exception to call for a constitutional referendum that, through "pressure from authorities" and "illegal circumstances," passed with 98.7 percent voting "yes" for the new constitution. This essentially allowed the king to concentrate power with the regime at the expense of parliament and did not tarnish his international image.

Morocco experienced mass protests both prior to and after the beginning of the pandemic. In contrast to much of the Middle East/North Africa (MENA) region, Morocco has historically made relative strides in human rights. For instance, Morocco was hailed as a leader in women's rights by passing one of the most progressive family law codes in the region. Moreover, Morocco was noted for its overwhelmingly concessionary and reformist stance to protests during the Arab Spring (Badran 2021). However, since the Rif Hirak Movement of 2016, the king has resorted to increased repression, and human rights in the country have deteriorated over the past several years, alongside increasing harassment of journalists and regime critics. Leaders of the Rif Hirak Movement have faced long prison sentences, journalists have been arrested and accused of being involved in the Rif Hirak Movement, and activists have had their phones and computers targeted by sophisticated spyware (Amnesty International 2020c).

In response to the emergence of COVID-19, the state of emergency in Morocco began with an emergency declaration by the Ministry of the Interior on March 19, 2020, and was later approved by the upper house of the Moroccan Parliament on May 8. Morocco's implementation of the emergency law (Decree Law No. 2.20.293) is notable given its specific focus on health. The state of emergency is generally referred to as a "state of health emergency," tying the law directly to the COVID-19 pandemic. Second, the emergency law is short, at only two pages, and vague, likely deliberately (Moroccan Parliament 2020). Here is a brief summary of the individual articles within the law:

1. Grants the government the ability to enforce the state of emergency when the health and safety of citizens are threatened.
2. Tasks the Ministries of the Interior and Health with carrying out the provisions of the state of emergency and enable the extension of the state of emergency.
3. Enables the government to use all necessary measures and means to protect the health and safety of citizens.
4. Declares violations of the law as punishable by fines and imprisonment from one to three months. Violations are specifically stated to include incitement of others through speech and other means of public distribution.
5. Broadens the government's ability to take any economic, financial, or social measures deemed necessary in the state of emergency.
6. The powers granted under the state of emergency will continue until the declared emergency is lifted.

Given the brevity and vague nature of the emergency law, how the government specifically used these broad powers is more relevant for analysis than the language within the law itself. Beginning in March 2020, the Moroccan government started taking steps to address the emerging COVID-19 pandemic. This began with a suspension of sea travel with Italy, the first European country to experience an outbreak. Over the following week, the Moroccan government continued implementing additional restrictions: international flights were suspended, schools and mosques were closed nationwide, and citizens were asked to dramatically curtail movement outside of the home.

With the declaration of a state of health emergency in March 2020, the Ministry of the Interior placed restrictions on movement, including a nightly curfew enforced by the military. The statement notified citizens that social gatherings were banned, and a permit was required to leave the house for nearly any activity, even going to work, shopping for groceries, or receiving medical care, with exceptions given to workers deemed essential. When the state of emergency was later approved by the Moroccan Parliament in May, accompanying monetary fines and penalties of up to three months' imprisonment were added. These measures were kept in place and strongly enforced until the Ministries of Health and of the Interior began a staged gradual exit from lockdown in June 2020. The government reversed this process at several points by reimposing travel restrictions on select cities when cases spiked.

Notably, despite the easing of the lockdown, the state of emergency itself has been extended multiple times and continues to be in effect as of September 2021 (Kasraoui 2020b, 2021). Alongside restrictions, government ministries took a number of measures to support businesses and individuals affected both by the virus itself and the resulting lockdown. In April, the military built a field hospital to host COVID-19 patients, the Ministry of Education established a website to host remote classes while schools were suspended, and international tourists were largely repatriated back to their home countries. A number of support programs were instituted by the government to provide support for families in need of food, shelter for the homeless, and stipends for workers in both the formal and informal economies who had lost their pay (Kasraoui 2020b).

Morocco has been combating misinformation and purported "fake news" concerning the pandemic since March 2020, when a social media personality with a large following was arrested for claiming that the pandemic was a hoax. Moreover, a unified Friday sermon was given by mosques across the country to encourage measures to curb the spread of the virus, officials with loudspeakers driving through the streets gave lockdown instructions, and the public prosecutor instructed courts nationwide to take action against fake news and a number of arrests followed.

On March 19, 2020, the government received backlash from civil society when it attempted to pass legislation (Draft Law 22.20) that would have enabled state-owned/affiliated telecommunication companies to restrict content and false information. The law governed access to information online, particularly on social media, and essentially allowed internet service providers to act as informants for the government. The Euro-Mediterranean Human Rights Monitor, a Geneva-based Human Rights NGO, reported that the law legitimized censorship and restricted freedom of expression (Euro-Mediterranean Human Rights Monitor 2020). The report also criticized the vague language used in the law that could easily be expanded to justify further restrictions on civil society. For instance, the law proposed to criminalize "fake news" without outlining what was deemed accurate or false. The legislation was so controversial that many publicly called on the ministers who introduced the bill to step down, and a petition to reject the amendment was signed by more than 25,000 Moroccans (Hekking 2020). Some claimed that the failed legislation, which could still be reintroduced, was an attempt to limit freedom of speech online and quell opposition voices under the guise of combating misinformation related to COVID-19.

Similar to Egypt's emergency "health" amendments, Morocco's draft legislation included many amendments that did not have an explicit public health focus. For instance, one article enabled the executive to arrest anyone who called for boycotting goods or services, and another stipulated jail time or a fine for sharing false information or undermining public order (Article 19 2020).

Regardless, under the existing emergency law, the General Directorate of National Security (DGSN) significantly enhanced its ability to track individuals. Anyone who wanted to go outside the home under lockdown had to request an exceptional movement permit using a smartphone app, Wiqaytna, that tracks individual movement. When downloaded, the app follows the user as they pass through police checkpoints and present a permit and ID number. The DGSN reported that the app was downloaded millions of times and used more than 400,000 times by May 2020 alone. Reportedly, the app was used to also track state of emergency violations to the DGSN, which then used the data to modify the implementation of restrictions across the country. The government's considerably enhanced ability to track citizens, alongside the large number of arrests and targeting of journalists, led to extensive criticism from several human rights groups. However, much of this criticism was countered by continued international praise for Morocco's COVID-19 response (Kasraoui 2020b).

Egypt

In contrast to Morocco, historically in Egypt the use of emergency laws to restrict dissent and curtail human rights has been the rule and not the exception. Emergency powers have been a routine part of Egyptian politics since 1958. Law 162 was enacted in 1958 and has been used since to arrest and imprison opposition members—without warrant—and intimidate participants in unapproved protests (Ghonim 2012). More recently, emergency powers were used to justify crackdowns during and after the Egyptian Revolution of 2011. Prodemocracy activists in Egypt have challenged the emergency law since the early 2000s and called for its abolishment in the years leading up to the Egyptian Revolution (Badran 2014).

Given that the emergency law was one of the main contentions of protestors in 2011, the law has since been more selectively and intermittently enforced in response, sometimes only for specific areas in Egypt. However, following a terrorist attack against Coptic churches in April 2017, President Sisi issued a decree to reinstitute the emergency law, which has been continuously renewed every three months since, with the parliament rubber-stamping the renewal annually (Ellaboudy 2020).

Since taking power in 2013, President Sisi has also expanded the role of the military in Egypt. Most notably, in 2014 Sisi issued a decree (Law No. 136) that placed public facilities under military control and therefore allows state prosecutors to "to refer any crimes at those places to their military counterparts, paving the way for further military trials of civilians" (Human Rights Watch 2014). This essentially allowed military courts to try protestors who illegally demonstrated in public areas. The expansion of military jurisdiction through the emergency law had been done before, but since 2014, "the new law greatly expands the jurisdiction of military courts, giving them their widest legal authority since the birth of Egypt's modern republic in 1952" (Human Rights Watch 2014). This created a powerful enforcement mechanism for the emergency law in Egypt, as protestors can be fast-tracked to the military courts, where they face fewer protections and stiffer penalties than they would in civilian courts.

Given the well-established precedent for emergency law, the Egyptian Parliament had a strong legislative foundation to build on following the outbreak of COVID-19 cases in Egypt. On April 21, 2020, parliament granted Sisi sweeping powers to curb the COVID-19 outbreak by amending the existing emergency law (Law 162 of 1958). The existing law had provisions that enabled extensive governmental restrictions on public demonstrations, but the new amendments, passed under Law No. 22 of 2020 (Egyptian Parliament 2020), greatly expanded the reach of the emergency law (Ali & Fakhry 2020; Al Watan News 2020). A summary of the key amendments in the 2020 law is presented below:

Amendments to Article 2:

1. The addition of Clauses 7 and 8 allows the government to shut down educational institutions and public offices to curb the spread of the virus.
2. Clauses 9, 10, 11, and 12 offer Egyptians an opportunity to delay or modify payments on their taxes, utilities, and other public services.
3. Clauses 13 and 14 prohibit public gatherings and demonstrations, which was applied even prior to the pandemic, and mandate a quarantine for those entering the country (Raghavan 2014).
4. Clauses 15, 16, and 17 give the government the ability to restrict the export, sale, possession, and price of unspecified goods.

5. Clauses 18, 19, 20, and 23 task the government with facilitating the collection and distribution of donations, financial assistance, and other support for individuals, families, the economic sector, and the healthcare system.
6. Clauses 21 and 22 grant the president discretion to require private hospitals and other medical centers to provide and fully staff their healthcare services, as well as impose additional restrictions on the scientific use of biological materials and waste.
7. Clause 24 allows public schools, centers, and business to be converted into temporary field hospitals.

Additionally, amendments to Article 4:

1. grant the president the power to shift jurisdiction for violations of the entire emergency law to military prosecutors;
2. clarify that public prosecutors have exclusive jurisdiction over the final result of investigations under the emergency law, as long as they do not violate the powers of the military prosecutors; and
3. specify the addition of military officers to the court tasked with adjudicating violations of the emergency law.

Although more specific and detailed than the Moroccan emergency law, the Egyptian modifications also intentionally provide significant space for interpretation when implemented by the regime. Therefore, again it is critical to analyze how the government put these new powers into practice. The next section delves into both the Moroccan and Egyptian emergency laws and compares them to the WHO recommendations.

Adherence to WHO guidelines

As noted, given the lack of detail within the emergency law itself, analysis of Morocco's use of emergency law in response to the pandemic must focus on the actions taken by the government under the authority granted by the emergency law. In general, most actions taken by the regime under the state of emergency followed WHO recommendations. Shutting down points of entry, the banning of all social gatherings, and permit requirements to leave the house were strict but largely fell within WHO guidance under Recommendation 4: Points of Entry and Recommendation 5: Infection Prevention. The government took a comprehensive approach to both support the healthcare system and keep the public informed by relying on multiple ministries, even the military, following Recommendation 1: Country-Level Coordination and Recommendation 6: Maintain Essential Services.

Where Morocco significantly deviates from WHO guidance falls under Recommendation 2: Risk Communication and Recommendation 3: Surveillance. The WHO strongly emphasizes the importance of strong lines of communication with the public to improve knowledge, encourage safer practices, and combat the spread of misinformation. As has been the global trend, laws passed to combat "fake news" are conveniently used to shut down the free press, particularly the more critical media outlets (Lees 2018).

During the pandemic, the Moroccan government used the emergency law to arrest individuals who claimed the pandemic was a hoax alongside the arrest of journalists who criticized the government's pandemic response (Amnesty International 2020a). Still, the government also informed the public on best practices to curb the spread of the virus via multiple outlets, such as Friday sermons and even loudspeakers in the street.

The WHO also recommends surveillance of citizens to ensure authorities can follow, and take actions against, the spread of the virus. This, unsurprisingly, opens the door to authoritarian exploitation. Based on the reportedly high use of the agency's tracking app, the DGSN designed a fairly effective means of tracking citizens. The incorporation of the permit system into the app was a clever means of improving public acceptance, as it appears that if individuals wanted to leave their homes, they had to use the app, because that was how they obtained and used the permit. This system received criticism from several human rights groups; but, given the tracking app's incorporation into social distancing enforcement, it is difficult to effectively argue that it went against WHO recommendations.

In the case of Egypt, many of the amendments instituted in 2020 resemble restrictions implemented by most governments during the pandemic: for instance, delaying tax payments and utilities payments, shutting down schools and public offices, and mandating a quarantine for those entering the country. These provisions were used to enact a partial lockdown from April through May of 2020; however, after June 2020, restaurants, stores, and cafes were opened with limited capacity (Mandour 2020). Along with the power to prohibit public gatherings, these measures generally meet WHO Recommendation 4: Points of Entry and Recommendation 5: Infection Prevention. Requiring healthcare centers to stay open and active during the pandemic, along with restricting the flow of goods and services, is broadly construed to fit Recommendation 6: Maintain Essential Services, as is the power to convert public places into field hospitals and the responsibility to coordinate financial support for affected individuals and institutions across society.

Simultaneously, these same provisions give the president significant leeway in targeting lockdowns, which enabled Sisi to clamp down on public activity in general, especially demonstrations. Notably, the prohibition on public gatherings and demonstrations applies even when there is not a public health emergency (Raghavan 2020). Most prominent are the addition of considerable judicial powers to the military in enforcing the emergency law. As with the Moroccan case, although the government could argue that these enhanced powers enable better surveillance of the infected following Recommendation 3, nothing in the WHO recommendation encourages an expansion to this degree, especially by the military. In contrast, the WHO actually recommends self-surveillance and reporting by citizens themselves as the most effective means of quickly ramping up an effective surveillance program, along with reliance on key civil society and religious groups to both monitor and communicate with the public (World Health Organization 2006).

Expectedly, multiple human rights organizations in Egypt have condemned the rollbacks on civilian judicial independence and the increased involvement of the military (Al Jazeera Arabic 2020). Most concerning to these organizations is the expansion of the emergency law allowing the military and its judicial officers to arrest and detain citizens, or even confiscate their property, without permission from the civilian court (special prosecutor's office; see Khalid 2020). Critically, these provisions are also not limited to the pandemic timeframe. These expansions enable the president to use military prosecutors to investigate and enforce the emergency law wherever and whenever it is applied. Civilians accused of crimes under this process often lose the right to stand before a civilian judge. Instead, the amendment forms an Emergency High Court for State Security staffed primarily by military judges. These changes give the president more control over the judicial process via the military, while "simultaneously undermining the civil and constitutional rights granted by the Egyptian constitution," which specifically states that civilians cannot be tried in a military court unless the crime targeted the military directly (Khalid 2020, para. 3). The degree to which each regime has been willing to put these expanded powers into practice are discussed in the next section.

Enforcement

Emergency measures were arguably used effectively to combat the pandemic in Morocco. Lockdown measures, closing borders, and social distancing were strong and are credited with lower infection and mortality rates from March 2020 onward (Abouzzohour 2020). Morocco has also led Africa in terms of vaccination rates (Drissi Bourhanbour and Ouchetto 2021). The rollout of the vaccine was praised by the international community and, as of April 2021, Morocco placed tenth globally in terms of vaccinations *per capita* (Abouzzohour 2020).

Early on, the government emphasized lockdown enforcement under the state of emergency. The police and military presence across the country was substantial, with military vehicles tasked with enforcing the state of emergency visible across neighborhoods. Despite restrictions, just two days after the emergency law was passed, Islamists flooded the streets of Morocco's major cities to protest the new measures (Kasraoui 2020c). However, authorities responded quickly with the new powers granted by the emergency law. Immediately following the emergency announcement in March 2020, five individuals were arrested in Fez for encouraging public demonstrations. Moroccan authorities soon expanded the targets of the emergency law beyond protestors. Soon after the arrests in Fez, the DGSN began investigating a nurse who recorded and shared allegations that the pandemic was worsening in Boujdour under the state of emergency's criminalization of misinformation sharing. Even a notable Moroccan YouTuber, "Mi Naima," was arrested and sentenced to one year in prison for spreading misinformation and encouraging people to not follow lockdown orders and preventive measures.

Activists and civil society organizations have also been targeted by this provision in Morocco. Authorities generally cite provisions within the emergency law that purportedly ban "offending public institutions" and "spreading false information" (Amnesty International 2020a). Amnesty International noted that popular citizen journalists with large social media followings have also been arrested. Most notably, Omar Naji, a local Rif leader of Morocco's largest human rights NGO, *l'Association Marocaine des Droits de l'Homme* (AMDH), was also arrested and prosecuted for spreading "false allegations and lies" (Kacha 2020).

Moreover, the Moroccan Association for Human Rights (AMDH), the country's most prominent human rights NGO, has been targeted. For instance, the organization's vice president was charged with defamation after challenging the targeting of street merchants by authorities in the city of Nador, and fellow AMDH member Siham el-Makrini was arrested in May of 2020 following a social media critique on the lack of government support for teachers' rights and charged with incitement (Freedom House Morocco 2021).

Since 2019, teachers' unions have frequently engaged in contentious politics and have often faced police repression. Roughly 15,000 members of teachers' unions took to the streets on March 15, 2021, and faced forced dispersion by police water cannons (Education International 2021). Similar demonstrations occurred on April 6–7, 2021. According to Amnesty International, 33 demonstrators were arbitrarily arrested and charged with "violating the health emergency law, as well as harming and insulting law enforcement officers," and two demonstrators were charged with "breaking the health emergency statutes law relating to Covid-19" (Amnesty International 2021a).

As an illustration of how intently Moroccan authorities have implemented the emergency law, arrest counts for violating the state of health emergency soared in the months following the imposition of lockdown, with more than 50,000 arrested in March and April 2020 alone, including at least five journalists (Kasraoui 2020a). Over 50% of these led to actual prosecutions, with the government even detaining more than 3,000 of these individuals until their court dates. Public statements from the Moroccan Interior Ministry noted that more than 1.5 million people have been arrested for lockdown breaches from July 2020 to April 2021, with 18 percent of those arrested facing trails (225,000 trials; see Odour 2021). Moreover, at least 30 activists were arrested for breaking the health emergency law and sentenced with jail terms (Karam 2020). Notably, despite the high number of arrests and significant curtailment of civil liberties early in the pandemic, the majority of citizens supported the arrest of those who publicly violated the emergency measures (Kasraoui 2020a).

As in Morocco, Egypt's quick response to the pandemic was arguably effective. Lockdown and social distancing measures were quickly implemented, and the government launched an online portal with a support center that effectively communicated pandemic-related information to the public. Additionally, a 24-hour hotline and phone app were made available for COVID-19-related information (Beschel 2021). In August 2020, cases dropped significantly throughout the country to around 200 cases a day before rising again in January 2021. The country also relies on a Chinese-made vaccine, Sinovac, which it imports and nationally produces. The WHO praised Egypt for producing over a million doses and planning to vaccinate 40 million citizens by the end of 2021 (Ahram Online 2021).

The emergency law has similarly been put to significant use; however, in contrast to Morocco, the pandemic did not mark as dramatic of an increase in arrests. But Egyptian authorities had been using the emergency extensively law to target opposition well before the pandemic. In 2019, various human rights organizations condemned Egypt's escalation in nationwide arrests of activists in what Amnesty International labeled a "chilling escalation" of crackdown on civil society (*BBC News* 2020b). Late September 2019 saw the largest wave of mass arrests since Sisi came into power, with more than 2,300 arrests of peaceful protestors, journalists, politicians, and activists (Amnesty International 2019). Executions of activists, many of whom are charged with terrorism, has also increased drastically since 2019 (Magdi 2021). After the pandemic began, arrests continued. Doctors and healthcare workers who criticized the regime's handling of the pandemic, specifically for lack of protective gear for healthcare workers, were charged with spreading false news or terrorism (Amnesty International 2020b) and even accused by the regime of being Muslim Brotherhood affiliates (Mandour 2020). As of July 2020, several NGOs estimated that at least 500 people had been arrested, including 11 journalists (Mandour 2020).

As of July 2021, the 2017 emergency law had been renewed 16 times. Egypt's emergency laws historically have been justified under the pretext of terrorism (as in 2017); however, the pandemic offered the regime a new public health pretext. As with terrorism, the pandemic has been used to expand presidential and military control. It is important to note that the pandemic, therefore, is not a critical juncture for the Egyptian consolidation of power but, rather, a continuation of authoritarian consolidation that began in 2014. The primary opportunity presented by the pandemic for the Egyptian regime is the ability to portray the continued use of the emergency law as necessary for public health in an attempt to shore up domestic support for the historically unpopular law. For example, since March 2020, various news websites and social media accounts have been blocked for spreading false news and one prominent Egyptian activist, Sanaa Seif, was sentenced to 18 months in prison for allegedly spreading "fake news" (Associated Press 2021). However, the laws and media regulatory bodies used to regulate the media were created in 2017 with parliamentary approval. Only the justification has changed.

Response

We know that international actors can encourage greater respect of human rights within authoritarian regimes by making the citizens of these regimes more aware of government abuse (Gruffydd-Jones 2019; Risse et al. 1999). Image matters as well. Scholars have noted how international image matters for authoritarian leaders and that a positive image abroad yields advantages at home (Dukalskis 2021). Notably, authoritarian states actively promote a good image abroad, often with the help of public relations firms, while also repressing dissident voices at home (Dukalskis 2021). International foreign pressure to improve human rights can create perceived threats for authoritarians at home by emboldening domestic activists (Kuran 1991). Keck and Sikkink's (2014) seminal work outlined how domestic activists often work with international actors to effectuate change domestically, even in democratizing states (Hawkins 1997). Similarly, Franklin (2008) found that international shaming of human rights abuses does force governments to reduce repression domestically, and this is especially true for states that have strong economic ties, like trade agreements, with other states. In essence, international criticism can influence authoritarian states.

During the age of social media, this constraint can be a key check on authoritarian consolidation. However, the COVID-19 pandemic demonstrated that, in many cases, critical international actors are willing to overlook repression if pandemic control measures are prioritized.

As a case in point, Morocco received extensive international praise from the beginning of the pandemic. Early on, the king took an active lead in developing a phased framework approach to help Africa manage COVID-19 more effectively across the continent as well as advocating for a more unified continental response targeting both the economic and social effects of international lockdowns. The government also started an initiative to donate medical supplies to 15 African countries.

These actions garnered praise from the WHO, the Pan-African Parliament, and the European Union. Given Morocco's unique position straddling both the African and European continents, the European Union commented on Morocco's key role to play in the European recovery as well as setting aside €450 million in financial aid for Morocco's pandemic response (Kasraoui 2020c).

Buttressing his reputation, the king set a personal example by wearing a face mask, maintaining social distance, and bringing a limited entourage as he presided over the *Laylat Al Qadr* and *Eid al-Fitr* prayers in 2020. These acts were generally positively covered by both domestic and international media and built a global image of Morocco's pandemic response as strong and effective. The World Bank singled out Morocco's low fatality rates for praise in a public statement in June 2020 (Gianaris 2020). Morocco's positive international image and success in curbing the pandemic led to its inclusion on the European Union's list of only 14 countries allowed to enter the Schengen Area in July 2020 (*BBC News* 2020a).

Domestically the response has been more mixed. Like his father, King Mohammed VI has witnessed multiple waves of protests, most prominently during the Arab Spring, and has maintained power by generally handling them deftly. Emergency powers, which historically had triggered strong negative reactions and protests, were never used by the regime during the Arab Spring. Notably, unlike the "state of exception" imposed by his father King Hassan II, which was very unpopular, citizens are overwhelmingly supportive of the current "state of health emergency" (Kasraoui 2020d). In fact, the 2020–2021 Arab Barometer survey on government responses to the pandemic found that 66 percent of Moroccan's believed that government limits on freedom of speech during the pandemic were justified; additionally, 79 percent agreed that freedom of movement should be limited, and 70 percent agreed that the media should censored when there is a public health emergency (Raz 2021; Al-Shami 2021). The regime's approval rating was 75 percent during July–September 2020 and increased to 86 percent during March–April 2020, the highest rating out of all MENA countries surveyed (Al-Shami, 2021; Raz 2021).

On the other hand, Egypt has received significantly more criticism than Morocco for its emergency law implementation. In March 2021, the United States and other Western nations issued a joint statement calling on Egypt to lift restrictions on freedom of expression and the right of assembly (Nebehay 2021). This was the first condemnation by the United States since 2014. Finland's ambassador even called on Egypt to lift travel bans and asset freezes of human rights activists (Nebehay 2021). The UN joint declaration was signed by 31 states and specifically called on Egypt to end the blocking of websites and independent media outlets, and expressed a deep concern for the "application of terrorism legislation" against human rights activists (United Nations Human Rights Council 2021).

NGOs from around the world praised the UN joint statement and, in February 2021, more than 100 NGOs wrote a joint statement to the United Nations outlining the deterioration of human rights in the country and the extensive use of "counterterrorism" legislation during the pandemic (Cairo Institute for Human Rights Studies 2021).

Although the statement does not explicitly mention Egypt's COVID-19 measures, the timing of the statement during the pandemic is noteworthy. The statement condemns many of the aforementioned powers that have been extended through the pandemic, like restrictions on media and digital freedom, intimidation of press and journalists, pretrial detention of opposition, and lack of due process. As outlined, all of these human rights have been curtailed through emergency legislation in Egypt, and the timing of this statement highlights the increasing deterioration of human rights since the onset of the pandemic in Egypt.

Domestically, prior to the pandemic, a poll conducted by the Egyptian Center for Public Opinion Research (Baseera) shortly after the 2017 terror attacks found that 63 percent of Egyptians supported the then three-month state of emergency (Noureldin 2017). A 2019 Arab Barometer poll found that most Egyptians trusted governmental institutions, "particularly institutions tasked with ensuring law and order" and "support for the army, government, and judiciary appears to be nearly unanimous" (Arab Barometer V: Egypt Country Report 2019). In fact, Egypt topped the list of Arab countries in terms of trust in institutions (66 percent) and trust in the judiciary (79 percent; see Kayyali 2020).

As with Moroccans, Egyptians also tended to support their government's response to the pandemic. An IPSOS survey conducted at the beginning of the pandemic (March–April 2020) found that 86 percent of Egyptians were satisfied with their government's response to the pandemic, with most supporting restrictions on public gatherings (Responding to COVID-19 2020). However, no polling has specifically focused on what Egyptians think about the current state of emergency. Still, based on the polls prior to the pandemic that show many Egyptians are comfortable with emergency measures, it is likely there is still fairly broad support for the current emergency, given its similarity to previous measures.

Discussion

Across governments, most authorities implemented the majority of the WHO recommendations to curb the spread of the virus. Borders were closed, social distancing mandates imposed, public gatherings discouraged, and health systems prioritized. The cases of Morocco and Egypt generally follow this trend. Both countries passed emergency laws containing most of these key provisions. However, within these emergency laws are two key considerations for the protection of human rights.

First is the inclusion of provisions without any real public health connection. These provisions are generally designed to strengthen the regime's ability to crack down on dissent using the security and judicial branches. Egypt provides the best example of this, with the inclusion of provisions that gave the president, via the military, a greater ability to prosecute citizens charged with violating the emergency law using the military judicial system, and the relative lack of defendant protections compared to the civilian system. No WHO recommendations hint at the need to use the military to enforce pandemic restrictions.

Second is the inclusion of provisions that fall into a grayer area. These provisions are, to a degree, supportive of pandemic mitigation but are also nebulous enough to enable their alternate use in curbing dissent against the regime. Morocco provides a good example of this with the use of a vague emergency law that placed considerable responsibility on the government to protect the health and safety of citizens but provided little guidance or critical restrictions on the measures to be used to accomplish that goal. The DGSN's rapid expansion of surveillance capabilities and the swift arrest of scores of lockdown violators served the purpose of curbing the spread of the virus by tracking its spread, restricting movement, and disincentivizing public gatherings, but it also hindered the public demonstrations against the regime that were active prior to the pandemic. This will continue to be a challenging discussion, given the global push to preserve human rights while also taking concrete steps to curb the pandemic. Freedom and the protection of human rights do not inoculate citizens against COVID-19. Following the findings of Cepaluni et al. (2021), as of August 2021, six out of the top 10 countries in *per capita* deaths from the virus are rated as free under the Freedom House rankings.[2]

Reviewing the implementation and use of emergency law powers across the Moroccan and Egyptian cases demonstrates how authoritarian regimes can use opportunities to institute emergency laws to consolidate or upgrade a regime's grip on power. In the case of Egypt, existing precedent in the form of the 1958 Emergency Law enabled the regime to expand on an already broad emergency law and use the pandemic to justify the law's implementation. In Morocco, a regime that had historically shied away from emergency powers upgraded to a powerful new set of tools to constrain contentious politics while preserving its domestic and international reputation. One of the most useful tools that has rapidly spread across authoritarian regimes and expanded dramatically during the pandemic response is the crackdown on the free press under the context of fighting misinformation and "fake news." A comparable tool added during the pandemic has been a similar restriction on public demonstrations justified by the need to enforce social distancing. Regular use of these dual-use tools is likely to continue to increase, given their public good pretext and effectiveness at curbing dissent.

In this comparison, the 2020 pandemic *does* represent a critical juncture for the progress of authoritarianism in Morocco. Prior to the pandemic, the regime had regularly threatened opposition protestors and carried out targeted arrests. However, the regime lacked the ability to engage in mass arrests and mass crackdowns. The emergence of the pandemic and the rapid expansion of powers under the emergency law gave it this capability, which it maximized. The implementation of extensive surveillance by the DGSN and the reports of truly remarkable arrest numbers—up to 1.5 million and more than 200,000 prosecutions by April 2021—are strong evidence that the regime in Morocco has embraced the new powers granted by the pandemic response.

Notably, history appears to matter. Morocco purposely framed its emergency law as a "state of *health* emergency." Prior to the pandemic, Moroccans did not have extensive experience under a state of emergency, and the brief experience with the "state of exception" in 1965 was very unpopular. Therefore, the regime likely tied the implementation of the emergency law specifically to the pandemic in order to ease the transition to a more restrictive *status quo* and encourage great acceptance of enhanced governmental powers. There is no reason to expect this to change as the pandemic eases, absent a powerful push by the public. On the other hand, Egyptians have extensive experience with a state of emergency given its regular use since 1958 and Egyptian regimes' regular use of the emergency law to consolidate power since 2014.

We know that image abroad matters, especially for autocrats who want to maintain their image as a liberalizing or democratizing state, while also balancing that image with a desire to maintain and consolidate power. The Moroccan regime received steady praise for a number of constitutional reforms made since 2011 that expanded parliamentary power and facilitated peaceful elections in 2012, while simultaneously maintaining exceptional stability. King Hassan II sought to protect his reputation as a "liberalizing autocrat" by packaging the emergency law as for the public good, while simultaneously using those newfound powers granted by the law to discourage public dissent against the regime.

The Moroccan regime's approach appears to have largely succeeded. The regime took this opportunity to consolidate power while simultaneously maintaining support and popularity at home and abroad. Despite a dramatic uptick in arrests and prosecutions of citizens, protestors, and journalists, along with the enactment of a pervasive surveillance program, the Moroccan regime leveraged its reputation well and continues to remain generally popular both in domestic polls and internationally. In contrast, Egypt entered the pandemic with strong majority domestic support but was very unpopular abroad due to extensive crackdowns on public dissent. The regime did little to improve this reputation and continued to receive considerable criticism from international actors. Notably however, although the emergency law specifically has always been unpopular domestically, polls indicated strong domestic approval of how the regime was handling the pandemic, at least early on. Future polls will show how stable this support is.

Consolidated autocracies, like Egypt, will use opportunities like the pandemic to enhance the regime's ability to quell dissent and further consolidate power. This is not surprising. However, the pandemic has allowed the president to pass emergency legislation and powers without inciting mass protests or rejection. This is surprising. As outlined, Egypt's emergency law has been and still is one of the main contentions of activists, especially since the Arab Spring. However, the pandemic has, at least temporarily, legitimized many of the same restrictions, but through the lens of fighting a public health crisis. The long-term implications of this domestic legitimization are unclear.

Similar to the difficulties inherent in sorting necessary pandemic restrictions from unnecessary crackdowns, how the international community responds to these restrictions needs to be considered. Regimes in both countries implemented harsh repressive measures and further consolidated authoritarian power during the pandemic, yet Morocco received general praise while Egypt received condemnation. This occurred despite the Moroccan regime blatantly touting colossal arrest numbers. This divergent response demonstrates both a prioritization by the international community for effective pandemic response over the protection of human rights and the partiality many key international actors have toward certain regimes. Favoritism by wealthy democracies toward useful autocrats and exclusive targeting of the less useful has been a frequent criticism in the past of these key backers of human rights and does not incentivize the prioritization of human rights by the regimes interested in staying in the good graces of the Western world. Markedly, both regimes received near-universal condemnation from both international and domestic NGOs.

Conclusion

The COVID-19 pandemic has important implications for authoritarian regimes and their respect of human rights. As expected by the literature, authoritarian regimes have used this crisis to consolidate power via creative dual-use tools designed for both pandemic control and restricting political opposition. There is no indication any of these regimes are interested in relinquishing these tools, even after the pandemic starts to subside. These tools have been used extensively to infringe on human rights. This slippery slope, particularly given the availability of a public health pretext, will likely lead to an expansion of these violations until these regimes receive real pushback (Goodhart 2020). We have seen this on display particularly in Egypt, where the human rights abuses under authoritarian consolation that started increasing in 2014 have continued during the pandemic. The intentions of the Moroccan regime are less clear, although the recent repression of the Hirak Rif and the massive expansion of mass arrests during the pandemic indicate an increasing willingness to violate human rights.

Both Egypt and Morocco have been accused of using the pandemic as a guise to consolidate power, and both regimes have justified the expansion of power under emergency laws as necessary to curb the spread of COVID-19. In both cases, the regimes enacted and enforced recommendations provided by the WHO to protect their citizens during the pandemic. These measures appear to have had some success in limiting the impact of the pandemic on the health of their citizens, economies, and society. Morocco, in particular, received extensive international praise for its actions.

However, both regimes have also gone far beyond WHO recommendations in the expansion of surveillance and arrest powers, both on paper and in practice. In the name of contact tracing and enforcing necessary restrictions on movement, they have implemented powerful and intrusive surveillance structures. Massive numbers of lockdown violators, protesters, journalists, and other oppositionists have been arrested and prosecuted. These arrests have been justified by the need to enforce social distancing and combat misinformation. Egypt took a step further and tacked on additional powers to its legacy emergency law that enable the president to circumvent the civilian judicial system in the prosecution of public dissent. Overall, pandemics of such a scale offer a significant window of opportunity for authoritarian regimes to consolidate power with a relatively lower risk of meaningful international and domestic pushback.

Morocco presents a notable example of the importance of reputation in international circles for autocrats. Despite a heavy rollback of personal freedom and civil protections, the international community has largely praised the regime for its actions during the pandemic and rewarded it with significant financial support. Egypt's poor preceding reputation and lack of democratic pretensions earned it primarily condemnation from comparable circles.

The pandemic experience has also shown these regimes that, during these times of crises, they can take heavy-handed actions against public demonstrations while also generally preserving or even improving their approval domestically, as long as those actions are perceived as targeting violators of the public good. Many of the actions taken by Moroccan authorities in 2020 to crack down on civil society would have drawn considerable public backlash in previous years but were seen as necessary during the pandemic. We expect that these lessons not only will be internalized by the regimes examined in this analysis but also will be incorporated by fellow autocrats looking to upgrade their own authoritarian toolkits.

Notes

1. We do not include an analysis of Algeria, which experienced a revolution in 2019; Tunisia, North Africa's only liberal democracy; or Libya, which is in a civil war.
2. For Freedom House Rankings, see Freedom House (2020); For COVID-19 deaths per 100,000 population, see Johns Hopkins University and Medicine (2020).

Funding

This work was supported by the American University of Sharjah Sir Easa Saleh Al-Gurg Honorarium.

ORCID

Sammy Badran http://orcid.org/0000-0002-6657-5697

References

Abouzzohour, Y. (2020a). Coping with COVID-19's cost: The example of Morocco. *Brookings Doha Center*. Retrieved February 13, 2022, from https://www.brookings.edu/research/coping-with-covid-19s-cost-the-example-of-morocco/

Abouzzohour, Y. (2020b). Policy and institutional responses to COVID-19 in the Middle East and North Africa: Morocco. *Brookings Doha Center*. Retrieved February 13, 2022, from https://www.brookings.edu/research/policy-and-institutional-responses-to-covid-19-in-the-middle-east-and-north-africa-morocco/

Ali, N., & Fakhry, N. (2020). The amendments to the emergency law to confront Corona after the approval of Parliament. Retrieved February 13, 2022, from https://www.youm7.com/story/2020/4/22/4737063/ ننشر-تعدي
لات-قانون-الطوارئ-لمواجهة-كورونا-بعد-موافقة-البرلمان

Al Watan News. (2020). *Legislature approves amendments to the emergency law.* Retrieved February 13, 2022, from https://www.elwatannews.com/news/details/4706149

Alon, I., Farrell, M., & Li, S. (2020). Regime type and COVID-19 response. *FIIB Business Review, 9*(3), 152–160. doi:10.1177/2319714520928884

Alrababa'h, A., & Blaydes, L. (2021). Authoritarian media and diversionary threats: Lessons from 30 years of Syrian state discourse. *Political Science Research and Methods, 9*(4), 693–708. doi:10.1017/psrm.2020.28

Al-Shami, S. (2021). COVID-19 in the Middle East and North Africa. *Arab Barometer.* Retrieved February 13, 2022, from https://www.arabbarometer.org/publication/covid-19-in-the-middle-east-and-north-africa/

Amnesty International (2019). *Egypt: Largest wave of mass arrests since President Abdel Fattah al-Sisi came to power.* 2 October. Retrieved February 13, 2022, from https://www.amnesty.org/en/latest/news/2019/10/egypt-largest-wave-of-mass-arrests-since-president-abdel-fattah-al-sisi-came-to-power/

Amnesty International (2020a). *Morocco and Western Sahara: End prosecution of activists under new health emergency law.* Retrieved February 13, 2022, from https://www.amnesty.org/en/latest/news/2020/06/morocco-and-western-sahara-end-prosecution-of-activists-under-new-health-emergency-law/

Amnesty International (2020b). *Egypt: Health care workers forced to make impossible choice between 'death or jail'.* Retrieved February 13, 2022, from https://www.amnesty.org/en/latest/news/2020/06/egypt-health-care-workers-forced-to-make-impossible-choice-between-death-or-jail/

Amnesty International (2020c). *Omar Radi: the Moroccan journalist who won't be silenced.* Retrieved February 13, 2022, from https://www.amnesty.org/en/latest/news/2020/06/omar-radi-moroccan-journalist-refuses-to-be-silenced/

Amnesty International (2021a). *Morocco: Drop charges against teachers who peacefully protested over workers' rights.* Retrieved February 13, 2022, from https://www.amnesty.org/en/latest/news/2021/05/morocco-drop-charges-against-teachers-who-peacefully-protested-over-workers-rights/

Arab Barometer V: Egypt Country Report (2019). *Arab Barometer.* Retrieved February 13, 2022, from https://www.arabbarometer.org/wp-content/uploads/ABV_Egypt_Report_Public-Opinion_Arab-Barometer_2019.pdf

Arabic, A.-J. (2020). *Egypt's el-Sisi expands powers, citing coronavirus pandemic.* Retrieved February 13, 2022, from https://www.aljazeera.com/news/2020/5/9/egypts-el-sisi-expands-powers-citing-coronavirus-pandemic

Article 19. (2020). *Morocco: Government must fully withdraw draft law on social media.* Retrieved February 13, 2022, from https://www.article19.org/resources/morocco-social-media/

Associated Press (2021). *Egyptian activist sentenced to 18 months for 'fake news.'* Retrieved February 13, 2022, from https://apnews.com/article/health-cairo-coronavirus-pandemic-arrests-egypt-569ae5471351b28d832be101e5c9a720

Badran, S. Z. (2014). The contentious roots of the Egyptian revolution. *Globalizations, 11*(2), 273–287. doi:10.1080/14747731.2014.887386

Badran, S. Z. (2021). Signaling reforms through election results: How a Moroccan opposition party demobilized protests. *British Journal of Middle Eastern Studies, 48*(3), 515–533. doi:10.1080/13530194.2019.1651634

Barceló, J., Kubinec, R., Cheng, C., Rahn, T. H., & Messerschmidt, L. (2020). Windows of repression: Using COVID-19 policies against political dissidents? *SocArXiv Papers, 59*(1), 1–51.

BBC News (2020a). *Coronavirus: EU to allow in visitors from 15 'safe' countries.* Retrieved February 13, 2022, from https://www.bbc.com/news/world-middle-east-54990177

BBC News (2020b). *Egypt arrests human rights group's staff in "chilling escalation."* Retrieved February 13, 2022, from https://www.bbc.com/news/world-middle-east-54990177

Beschel, R. (2021). Policy and institutional responses to COVID-19 in the Middle East and North Africa: Egypt. *Brookings Doha Center.* Retrieved February 13, 2022, from https://www.brookings.edu/research/policy-and-institutional-responses-to-covid-19-in-the-middle-east-and-north-africa-egypt/

Brysk, A. (2022). Pandemic patriarchy: The impact of a global health crisis on women's rights. *Journal of Human Rights, 21*(3), 283–303.

Cairo Institute for Human Rights Studies (2021). *Egypt | Human Rights Council: Countries should take bold action.* Retrieved February 13, 2022, from https://cihrs.org/egypt-human-rights-council-countries-should-take-bold-action/?lang=en

Cavatorta, F. (2009). 'Divided they stand, divided they fail': Opposition politics in Morocco. *Democratization, 16*(1), 137–156. doi:10.1080/13510340802575882

Cepaluni, G., Dorsch, M. T., & Branyiczki, R. (2021). Political regimes and deaths in the early stages of the COVID-19 pandemic. *Journal of Public Finance and Public Choice, 37*(1), 1–27. doi:10.33774/apsa-2020-5lhhc

Cheibub, J. A., Hong, J. Y. J., & Przeworski, A. (2020). *Rights and deaths: Government reactions to the pandemic* [Unpublished manuscript]. Retrieved February 13, 2022, from https://papers.ssrn.com/sol3/papers.cfm?abstract_id=3645410

Chenoweth, E. (2022). Can nonviolent resistance survive COVID-19? *Journal of Human Rights, 21*(3), 304–316.

Chiozza, G., & Goemans, H. E. (2011). *Leaders and international conflict.* Cambridge University Press.

Chiozza, G., & King, J. (2022). Introduction to a special issue on "beyond complacency and acrimony: Studying human rights in a post-COVID-19 world." *Journal of Human Rights*, *21*(3), 245.

Clay, C., Abdelwahab, M., Bagwell, S., Barney, M., Burkle, E., Hawley, T., Rowden, T., LaVelle, T., Parker, A., & Rains, M. (2022). The effect of the COVID-19 pandemic on human rights practices: Findings from the Human Rights Measurement Initiative's 2021 Practitioner Survey. *Journal of Human Rights*, *21*(3), 317–333.

Davidson, H. (2020, April 20). Hong Kong using Covid-19 crisis as 'golden opportunity' for crackdown, says arrested leader. *The Guardian*. Retrieved February 13, 2022, from https://www.theguardian.com/world/2020/apr/20/hong-kong-using-covid-19-crisis-as-golden-opportunity-for-crackdown-says-arrested-leader.

Drissi Bourhanbour, A., & Ouchetto, O. (2021). Morocco achieves the highest COVID-19 vaccine rates in Africa in the first phase: what are reasons for its success? *Journal of Travel Medicine*, *28*(4), 1–2. doi:10.1093/jtm/taab040

Dukalskis, A. (2021). *Making the world safe for dictatorship*. Oxford University Press.

Eck, K., & Hatz, S. (2020). State surveillance and the COVID-19 crisis. *Journal of Human Rights*, *19*(5), 603–612. doi:10.1080/14754835.2020.1816163

Economist Intelligence Unit. (2020). *Democracy Index 2020. In sickness and in health?* EIU. Retrieved February 13, 2022, from https://www.eiu.com/n/campaigns/democracy-index-2020/

Education International (2021). *Morocco: Strikes and demonstrations demand better conditions for contract teachers*. 24 March. Retrieved February 13, 2022, from https://www.eiie.org/en/item/23722:morocco-strikes-and-demonstrations-demand-better-conditions-for-contract-teachers

Egyptian Parliament. (2020). *Law No. 22 of 2020 amending the Emergency Law No. 162 of 1958*. Retrieved February 13, 2022, from https://www.ilo.org/dyn/natlex/docs/ELECTRONIC/111244/138541/F-2028363771/EGY111244.pdf

Ellaboudy, A. (2020, May 19). Emergency law amendments to fight covid-19 in Egypt: Putting the poison in the honey. *Verfassungsblog*. Retrieved February 13, 2022, from https://verfassungsblog.de/emergency-law-amendments-to-fight-covid-19-in-egypt-putting-the-poison-in-the-honey/

Euro-Mediterranean Human Rights Monitor (2020). Draft law would violate right to freedom of expression in Morocco. Retrieved June 17, 2022, from https://euromedmonitor.org/uploads/reports/moroccoen.pdf.

Franklin, J. C. (2008). Shame on you: The impact of human rights criticism on political repression in Latin America. *International Studies Quarterly*, *52*(1), 187–211. doi:10.1111/j.1468-2478.2007.00496.x

Freedom House. (2020). *Countries and Territories*. Retrieved February 13, 2022, from https://freedomhouse.org/countries/freedom-world/scores?sort=desc&order=Total%20Score%20and%20Status

Freedom House. (2021). *Freedom in the World: Morocco*. Retrieved February 13, 2022, from https://freedomhouse.org/country/morocco/freedom-world/2021.

Frey, C. B., Chen, C., & Presidente, G. (2020). Democracy, culture, and contagion: Political regimes and countries responsiveness to Covid-19. *Covid Economics*, *18*(1), 1–20.

Ghonim, W. (2012). *Revolution 2.0: The power of the people is greater than the people in power: A memoir*. Houghton Mifflin Harcourt.

Gianaris, K. (2020). World Bank spotlights Morocco's 'effective' COVID-19 response. *Morocco World News*. Retrieved February 13, 2022, from https://www.moroccoworldnews.com/2020/06/306131/world-bank-spotlights-moroccos-effective-covid-19-response

Goodhart, M. (2020). Revisiting interdependence in times and terms of crisis. *Journal of Human Rights*, *19*(5), 520–527. doi:10.1080/14754835.2020.1814709

Gruffydd-Jones, J. J. (2019). Citizens and condemnation: Strategic uses of international human rights pressure in authoritarian states. *Comparative Political Studies*, *52*(4), 579–612. doi:10.1177/0010414018784066

Hawkins, D. G. (1997). Domestic responses to international pressure: Human rights in authoritarian Chile. *European Journal of International Relations*, *3*(4), 403–434. doi:10.1177/1354066197003004001

Hekking, M. (2020, May 4). Justice minister requests delay in controversial social media law. *Morocco World News*. Retrieved February 13, 2022, from https://www.moroccoworldnews.com/2020/05/301497/justice-minister-requests-delay-in-controversial-social-media-law

Heydemann, S., & Leenders, R. (2011). Authoritarian learning and authoritarian resilience: Regime responses to the 'Arab Awakening'. *Globalizations*, *8*(5), 647–653. doi:10.1080/14747731.2011.621274

Human Rights Watch (2014). *Egypt: Unprecedented expansion of military courts: decree broadens jurisdiction over civilians*. Retrieved February 13, 2022, from https://www.hrw.org/news/2014/11/17/egypt-unprecedented-expansion-military-courts

Hungarian Helsinki Committee (2020). Hungary: Illiberal Highlights of 2020. Retrieved June 17, 2022, from https://helsinki.hu/en/illiberal-highlights-of-2020/.

Ismangil, M., & Lee, M. (2021). Protests in Hong Kong during the Covid-19 pandemic. *Crime, Media, Culture: An International Journal*, *17*(1), 17–20. doi:10.1177/1741659020946229

Johns Hopkins University and Medicine. (2020). *Coronavirus Resources Center: Mortality in the most affected countries* Retrieved February 13, 2022, from https://coronavirus.jhu.edu/data/mortality

Kacha, Y. (2020, May 29). In a post-COVID-19 world, "fake news" laws, a new blow to freedom of expression in Algeria and Morocco/Western Sahara? *Amnesty International.* Retrieved February 13, 2022, from https://www.amnesty.org/en/latest/news/2020/05/in-a-post-covid19-world-fake-news-laws-a-new-blow-to-freedom-of-expression-in-algeria-and-morocco-western-sahara/

Karam, S. (2020). Morocco rolls back democracy under cover of Covid-19. *Bloomberg News.* Retrieved February 13, 2022, from https://www.bloomberg.com/news/articles/2020-07-24/covid-crackdown-snuffs-out-flickering-embers-of-the-arab-spring

Kasraoui, S. (2020a, March 19). Coronavirus pandemic: A timeline of COVID-19 in Morocco. *Morocco World News.* Retrieved February 13, 2022, from https://www.moroccoworldnews.com/2020/03/296727/coronavirus-a-timeline-of-covid-19-in-morocco

Kasraoui, S. (2020b). Moroccan police USE DGSN tracking app for 426,072 control operations. *Morocco World News.* Retrieved February 13, 2022, from https://www.moroccoworldnews.com/2020/05/301702/moroccan-police-use-dgsn-tracking-app-for-426-072-control-operations

Kasraoui, S. (2020c). EU convinced of Morocco's crucial role in African COVID-19 response. *Morocco World News.* Retrieved February 13, 2022, from https://www.moroccoworldnews.com/2020/04/301101/eu-convinced-of-moroccos-crucial-role-in-african-covid-19-response

Kasraoui, S. (2020d). Moroccans slam demonstrations defying Morocco's state of emergency. *Morocco World News.* Retrieved February 13, 2022, from https://www.moroccoworldnews.com/2020/03/297155/moroccans-slam-demonstrations-defying-moroccos-state-of-emergency

Kasraoui, S. (2021). Morocco extends state of emergency until September 10. *Morocco World News.* Retrieved February 13, 2022, from https://www.moroccoworldnews.com/2021/07/343616/morocco-extends-state-of-emergency-until-september-10

Kayyali, A.-W. (2020). The Arab World's trust in government and the perils of generalization. *Arab Barometer.* Retrieved February 13, 2022, from https://www.arabbarometer.org/2020/06/the-arab-worlds-trust-in-government-and-the-perils-of-generalization/

Keck, M. E., & Sikkink, K. (2014). *Activists beyond borders: Advocacy networks in international politics.* Cornell University Press.

Khalid, M. (2020). Egypt's emboldened military courts. *Carnegie Endowment for International Peace.* Retrieved February 13, 2022, from https://carnegieendowment.org/sada/82146

Kuran, T. (1991). Now out of never: The element of surprise in the East European revolution of 1989. *World Politics, 44*(1), 7–48. doi:10.2307/2010422

Lahbib, M. (2020). Magreb:¿ el regreso del autoritarismo después de las revoluciones. In Breno Bringel & Geoffrey Pleyers (Eds.), *Alerta Global: políticas, movimientos sociales y futuros en disputa en tiempos de pandemia* (pp. 168–177). Clacso.

Lees, C. (2018). Fake news: the global silencer: The term has become a useful weapon in the dictator's toolkit against the media. Just look at the Philippines. *Index on Censorship, 47*(1), 88–91. doi:10.1177/0306422018769578

Liu, J., & Zhao, H. (2021). Privacy lost: Appropriating surveillance technology in China's fight against COVID-19. *Business Horizons, 64*(6), 743–756.

Magdi, A. (2021). Egypt's execution Frenzy has to stop. *Human Rights Watch.* Retrieved February 13, 2022, from https://www.hrw.org/news/2021/06/28/egypts-execution-frenzy-has-stop

Mandour, M. (2020). Repression and coronavirus response in Egypt. *Carnegie Endowment for International Peace.* Retrieved February 13, 2022, from https://carnegieendowment.org/sada/82304

Moroccan Parliament. (2020). *Decree Law No. 2.20.293.* Retrieved February 13, 2022, from https://covidlawlab.org/wp-content/uploads/2020/06/De%CC%81cret-loi_n%C2%B02-20-292_AR.pdf

Murdie, A. (2022). Hindsight is 2020: Lessons from the COVID-19 pandemic for future human rights research. *Journal of Human Rights, 21*(3), 354–364.

Nebehay, S. (2021). U.S. joins West in rare criticism of Egypt on human rights abuses. *Reuters.* Retrieved February 13, 2022, from https://www.reuters.com/article/egypt-rights-un-int/u-s-joins-west-in-rare-criticism-of-egypt-on-human-rights-abuses-idUSKBN2B4174

Noureldin, O. (2017). 63% of Egyptians agree that Emergency Law should be imposed: Baseera poll. *Egypt Independent.* Retrieved February 13, 2022, from https://egyptindependent.com/63-egyptians-agree-emergency-law-should-be-imposed-baseera-poll/

Odour, M. (2021). Morocco: More than 1.5 million people arrested for Covid breaches. *African News.* Retrieved February 13, 2022, from https://www.africanews.com/2021/04/28/morocco-more-than-1-5-million-people-arrested-for-covid-breaches//

Online, A. (2021). *WHO praises Egypt for producing 1 million coronavirus vaccine doses.* Retrieved February 13, 2022, from https://english.ahram.org.eg/NewsContent/1/64/416800/Egypt/Politics-/WHO-praises-Egypt-for-producing–million-coronavir.aspx

Raghavan, S. (2020, May 10). As coronavirus spreads in Egypt, Sisi sees opportunity to tighten his grip. *The Washington Post*. Retrieved February 13, 2022, from https://www.washingtonpost.com/world/africa/as-coronavirus-spreads-in-egypt-sissi-sees-opportunity-to-tighten-his-grip/2020/05/10/11a840be-92a5-11ea-87a3-22d324235636_story.html

Raz, D. (2021). Is COVID-19 compelling Arab citizens to surrender freedoms to their governments? *Arab Barometer*. Retrieved February 13, 2022, from https://www.arabbarometer.org/2021/05/is-covid-19-compelling-arab-citizens-to-surrender-freedoms-to-their-governments/

Responding to COVID-19. (2020). IPSOS: Retrieved February 13, 2022, from https://www.ipsos.com/sites/default/files/ct/publication/documents/2020-05/egypt_report_0.pdf

Risse, T., Ropp, S. C., & Sikkink, K. (1999). *The power of human rights: International norms and domestic change*. Cambridge University Press.

Spadaro, A. (2020). COVID-19: Testing the limits of human rights. *European Journal of Risk Regulation*, *11*(2), 317–325. doi:10.1017/err.2020.27

Tamburini, F. (2021). The COVID-19 outbreak in North Africa: A legal analysis. *Journal of Asian and African Studies*, *56*(7), 1738–1754. doi:10.1177/0021909620983586

United Nations Human Rights Council. (2021). General debate item 4: Human rights situations that require the Council's attention: Joint statement on Egypt. https://cihrs.org/wp-content/uploads/2021/03/HRC46-JST-on-Egypt-item-4.pdf

Witt, J. F. (2020). *American Contagions*. Yale University Press.

World Health Organization (2006). *Communicable disease surveillance and response systems, guide to monitoring and evaluating*. World Health Organization. Retrieved February 13, 2022, from https://www.who.int/csr/resources/publications/surveillance/WHO_CDS_EPR_LYO_2006_2.pdf

Yao, L., Li, M., Wan, J. Y., Howard, S. C., Bailey, J. E., & Graff, J. C. (2021). Democracy and case fatality rate of COVID-19 at early stage of pandemic: A multicountry study. *Environmental Science and Pollution Research*, *29*(6), 1–11.

Zartman, I. W. (2015). Opposition as support of the state. In G. Luciani (Ed.), *Beyond coercion* (pp. 61–87). Routledge.

Fighting COVID-19, maintain human rights: Challenges and tradeoffs

Pandemic patriarchy: The impact of a global health crisis on women's rights

Alison Brysk

ABSTRACT
The COVID-19 pandemic has brought a surge in patriarchal repression for women worldwide, with marked increases in gender violence, gendered job loss and deterioration in labor conditions, regression in health care access and reproductive rights, and backlash against feminist consciousness. Beyond intensifying chronic rights gaps and the preexisting conditions of patriarchy, the global health crisis has increased the gendered impact of interdependence across the social-civil-security rights domains, the public-private divide, and intersecting identities of gender, race, and class. The cumulation of these shifts constitutes a new phase of pandemic patriarchy that sets new parameters for the fulfillment of women's rights in the international rights regime. The uneven rights regime response to the panoply of rights challenges under conditions of pandemic patriarchy shows that an adequate global response must move beyond the recognition of women's rights as human rights to incorporate feminism as an ethic of care, struggle for systematic gender equity, and feminist reconstruction of global governance.

Introduction: Pandemic patriarchy

Pathogens and the human insecurity they generate have always been intertwined with social pathologies and the struggle for empowerment. This special issue aims to map, analyze, and strategize the relationship between rights and the COVID-19 crisis (Chiozza & King, 2022a)—including its gendered dimension. The pandemic has brought a surge in patriarchal repression for women worldwide, with marked increases in gender violence, gendered job loss and deterioration in labor conditions, regression in reproductive rights, and backlash against feminist consciousness (Lewis, 2020). The global health crisis has revealed broader patterns of the relationship between women's rights and global public health that will extend beyond this crisis, with implications for 21st century global governance (Vogelstein, 2021). Health rights advocates have long recognized that "women remain disproportionately affected by infectious disease as a result of their greater vulnerability to violence of all kinds, their traditional role as care workers in the home and the health system, and the endemic discrimination that blocks their access to adequate treatment and prevention systems" (Sekalala & Harrington, 2020, p. 235).

As Chiozza and King (2022b) explain the post-COVID-19 condition of human rights, exogenous shocks reveal the fissures in social systems and both the crisis conditions and social response lead to critical junctures and tradeoffs. The perfect storm of COVID-era rights challenges results in *pandemic patriarchy: a global cumulative deterioration in women's rights conditions with increased interdependence among them.* The global health crisis has intensified chronic gaps in women's rights—and the pandemic has increased interdependence across the domains of social and security rights, labor and health rights spanning the public-private divide, and the impact of intersecting identities of race, class, and migration status on women's rights. Pandemic patriarchy constitutes a qualitative shift in the conditions for the fulfillment of women's rights that cuts across regions and gender regimes but appears most at risk in illiberal nationalist polities.

Human rights regime gaps + preexisting patriarchy x health crisis = Pandemic patriarchy

The gendered impact of COVID-19 shows how exogenous rights challenges intersect with long-standing shortfalls of the human rights regime (Chiozza & King, 2022b) plus the preexisting condition of patriarchy. Thus, pandemic patriarchy systematically undermines women's rights as it renders women more vulnerable to physical and economic insecurity; loss of self-determination over mobility, labor conditions, and reproduction; deterioration in health rights through greater disease burden and displacement of health care access; and declining access to water, food, and education. Women's rights are affected by the pandemic worldwide, but the impact is stronger at the intersections of vulnerability: in developing countries and marginalized communities where women are already more economically, legally, and socially disadvantaged (United Nations Human Rights, 2020). The combination of regime gaps, preexisting patriarchy, and health inequities in pandemic patriarchy sets new parameters for women's rights that will require a new kind of multi-dimensional response based in a feminist expansion of rights.

This article will map the emergence of pandemic patriarchy and analyze the implications of these gendered shifts in the dynamics of rights for a feminist response. Building on prior human rights scholarship can allow us to map trends, mark qualitative and systemic change, and derive lessons for the new environment (Murdie, 2022). As we will discuss below, the baseline analysis of chronic human rights regime gaps and the struggle for health rights developed further in this special issue suggest the following frameworks for assessment (Clay et al., 2022):

1. Contested tradeoffs between security and health rights in the face of external threat (Chenoweth, 2022);
2. Lagging accountability for violations by non-state actors, especially in the private sphere (Brysk, 2018a);
3. Discriminatory fulfillment compounded at intersections of multiple forms of disadvantage (Koo, 2022);
4. Increased vulnerability to discrimination and disease in illiberal nationalist regimes (Badran & Turnbull, 2022);
5. Backlash at the boundaries between the public and private spheres (Brysk, 2018b).

While there has been some institutional acknowledgement and rights regime response to the increase in gender-based violence and some women's COVID-related health needs, more structural gendered economic vulnerability and barriers to health care access and reproductive rights are less attended by the international human rights regime or national authorities. Because this uneven capacity for response is based in the chronic shortfalls of the international rights regime, the impact of pandemic patriarchy shows that an adequate global response must incorporate additional elements: a rights-based approach to health and a feminist expansion of the domain and protagonists of rights.

Response to pandemic patriarchy = rights–based health × feminist empowerment

The article will proceed as follows. First, we will review scholarly understandings of the constituents of pandemic patriarchy–human rights regime gaps, preexisting patriarchy, and health rights crisis–to derive frameworks for assessing trends. Then, we will map the worldwide pattern of cumulative decline and rising interdependence of women's rights in the areas of gender violence, labor and social rights, and health and reproductive rights. Finally, we will derive lessons for a rights-based response based in expanding understandings of health rights, a feminist ethic of care, and systemic gender equity.

Human rights at the crossroads

Human rights are a combination of norms, institutions, and practices for the promotion, protection, and fulfillment of human freedom, dignity, and equality relative to the authority of states, markets, and global governance. Rights are articulated in manifestos, treaties, laws, and national charters; claimed in courts, protests, and campaigns; and constructed on battlefields, at borders, in prisons, streets, workplaces, schools, and homes. Rights may transform social recognition, legal entitlements, citizenship conditions, resource allocation, social solidarity, and political contention—and ultimately secure the protection and empowerment of rights claimants. However, struggles for human rights claims always face countervailing norms and interests (from religious identities to economic logics to health emergencies) and even tradeoffs among different kinds of rights.

At the threshold of the COVID-19 pandemic, human rights stood at a contested crossroads, "between complacency and acrimony" (Chiozza & King, 2022b). The United Nations' Vienna World Conference on Human Rights declared in 1993 an international consensus that rights are universal, indivisible, and interdependent. While rights norms are inherently universal in principle, rights *access* and *fulfillment* are highly conditioned by intersecting identities of gender, race, class, and migration status, among others. Indivisibility of rights is undermined by long-standing differential patterns of international human rights: gaps in enforcement of human rights for "private wrongs" committed by nonstate actors in contexts such as domestic violence and unfair labor conditions, and systematic challenges to fulfillment of positive social and economic rights such as access to sustainable work and health care (Whelan, 2010).

In the first generation of the twenty-first century, the international regime for human rights was characterized by an uneasy combination of expanding principles, pathways and protagonists for new rights—including the right to health—contrasting with historic lags in access and accountability, especially for securitized crises and venues above and below the state. Moreover, a rising constellation of populist regimes and counter-cosmopolitan forces sought to contract the liberal international rights regime (Brysk, 2018a). In particular, the rights and security of people out of place (migrants, refugees, and asylum-seekers) are more vulnerable to any exogenous shock or repressive political regime. The impact of COVID-19 and state responses on the rights and security of migrants reveals and deepens this shortfall (Ramji-Nogales & Goldner Lang, 2020).

The crossroads of human rights carried particular potential and challenges for women. The 1995 Beijing Conference on Women marked global recognition of women's rights as human rights. Women's rights include equal access to all of the political and social rights outlined in the Universal Declaration of Human Rights, ICCPR, and ICESR. Beyond this, the CEDAW Convention and the Declaration on the Elimination of Violence Against Women require equitable treatment in gendered reproductive and social roles. Women and people with minority status based on sexual orientation and gender identity (SOGI) are systematically disadvantaged in fulfillment of universal rights to physical integrity, political freedoms and participation, labor and social rights—as well as self-determination in marriage, sexuality, and reproduction. Within these gendered patterns of rights shortfalls, race, class, origin, and citizenship status compound vulnerabilities and complicate responses (Bunch & Reilly, 2019; Theidon, 2020).

Patriarchy as preexisting condition

The parameters for the fulfillment of women's rights follow issue-specific patterns rooted in reproductive relations, and gender relations are the first political order that underlies the distribution of all power (Hudson et al., 2020)—including the international human rights regime. Patriarchy is a preexisting condition that articulates with additional vectors of vulnerability: political regimes, poverty, citizenship status, and intersectional identity. These disadvantages are linked through social structures of patriarchal dominance institutionalized in regimes of law, markets, mobility, and disciplinary violence: gender regimes. Gender regimes are configurations of structural patriarchy that manifest as patterns of gender rules, roles and beliefs specific to a region, political economy, and/or historical period (Brysk, 2018b).

Gender regimes shape the rights at risk from any exogenous challenge and filter the rights repertoires available to respond. One contemporary analysis characterizes the rights repertoires of gender regimes across regions according to political economy: patrimonial, liberal/neo-liberal, and semi-liberal. In the middle-income semi-liberal gender regimes that include some of the societies most affected by the global health crisis—such as Brazil and India–women's rising public political and economic empowerment are systematically undermined by high levels of disciplinary gender violence and backlash in the private sphere (Brysk, 2018b).

The intersection of gender regimes with political regimes will further shape the incidence and impact of the new wave of pandemic patriarchy unleashed by the global health crisis. Women's security and social rights are at greater risk under nationalist populist regimes due to their tendency to mobilize the masses by heightening ethnic conflict, suppressing political challenges from civil society movements, seeking control of reproduction, and mismanaging public health. Most—although not all—nationalist populist political regimes arise in middle-income illiberal societies with corresponding semi-liberal gender regimes. Backlash in gender ideology, gender violence, and reproductive rights is most common in semi-liberal gender regimes facing an external crisis—as in Brazil, Russia, Turkey, the Philippines, Poland, and Mexico (Korolczuk & Graff, 2018). However, some fully liberalized developed democracies—such as the United States—have also experienced a surge of nationalist populism generating gender backlash and failures of health governance, which feeds back to a decline in democracy itself (Institute for Democracy & Election Assistance [IDEA], 2021).

Global health crisis and human rights

As we have seen across this special issue, health crises pose systematic challenges for civil, social, and collective rights across all populations (Chiozza & King, 2022b). The gendered impact of a global health crisis is intertwined with the status and struggle for health as a human right, defined as equitable and self-determined access to the *highest attainable standard of health care*. Access to health is an interdependent enabling right for the pursuit of most forms of political and economic rights, a vector of discrimination, and an indivisible right that bridges individual and collective conditions (Meier & Gostin, 2018). Differential access to health rights is an indicator of political pathologies (Farmer, 2005), which have intensified with the rise of authoritarian populism. Throughout the twenty-first century, norms and mechanisms to claim the human right to health have expanded, empowered by transnational advocacy for access to essential medicines, patients' rights, privacy, disability rights, and reproductive justice (Brysk, 2018a). But in every type of society, preexisting patriarchy has produced chronic discrimination in women's self-determination and access to health care, especially in the area of reproductive rights.

The impact of a global health crisis on human rights comes from a combination of the direct consequences of the disease or condition itself for human well-being and capabilities; abusive or discriminatory international, state, and civic health management responses; and manipulation of public health insecurity to consolidate state or corporate power at the expense of vulnerable populations (Sekalala & Harrington, 2020). The social response to communicable disease began as governance and management of public health, but throughout the twentieth century, alternative rights-based and securitized approaches have been in contest (Sekalala & Harrington, 2020, p. 221). With the turn to a rights-based public health response to the AIDS epidemic, Director of the WHO Global Programme on AIDS Jonathan Mann depicted the disease as three "distinct yet intertwined" epidemics: infection, illness, and the "social, cultural, economic and political reaction" thereto (Sekalala & Harrington, 2020, p. 224).

Health crises challenge states to safeguard individual rights as parameters of transparent and accountable public health response, assure the right to health and nondiscriminatory equitable access, guarantee participation and inclusion of affected and vulnerable populations, and maintain international obligations of cooperation and assistance (Bustreo & Doebbler, 2020). Rights-based health experts affirm that the limitations of individual rights in emergency health response must be necessary, proportionate, and nondiscriminatory. They point out that social and economic inequalities in the incidence and impact of COVID-19 show that human rights to health and economic and social rights are indivisible and interdependent (Sekalala et al., 2020). All of these challenges are filtered by the preexisting condition of patriarchy and gender regimes—and we will map the gendered impact of disease, discrimination, insecurity, and inequality on women's rights.

A global health crisis increases the interdependence between political and civil rights with health rights (Clay et al., 2022). In particular, populist nationalist regimes challenge health rights through rejection of the universalism and interdependence of rights as a public good, reactionary resistance to scientific expertise, and resistance to global governance (Gostin et al., 2020; Cooper & Atchison, 2020). Illiberal regimes' COVID-19 response also heightens threats to interdependent civil, political, and equity rights—with special salience for women's rights:

> Although many states' public health efforts have infringed rights, populist nationalist responses are deliberately repressive: they scapegoat marginalized groups, exploit chaos to consolidate power, and punish those who dare counter official positions. Politicians from the United States to Poland have expressly encouraged racism, xenophobia, and homophobia, fomenting discrimination and violence in the pandemic response. Abusing emergency powers, populist leaders in Hungary and India have sought to entrench authoritarian governance structures, further restricting rights and freedoms. (Williams et al., 2020, p. 1767)

We will see discriminatory restrictions on women's self-determination in mobility, labor, and reproduction below intensified under such illiberal regimes. Feminist scholars depict the intersectional impact of COVID-19 as a forecasted failure, based on the historic pattern of discriminatory impact of previous pandemics such as the 1918 flu (Theidon, 2020). More recently, observers of the smaller and more regionally limited Ebola epidemic outlined strikingly similar gendered effects to the current pattern of pandemic patriarchy:

> School closures affected girls' life chances, because many dropped out of education. (A rise in teenage-pregnancy rates exacerbated this trend.) Domestic and sexual violence rose [emphasis original]. And more women died in childbirth because resources were diverted elsewhere. "There's a distortion of health systems, everything goes towards the outbreak," said Wenham, who traveled to west Africa as a researcher during the Ebola crisis. "Things that aren't priorities get canceled. That can have an effect on maternal mortality, or access to contraception." (Lewis, 2020: online)

While these effects of Ebola occurred mostly in traditional gender regimes, the COVID-19 pandemic globalized these rights impacts across all types of gender regimes—a marker of the new parameters of pandemic patriarchy. As Theidon predicts from the initial pattern of the pandemic and the lessons of masculinist responses to past pandemics, "although more men are dying from the direct medical effects, more women and girls will die from the socioeconomic legacies and the spike in domestic and intimate partner violence" (Theidon, 2020, p. 528).

Pandemic patriarchy: The impact of the COVID-19 crisis on women's human rights

The overall impact of the COVID-19 crisis on women's rights has been a cumulative deterioration of conditions with increasing interdependence among types of rights and vulnerable populations. As predicted by the literatures on the human rights regime, patriarchy, and health rights, we have seen increasing tradeoffs of women's security to public health emergencies, declining accountability for lagging social and private sphere rights, growing discrimination in mobility, informal labor, and health care, exacerbated vulnerability of migrants and minorities, and shrinking reproductive rights in illiberal nationalist regimes.

A global panorama illustrates the overall trends, which will be followed by specific tracking of gendered patterns of deterioration in security, labor, and health rights. In the first year of the COVID-19 pandemic, the Global Gender Gap *regressed* more than half a percentage point, led by a 2.4% decrease in women's political empowerment and a gender gap in economic participation and opportunity that is estimated to take over 200 years to close (World Economic Forum, 2021). Gendered vulnerability to the impact of the pandemic includes a preponderance of female health workers at greatest risk from direct contact, migration restrictions differentially targeted at domestic workers, closure of schools which has in turn increased childcare demands on women, and inadequate women's health resources in lockdown and quarantines (Wenham et al., 2020). Moreover, women are especially at risk of loss of employment, health care, and income as informal sector, migrant, service sector, and sex workers (Amnesty International et al.). Rights regressions in the response to COVID-19 can be seen in gendered curfews and selective harassment of marginalized populations for breaking restrictions, women displaced from precarious employment, the increase in women's uncompensated care work, and gendered vulnerability to domestic abuse—with declining access to state services such as shelters (Sekalala et al., 2020; Dlamini, 2020. These new challenges articulate with chronic vulnerabilities and gender discrimination in respect and protection of women's rights to life and safety, to free and fair working conditions, health, and to reproductive self-determination (Smith-Ramakrishnan, 2021).

Gender based violence: Increasing tradeoffs, declining accountability

Gender based violence is a threat to women's rights to life, bodily integrity, security, equality, and health. It is condemned as such by the anti-discrimination CEDAW Convention, the United Nations' Declaration on the Elimination of Violence Against Women, the Council of Europe's Istanbul Convention on Preventing and Combatting Violence Against Women and Domestic Violence (signed by 45 countries and the EU), and the Inter-American Convention on the Prevention, Punishment, and Eradication of Violence against Women (signed by 32 countries). The regional conventions are binding and include monitoring provisions and complaint procedures, which have resulted in state remedies including adoption of new legislation and protection mechanisms. This ensemble of treaties, recommendations, and adjudication has shaped a growing international jurisprudence affirming the due diligence obligations of states for protection from violence by non-state actors. Moreover, there are prevention and assistance programs from UN Women, the Council of Europe, and the Organization of American States. All of these entities have tracked the impact of the COVID-19 pandemic on gender violence which is marked by increasing tradeoffs of women's security and collective health rights, along with declining accountability of perpetrators during lockdowns and with closed or backlogged courts.

COVID-19 lockdowns have been associated with a worldwide increase in reports of domestic violence, as well as increased vulnerability of women cut off from state services such as shelters and police. The global pattern of an immediate surge is striking and consistent. In one of the COVID-19 areas of origin, Chinese cases of gender violence tripled; Brazilian authorities report an increase of 40 to 50% (Graham-Harrison et al., 2020). Calls to the UK Domestic Violence

Helpline increased 25% within a week of the initial lockdown (Bradbury-Jones & Isham, 2020). UN Women has tracked similar increases of 20–30% in reporting and demands for emergency shelter in Argentina, Canada, France, Germany, Spain, the United Kingdom, Australia, and the United States, concluding that "Singapore and Cyprus have registered an increase in calls by more than 30 per cent" (UN Women, 2020, April 6).

A longitudinal regression study from the U.S. shows a 22% greater likelihood of residential domestic violence during the pandemic period compared with the previous year, with a 64% increase following lockdown (Mclay, 2021). One study in India (with one of the worst preexisting rates of gender violence in the world) finds that districts with the most restrictive lockdowns see an increase of .47 standard deviation in domestic violence reports (Ravindran & Shah, 2020). Tracking the social relations that produce this impact, U.N. agencies and their NGO partners in India report characteristic surges in violence along with pandemic losses, draconian government responses, and economic displacement (United Nations Sustainable Development Group, 2020). In a dozen countries of Eurasia, field accounts show how chronic gender inequity and legal lags have similar effects of locking women in with abusers and curtailing access to reporting or protection (Equality Now, 2020). Some governments have adopted tailored responses, from banning alcohol sales in Greenland to setting up alternative reporting channels in grocery stores and pharmacies in France to facilitating court filings for restraining orders during shutdowns in Australia (Berger, 2020). Grassroots women's organizations worldwide have responded by increasing direct services such as hotlines, mobilizing government attention, providing resources for protective equipment in shelters, and facilitating online access.

Pandemic conditions have also been implicated in an increase in human trafficking and forced/child marriage. As a public health study summarizes the increased risk factors and response limitations, "Social isolation of families and severe economic distress amplify the risk of interpersonal violence, unemployment and homelessness, as well as increased internet use by under-supervised children. Aggravating the situation are overwhelmed health systems, severe limitations in activities of social service organizations, and decreased contact of healthcare professionals with children" (Greenbaum et al., 2020, Abstract). The U.N. Office of Drugs and Crime is tracking how loss of livelihood and increases in indebtedness in subsistence informal sectors increases vulnerability to all forms of labor trafficking in several African countries—including how school closures may trigger the exploitation of children denied shelter and food at school sites. Meanwhile, COVID-19 restrictions decrease monitoring of labor rights and trafficking and access to shelters, especially for at-risk populations such as domestic workers. Pandemic shutdowns of police, protective services, and migration processing further isolate trafficking victims (United Nations Office of Drugs & Crime).

At a more structural level, UNFPA studies model the combined effect of declines in family income and interruptions of prevention and intervention programs linked to resource loss and social distancing requirements to increase gender-based violence, child marriage, and FGM/C (female genital mutilation/cutting) in similar ways. For example, one study shows that decline in family income accounts for about 30% of the risk of child marriage in the poorer quintiles of the population and projects average 20% declines in developing world national economies due to the COVID-19 crisis (UNFPA, 2020). A rapid assessment by Save the Children worldwide estimates that COVID-19 economic declines, school closures, and mobility restrictions have put an additional 500,000 girls at risk of forced early marriage that year alone. The majority of those newly at risk are in India, where the economy contracted over 20% and lockdowns displaced migrant laborers and family wage-earners to the most impoverished regions (Cousins, 2020).

Migrants are especially affected by the increase in all of these forms of gender violence, as the analysis above of long-standing gaps in the human rights regime and the intersectional incidence of preexisting patriarchy would suggest. In 2020, a study of the impact of pandemic conditions on displaced women from 15 African countries found that almost three-quarters experienced increased intimate partner violence, over half reported sexual violence, and one-third cited an upsurge in child marriage (Lee, 2021).

The pandemic-era surge in gender-based violence is a reflection and driver of women's loss of political empowerment, labor market participation, and health rights that has a multiplier effect on gender roles and rules going forward. Women disabled, displaced, and disempowered by socially sanctioned abusive relationships suffer life-long consequences that extend to their families and communities—and pandemic-related state suppression of social mobilization diminishes the capacity of women's movements to contest the declining gender regime. The international rights regime that has struggled to expand norms and responsibilities for violence by non-state and transnational actors has declined further with the diminished capacity and resources of states and international institutions alike.

Labor and social rights: Discrimination, displacement, and invisibility

Women worldwide are chronically constrained in social and economic rights through the feminization of poverty, unequal access and treatment in both the formal and informal labor market, vulnerability to sexual harassment, and interdependent constraints on working conditions linked to the double shift of domestic and care work. The pandemic itself and associated response has intensified these conditions—and also introduced new challenges for employment and labor conditions through lockdowns, school and business closures, and migration restrictions. Although labor rights are enumerated in the International Convention on Economic, Social and Cultural Rights (ICESCR) and International Labor Organization (ILO) Conventions—including a recent Convention on the rights of Domestic Workers—implementation occurs unevenly almost exclusively at the national level, and World Bank studies suggest that women are systematically disadvantaged in access to paid employment and working conditions (Buvinic & Furst-Nichols, 2014).

In the era of COVID-19, women worldwide have suffered discrimination and displacement from losses in employment, declining access to income and social goods, and vulnerability to infection as women are disproportionately "essential yet expendable" workers (Neely, 2020). Although cyclical economic recessions typically affect male employment more, the lockdowns of Spring 2020 affected female-dominated service sector jobs—and especially women of color in the lowest-paid and most insecure jobs like domestic workers. Women worldwide experienced relatively higher unemployment and reduced labor market participation, delays in reemployment, increase in the double-shift of care work due to school and childcare closures, and consequent increase in wage gap and regression in professional leadership positions (World Economic Forum, 2021). By 2021, the ILO estimated that during 2020 at least 45 million women left the formal workforce—at least half in Asia (International Labor Organization [ILO], 2021).

The level of gendered impact was most severe in the most unequal developing countries, but also notable in neo-liberal political economies like the U.S., and transitional gender regimes with large numbers of precarious and first-generation women workers. For example, the UNDP Gender Tracker survey of Europe showed that in Turkey, in the first year of the pandemic women took on four times as much unpaid care work as men, while suffering over 50% loss in income (UNDP, 2020). Similarly, in Spain, women were more likely to lose employment and income due to concentration in the service sector. Moreover, "Employment rates were higher for men before the lockdown … . As a result, at the time of the survey, 63.5% of men were working, compared with 46% of women" (Farre et al., 2020, p. 12).

The differential impact of the pandemic on women's job loss, wages, and double shift in the U.S. was labeled a "shecession" (Haradasani Gupta, 2020). Women's unemployment exceeded men's in the U.S., with Latinx women most affected with an estimated 20% unemployment rate. "Women account for two-thirds of workers who make less than $11 an hour, and women of color are overrepresented in these jobs. For example, 90% of domestic care workers are women, and women of color and immigrants compose 58% and 35% respectively of workers in these fields … " (Neely, 2020). Poor women and women of color are even more dependent on low-wage employment for household income, and are disproportionately single mother breadwinners (Frye, 2020). Women at all levels of the income scale are dependent on childcare removed by lockdowns and school closures, and it is estimated that millions of working mothers involuntarily left the workforce in 2020 due to lack of childcare—at levels several times greater than men—suffering billions of dollars in lost wages (Kashen et al., 2020).

At the same time, women's occupational patterns concentrate them as essential workers more vulnerable to health risks—and lower-wage service workers typically lack access to sick leave and adequate health insurance. One of three jobs held by women has been considered "essential"; women comprise a majority of primary care doctors, nurses, health aides, pharmacists, and grocery store cashiers (Robertson & Gebeloff, 2021). As Powell (2020) explains:

> Within this new ecosystem, a "racial justice paradox" has emerged: Blacks and Latinxs are more likely to be unemployed due to the impacts of the pandemic on the labor market, but they are also overrepresented among essential workers who must stay in their jobs, particularly lower-skilled positions, where they are at greater risk of exposure to the virus … . and women of color are more likely to have essential jobs.

In the global South, women's economic vulnerability and concentration in low-wage, precarious, high-risk sectors like crowded sweatshops threatens livelihoods and family access to essential needs. Widespread observations of growing food insecurity in Asia and Latin America due to the gendered impact of economic disruption are echoed in a report on women garment workers in Bangladesh:

> Bangladesh's garment industry is the second-largest in the world, behind China's. It accounts for about 84% of Bangladesh's export revenue and is so critical to the economy that sewing machine operators like Akter were declared essential workers, exempt from a lockdown. Some operations closed anyways … . At least 1 million garment workers [were] fired or furloughed by early April — about a quarter of the industry's Bangladeshi workforce … . Four out of five garment workers are women, who in many cases support several relatives and live from paycheck to paycheck — in a country with no unemployment benefits … . For those workers, a prolonged global recession may prove more deadly than the coronavirus, workers and union representatives say. (Frayer, 2020: online)

Within this pattern of "essential yet expendable" low-wage labor (Neely, 2020), several informal sector gendered job categories are even more vulnerable because they are invisible in the private sphere: domestic workers and sex workers. The ILO estimates that at least 55 million domestic workers lost their jobs in the immediate aftermath of the pandemic, and over 70% suffered major loss of income (ILO, 2021). Domestic workers worldwide are often unregistered, work part-time with multiple employers, lack access to formal health care and social security systems, and many are migrants (Wolfe, 2020).

Sex workers worldwide are unable to work during quarantines and social distancing. In countries where sex work is criminalized, women may be pushed into dangerous endeavors, punished for defiance of lockdowns, and/or ineligible for pandemic relief programs. Even in developed democracies, sex workers report economic crisis and exclusion from government assistance in Europe and Canada (Wheeler, 2020). In developing countries, reports from Asia, Africa, and Latin America show that quarantines of sex workers may threaten food supplies and access to health care—including closure of HIV prevention and treatment programs and facilities (Quarantined to Starvation, 2020; Namubiru et al., 2020). Even states that do not criminalize sex work have generally failed to include women sex workers in medical or social COVID-19 response. Later in the pandemic, sex workers at high risk of COVID-19 due to intimate contact work were often denied priority or eligibility for vaccines—leading to protests in Brazil in March 2021 (Brazil Prostitutes Strike, 2021).

The most vulnerable migrant women's labor and livelihood has also been especially affected by pandemic disruptions of mobility and the informal service economy. Across the developed countries in Europe and North America, immigrants are concentrated in precarious, low-wage, service sector, and unsafe employment and have been disproportionately affected by job loss due to hospitality business closures, COVID-19 morbidity and mortality, and loss of access to health care and education (Organization for Economic Cooperation & Development [OECD], 2020). Migration flows and impacts are also centered in both sending and receiving countries of high COVID-19 incidence, multiplying the economic effects and social costs of the pandemic. According to the International Organization for Migration's Data Analysis Centre–based on World Bank, WHO, and UN Department of Economic and Social Affairs data spanning 2020-2021:

> As of 10 October 2021, emigrants from the 20 countries with the highest number of COVID-19 cases accounted for 33 per cent of the total international migrant stock and they had sent an estimated 41 per cent of all remittances globally to their countries of origin in 2020 (GMDAC analysis based on UN DESA, 2020; World Bank 2021a; WHO, 2021). Immigrants accounted for at least 3.7 per cent of the population in 13 of the 20 countries with the highest number of COVID-19 cases, and this share is more than 8 per cent in 9 of these countries (GMDAC analysis based on UN DESA, 2020; WHO, 2021). Compared to the global share of international migrants making up 3.6 per cent of the total population, international migrants are overrepresented in these countries. (Migration Data Portal, 2021)

An unprecedented intensification in migration restrictions during 2020 further disrupted economic and human flows—and curtailed the operations of humanitarian organizations that assist migrants with social services and resettlement (Ramji-Nogales & Goldner Lang, 2020).

Around half of migrant workers are women, comprising over 66 million women; at least 8.5 million migrants are domestic workers. For women migrants, the pandemic has had a deeper impact on loss of livelihoods and remittances, increase in care work, lack of social protection, limited freedom of movement, and vulnerability to violence. According to UN Women, female migrants are systematically disadvantaged in access to international money transfer services, resulting in increased fees and reduced net remittances, and their remittances are usually dedicated to support for children's education and for the care and health of children and elders—substituting for their domestic gender roles. Migrant women are even more likely than their male counterparts to work in the informal sector—including domestic and sex work–which brings precarious employment, lack of access to health and social services, and increased vulnerability to gender-based abuse and harassment. Women workers are also more likely than males to be undocumented, intensifying their economic and physical insecurity, dependency on exploitative or abusive employers, brokers, and partners, and consequent isolation from health services critical in the pandemic. While some host countries and localities—such as Thailand and California—facilitated universal access to COVID-19 testing and treatment regardless of migration status, and several European states suspended deportations, Trump administration migrant detention policies in the U.S. increased migrants' exposure and infection rate (UN Women, 2020)—with only modest improvement under the Biden Administration.

The World Economic Forum Gender Gap report warns that the ensemble of these declines in women's wages, employment, professional placement, and double shift will have long-term effects, which it labels "labor market scarring" (World Economic Forum, 2021). COVID-19-era regression in economic empowerment is also interdependent with women's insecurity, lack of health care access and reproductive self-determination. Women's economic displacement is abetted by gender regimes that police and privatize women's productive roles, while informalization and occupational stratification of women's labor intersects with marginalization of minorities and migrants—and feeds back to increased care work and declining opportunities in high-wage and emerging sectors.

Women's health and reproductive rights: Discrimination, vulnerability, and backlash

As in other areas, the challenges for women's health rights are a combination of equitable access to universal health rights and gender-specific reproductive rights. The generic right to the highest attainable standard of health and prohibitions on discrimination in health care are enumerated in every major human rights document, including the Universal Declaration of Human Rights; International Covenant on Economic Cultural and Social Rights, Convention on the Elimination of Racial Discrimination (CERD); Convention on the Elimination of Discrimination Against Women (CEDAW); and the Convention on the Rights of Persons with Disabilities. However, rights to health care are notoriously difficult to implement, with limited justiciability relative to states and numerous influences of non-state actors. More specific health-related international jurisprudence and practice has established a right to access to essential medicines, as well as responsibilities of medical professionals relative to torture, children's rights, discrimination, and privacy. Pandemic conditions have directly affected women's vulnerability to COVID-19, discrimination in differential access to health care, and gender-specific restrictions in reproductive health rights (McGovern & Ahmed, 2020).

As the United Nations Office of the High Commissioner on Human Rights outlines reproductive rights norms,

> CEDAW Article 16 guarantees women equal rights in deciding "freely and responsibly on the number and spacing of their children and to have access to the information, education and means to enable them to exercise these rights.... The Beijing Platform for Action states that "the human rights of women include their right to have control over and decide freely and responsibly on matters related to their sexuality, including sexual and reproductive health, free of coercion, discrimination and violence." The CEDAW Committee's General Recommendation 24 recommends that States prioritize the "prevention of unwanted pregnancy through family planning and sex education." The CESCR General Comment 14 has explained that the provision of maternal health services is comparable to a core obligation which cannot be derogated from under any circumstances, and the States have to the immediate obligation to take deliberate, concrete, and targeted steps towards fulfilling the right to health in the context of pregnancy and childbirth. (United Nations Office of the High Commissioner of Human Rights, "Sexual & reproductive health & rights")

The right to safe abortion as integral to health has been progressively recognized by international norms, most recently in the 2016 General Comment by the UN Committee on Economic, Social and Cultural Rights (United Nations Human Rights Committee, General Comment No. 36 (2018) on Article 6 of the International Covenant on Civil and Political Rights, on the Right to Life) (McGovern & Ahmed, 2020).

The COVID-19 pandemic has increased women's vulnerability to illness and need for access to health care. Although male mortality rates from COVID-19 are higher, women in many places are more exposed to COVID-19 due to the concentration of women workers in front-line health and caretaking roles with generally lower access to protective equipment. In Europe, for example, women comprise 83% of nurses and 84% of health care aides for disabled and elderly persons, with documented increased risk of contracting and transmitting COVID-19 (Amnesty International et al., 2020). By mid-2020, the U.S. Centers for Disease Control reported that almost three-fourths of the health workers infected were female (CDC, 2020). Similarly, in Spain women comprised over 75% of health care workers infected with COVID-19 (UN Women, 2020). This vast disproportion of numbers infected means that even with lower mortality rates for females, a larger number of women are likely to perish, suffer acute illness, or struggle with chronic legacies of COVID-19 infection. This observation of differential exposure and infection rates for women in well-documented Northern societies is likely to represent an even greater imbalance in the developing world.

Meanwhile, pandemic-related diversion of medical resources, closures of medical facilities, and lockdowns also deepen women's chronic disadvantage in access to medical care for preventative services and chronic conditions—especially in the developing world. Women worldwide face a panoply of barriers to medical treatment including the feminization of poverty, precarious employment without medical coverage or sick leave, and cultural barriers to access in patriarchal regimes. A U.N. survey in Asia shows that during the pandemic more than half of women surveyed lacked access to medical care, while women in Pakistan, Bangladesh and Thailand waited longer to see a doctor than their male counterparts (UN Women, 2020).

Gendered inequity in health care access is compounded by intersectional discrimination for women of color and migrants. In one representative best-case scenario of a developed country with a national health care system, nevertheless researchers find that "the COVID-19 pandemic has amplified existing barriers to healthcare in England for ethnic minority and migrant women" (Germain & Yong, 2020, Introduction). They trace this disparity to pandemic-related shifts within the healthcare system that interact with long-standing issues in the broader society. In response to COVID-19, the health care system allocates resources away from non-COVID-19 patients and institutes patient ranking systems that result in disproportionate ethnic minority deaths and pregnancy vulnerability. These patients already face lower access to preventative and mental health care, biased medical perceptions, and gendered cultural norms that discourage women from seeking care or prioritizing their own health within the family that are exacerbated by pandemic conditions.

In the broader society, minority and migrant women's access to health care is impaired by less exposure to health and healthcare information and lower internet access, legal barriers and tiered medical payment requirements for migrants—who are often lower-wage women and single mothers–and in some cases, dependency on abusive partners to get medical care and/or migration status. A similar pattern is seen for the U.S., where the highest maternal mortality rates in the developed world manifest extreme racial disparities, and both COVID-19 itself and discriminatory health system response have further undermined maternal health care (Center for Reproductive Rights, 2020, 2021; Chosid, 2021).

Pandemic policies threaten reproductive rights in new ways, including increased vulnerability to unwanted pregnancy; lack of access to contraception, prenatal care and abortion services due to mobility restrictions and resource diversion; and deepening government restrictions on contraception and abortion adopted under cover of the crisis (Brysk & Fuentes Carreño, 2020a, Chosid, 2021). COVID-19 has disrupted women's access to family planning through closures of health facilities, supply chain disruptions, and mobility restrictions. The U.N. projects that 47 million women with unmet need for family planning in developing countries may lose access due to lockdowns, with a resulting seven million unintended pregnancies in six months (UNFPA, 2020). As one global analysis put it, "the sexual-health supply chain is broken"—with detailed examples of the scope and impact of interruptions of supplies of condoms in several major African countries (Sussman, 2020). Because manufacturing in Asia was hit hard by COVID-19, severe lockdowns and restrictions on pharmaceutical exports and imports made women vulnerable who depend on low-cost supplies of abortion medication that originate in China. For example, Kenya and Uganda have been facing a shortage of medical abortion pills and other contraceptive supplies because they depend on imports (Wadekar, 2020). In Latin America, where abortion is mostly illegal but the use of pharmaceuticals rather than surgical abortion is often tolerated, activists have struggled to overcome pandemic intensification of barriers to access misoprostol due to lockdowns, mobility restrictions in rural areas, increasing domestic violence, and legal bottlenecks (Salomon & Alford, 2020).

Access to abortion is even more affected due to its contentious legal status. Poland, with one of the most restrictive abortion laws in Europe, took advantage of the crisis to push through a near total ban (Krajewska, 2020). Even where access is legal, it may be effectively limited by restricted mobility due to pandemic measures. For example, in Mexico, women who need surgical abortions are denied access because they cannot travel to Mexico City or Oaxaca where these services are available, while local restrictions on movement make it almost impossible for women in urban areas to get the pills for medical abortions from pharmacies.

Women's lack of health care access and reproductive self-determination is interdependent with vulnerability to gender-based violence, limitations in the labor market, and gender roles in the household. Declining fulfillment of women's health rights weighs most heavily on the lower-resourced Global South and the poor worldwide. Gendered patterns of COVID-19 morbidity, maternal mortality, and unplanned reproduction have inter-generational consequences for gender roles and family structure. Moreover, regressions in reproductive rights are often impelled by and reinforce populist nationalist regimes that manifest poor pandemic governance—and may even use "culture wars" on gender modernization to distract from health crisis.

Responding to pandemic patriarchy: Feminist empowerment

Responsibility for responding to pandemic patriarchy is clearly identified in the human rights regime by the norms cited in each area, but the parameters of pandemic patriarchy have exacerbated chronic rights gaps and gender inequity. In response to the COVID-19 crisis, human rights monitors and advocates quickly called for gender-sensitive-monitoring of the impacts and women's inclusion in designing health measures and social policies. They identified concrete measures states can undertake to ameliorate gender violence, economic insecurity, and health needs—and disseminated some model responses (United Nations Human Rights, 2020). For example, Amnesty International, International Planned Parenthood Federation, and Women's Link Worldwide provided a detailed guide for high-capacity European states on their rights obligations and recommendations for the enhancement of state support services and due process during pandemic conditions of lockdown, quarantines, and travel limitations in the areas of gender violence; trafficking; access to contraceptives, abortion, and reproductive health services; protection for migrants, refugees, and asylum-seekers (Amnesty International et al., 2020). These worthwhile measures to promote women's human rights are a necessary but by no means sufficient response to a cumulative, structural crisis of pandemic patriarchy—and "rights as usual" policies have not been consistently adopted even in the best-resourced and governed regions.

As we have seen above, there has been some increased global awareness of the gendered impact of this pandemic and best practices to restore rights but state policy response has been inadequate and unbalanced—worldwide and especially in areas of stronger preexisting patriarchy. (UN Women, 2021) The UNDP tracks shortfalls in Gender Policy responses to COVID-19 worldwide as well as in-depth regional profiles in the areas of violence against women, social protection and labor market policies to safeguard women's economic security, and policy support for unpaid care work. For example, the Arab States region shows highly variable state response impaired by poverty, conflict, and limited COVID-19 monitoring and funding. Throughout the MENA region, women are greatly underrepresented in pandemic decision-making bodies such as COVID-19 task forces. Less than half the 22 states adopted measures responding to gender-based violence, and the region's response is the lowest in the world—but countries such as Egypt, Bahrain, Jordan, Palestine, and Lebanon did support increased services for survivors of violence. While most Arab states have adopted social protection policies in response to the pandemic, only about one-quarter are ranked by this U.N. assessment as gender-sensitive, defined as attending to the impact of the pandemic on women's labor market and social resource needs. Specifically, there has been very little response to the impact of COVID-19 on care work, which is especially salient for women in the region heavily concentrated in that sector (United Nations Development Programme [UNDP], 2021). Similarly, in the Europe Central Asia region (Western Balkans, South Caucasus, and Central Asia) most states took some measures to strengthen services for gender-based violence, but there was little gender-sensitive social policy (UNDP, 2021).

Our analysis of the changing scenario of pandemic patriarchy suggests that a reorientation of response is needed, based in a more systematic incorporation of feminist insights on human rights. Feminism as a strategy of global governance, program of national gender equity, ethic of care, and movement toward women's empowerment contributes to addressing the preexisting patriarchy and lagging health rights that drive pandemic patriarchy.

Women's empowerment shapes a successful response to the pandemic and the attendant social consequences. In every region and at every level of development, female-headed countries have

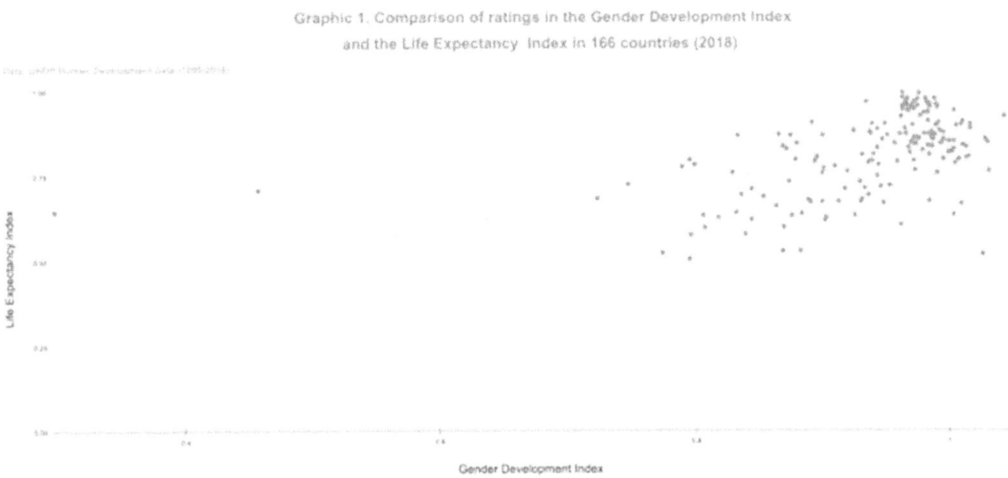

Figure 1. Comparison of ratings in the gender development index and the life emergency index in 166 countries (2018). *Source.* UNDP Human Development Data (1990–2018), graphic courtesy of the authors (Brysk and Fuentes 2020b).

managed the COVID-19 crisis more effectively, with fewer fatalities and less livelihood loss than others: from Germany to Taiwan to Sint Maarten, from Norway to New Zealand to Namibia (Ayene, 2020; Hassan & O'Grady, 2020; Wittenberg-Cox, 2020; Yancey-Bragg, 2020). Even more gender-balanced societies headed by men—like Canada—do better in health crises compared to their less gender equitable peers and neighbors—like the United States. On the other hand, the most patriarchal countries headed by nationalist strongmen do worse; in the case of COVID-19, Iran, Russia, and Brazil stand out for the costs of pandemic patriarchy. In Brazil, we can even compare longitudinally the current COVID-19 denial and Bolsonaro's disastrous mismanagement with a positively evolving response to the AIDS and Zika health crises under less masculinist leadership that was engaged with improving gender equity (Londono et al., 2020). A mid-2020 economists' study that compares COVID-19 cases and deaths by matching female-led countries to their sociologically similar neighbors and peers and tracking differences in policy response such as the length of lockdowns concludes that COVID-19 outcomes are systematically better in countries led by women. The study links better outcomes to differences in policy measures (Garikipati & Kambhampati, 2020).

Feminist leadership is a proxy for a broader positive association between gender equity and human rights that is particularly strong for health rights. In "Why Feminism Is Good for Your Health," we sketch this suggestive pattern with a simple scatter plot and a Pearson correlation of the Gender Development Index and the Life Expectancy Index that shows a positive linear relationship between them (Brysk & Fuentes Carreño, 2020b) (Figure 1).

The overall association depicted incorporates many additional elements—but we can trace a connection between women's rights and health more systematically through literature on the sociological impact of women's empowerment and equity on development and governance. Long-standing research shows that gender equity is associated with more and better distributed development, which leads to better state capacity and fulfillment of social rights (Lawson-Remer, 2012). Women's empowerment generally fosters more rights-based development, better personal and international security, and more sustainable population growth as lower levels of hierarchy provide political incentives to invest in the broader population (Hudson et al., 2020). At the same time, broader political participation by women tends to drive more spending on public health, education and children's needs (Doepke et al., 2012). Societies with higher levels of women's rights and empowerment are usually better for overall rights fulfillment and broader political participation because they tend to be more collaboratively and more effectively governed (Muntaner

& Ng, 2019). This ensemble of tendencies suggests that more gender equitable societies have been relatively resilient in the current pandemic because they have more equitable access to social welfare such as health care, more effective and accountable governments, more diversified economies with better social safety nets for economic impacts, along with more global cooperation for expertise and management (Vogelstein, 2021; Greer et al., 2021).

In one outstanding example, Taiwan's record as a COVID-19 champion illustrates how feminist governance is an alternative to pandemic patriarchy. Through a combination of Taiwan's democratization pathway, an empowered women's movement, and a cosmopolitan global role of "soft power" to break its diplomatic isolation, Taiwan has achieved the highest level of gender equity in East Asia—by the metric of the United Nations Gender Inequality Index (Li, 2020; "Taiwan No. 1," 2021). As the general trends above suggest, Taiwan's feminist governance has built from and reinforced the lowest level of economic inequality in the region, a rapid voluntary population transition, an increasingly information-based economy, and marked investments in public health and education (Brysk, 2020a).

Turning to the global level and health cooperation, more gender-balanced states tend to have more multilateral and humanitarian foreign policies—they invest in global institutions and programs that support global health at home and abroad (Brysk & Mehta, 2014). Such globalist countries are better positioned to tap into international knowledge, networks, and resources to manage a border-crossing health crisis. By contrast, macho nationalists operating in isolation from global cooperation in the United States, the United Kingdom, Iran, and Russia visibly failed to protect their citizens—and lagged in adjusting their supply chains for medical supplies and citizen consumption of essential goods alike. At the global level, leading gender equitable societies such as Canada and Sweden and some feminist leaders have long proposed a "feminist foreign policy" that would enhance all aspects of interdependent international human rights. A feminist foreign policy pursues a combination of representational gender equity in diplomatic leadership, international institutions, and conflict resolution venues–as well as prioritizing women's rights issues in all aspects of international political economy, security, humanitarian, environment, and global health governance (Thompson & Clement, 2019).

At the level of human rights norms, this suggests that we must move toward a rights ethos imbued with a feminist ethic of care—and that this broader vision may also improve responses to pandemic patriarchy. The ethic of care can expand our notions of inclusion, solidarity, and empowerment across the public-private, civil-social, and national-global divides that bedevil the current human rights regime. A more relational vision of rights broadens the "responsibility to protect" from states to societies and across social systems—including the evolving forms of structural patriarchy (Brysk, 2021). The Economic Commission on Latin America (CEPAL) combined efforts with UN Women at the onset of the pandemic to document the impact and needs of the care economy in the region and to highlight emerging planning and policy modalities for the chronic care crisis in Uruguay, Costa Rica, Colombia, Mexico, Chile, and Paraguay. The report documents model state policy responses to the care economy: protection of domestic workers enacted in Argentina, Chile, and Peru; extended family leave in Argentina, Cuba, and Trinidad; relief funding for home and care workers in Argentina, Ecuador, Dominican Republic, Uruguay; and public education campaigns on gender equity, women's rights, and household labor in Argentina, Ecuador, El Salvador, Mexico, and the Dominican Republic (CEPAL/UN Women, 2020). In Argentina, the Women's Ministry has convened an Inter-Ministerial planning process for the care economy with the Ministries of Economy, Labor, Health, Education, and Social Development. This body met at the initial declaration of a health emergency in March 2020, and enacted gender-sensitive policies such as paid leave for caretakers of minor children, registration of domestic workers for emergency relief funds, and expansion of reporting channels for gender-based violence. The national slogan was #CuarentenaconDerechos [Quarantine with rights] (Argentina, 2020).

Thus, a UNDP study of pandemic effects on gender inequity through the care work burden concludes that a profound and coordinated investment in gender equity in policy, the private sector, and attitudinal change will yield benefits for women—and also the recovery of overall growth and employment:

> In conclusion, the pandemic's profoundly negative impacts on women's work have also had the effect of bringing the phenomenon of unpaid care to the forefront of public and policy discourse. We now have incontrovertible evidence of the costs of women's unpaid caring labour and its value to economies and societies, along with policy tools and innovative community-based and business initiatives to make investing in a care economy a reality. (Mariotti et al., 2021, p. 4)

Conclusion

This survey of the gendered impact of COVID-19 suggests key findings of the impact of public health on women's private sphere vulnerability to gender violence, the interdependence between gendered economic roles and health rights, and the dangers of reproductive rights regression. At the same time, women's empowerment and political participation at all levels has special significance for the management of global health. The deterioration in gendered power relations articulates with long-standing gaps in the international human rights regime in the areas of rights interdependence, intersectional vulnerability, and accountability for "private wrongs" committed by non-state actors.

The struggle to overcome pandemic patriarchy reinforces some long-standing guidance for the international human rights regime—and suggests greater emphasis on some emerging challenges. In an era of global health crisis, human rights are ever more indivisible, interdependent, and intersectional. Now more than ever, for women's rights as human rights, the personal is political and the gendered body is a site of struggle. But there are differences in the character of pandemic patriarchy that warrant further research on the intervening impact of patriarchal gender regimes, intersectional vulnerability, and illiberal nationalism on health governance, reproductive rights, and women's empowerment.

Successful responses to pandemic patriarchy go beyond women's leadership to deepening gender equity and a feminist approach to global governance. A feminist ethos of rights as care carries the potential to heal—and perhaps prevent—the harms of pandemic patriarchy in the COVID-19 crisis and beyond.

References

Amnesty International, International Planned Parenthood Federation, Women's Link Worldwide (2020). *A guide for Europe: Protecting women's rights in the time of COVID*. May 26, 2020, Index Number: EUR 01/2360/2020.

Argentina. Ministerio de las Mujeres, Generos y Diversidad (2020). *Políticas de Cuidado frente al COVID-19: Segundo Encuentro de la Mesa interministerial de Políticas de Cuidado*. March 2020. Políticas de cuidado frente al COVID-19 - Argentina.gob.ar https://www.argentina.gob.ar›sites›default›files

Ayene, T. (2020, May 27). Coronavirus: Namibia praised for containing the virus. The Africa Report. https://www.theafricareport.com/28840/coronavirus-nambia-praised-for-containing-the-virus/

Badran, S., & Turnbull, B. (2022). COVID-19 and authoritarian consolidation in North Africa. *Journal of Human Rights, 21*(3).

Berger, M. (2020). Measures to combat COVID are a nightmare for victims of domestic violence. *The Washington Post.* https://www.washingtonpost.com/world/2020/04/01/measures-control-spread-coronavirus-are-nightmare-victims-domestic-violence-advocates-are-demanding-that-governments-step-up/

Bradbury-Jones, C., & Isham, L. (2020). The pandemic paradox: The consequences of COVID-19 on domestic violence. *Journal of Clinical Nursing, 29*(13–14), 2047–2049. https://doi.org/10.1111/jocn.15296

Brazil prostitutes strike for first-line COVID shots (2021, April 7). *France 24.* https://www.france24.com/en/live-news/20210407-brazil-prostitutes-strike-for-first-line-covid-shots

Brysk, A. (2021). Making rights rhetoric work: Constructing care in a post-liberal world. In A. Brysk, H. Mahmoudi, & K. Seaman (Eds.), *The changing ethos of human rights.* Edward Elgar Publishing.

Brysk, A. (2020a). Constructing rights in Taiwan: The feminist factor, democratization, and the quest for global citizenship. *The Pacific Review, 34*(5), 838–870. https://doi.org/10.1080/09512748.2020.1784985

Brysk, A. (2020b). Global dynamics of authoritarian populism. https://www.21global.ucsb.edu/global-e/february-2020/global-dynamics-authoritarian-populism

Brysk, A. (2018a). *The future of human rights.* Polity Press.

Brysk, A. (2018b). *The struggle for freedom from fear: Contesting violence against women at the frontiers of globalization.* Oxford University Press.

Brysk, A., & Mehta, A. (2014). Do rights at home boost rights abroad? Sexual equality and humanitarian foreign policy. *Journal of Peace Research, 51*(1), 97–110. https://doi.org/10.1177/0022343313500805

Brysk, A., & Fuentes Carreño, M. (2020a, September 2020). Pandemic patriarchy and threats to reproductive rights. *Open Global Rights.* https://www.openglobalrights.org/pandemic-patriarchy-regulation-access-and-governance-in-reproductive-rights/

Brysk, A., & Fuentes Carreño, M. (2020b, August 2020). Why feminism is good for your health. *New Security Beat.* https://www.newsecuritybeat.org/2020/08/feminism-good-health/?utm_source=feedburner&utm_medium=email&utm_campaign=Feed%3A+TheNewSecurityBeat+%28New+Security+Beat%29

Bunch, C., & Reilly, N. (2019). Women's rights as human rights: Twenty-five years on. In N. Reilly (Eds.), *International human rights of women.* Springer. https://doi.org/10.1007/978-981-10-8905-3_2

Bustreo, F., & Doebbler, C. (2020). The rights-based approach to health. In L. O. Gostin & B. M, Meier (Eds.), *Foundations of global health & human rights* (pp. 89–110). Oxford University Press.

Buvinic, M., & Furst-Nichols, R. (2014). Promoting women's economic empowerment: What works? Policy Research Working Paper No. 7087. World Bank Group. https://openknowledge.worldbank.org/handle/10986/20629.

Centers for Disease Control (2020). *Characteristics of Health Care Personnel with COVID-19* — United States, February 12–April 9, 2020. *MMWR Morbidity and Mortality Weekly Rep, 69*, 477–481. http://dx.doi.org/10.15585/mmwr.mm6915e6

Center for Reproductive Rights. (2020). *The COVID-19 pandemic is exacerbating a human rights crisis in U.S. maternal health.* (2020, September 9). https://reproductiverights.org/covid-19-resources/

Center for Reproductive Rights. (2021). *COVID-19 resources: Reproductive rights in the time of COVID, abortion is essential healthcare, COVID-19 is exacerbating a crisis in maternal health care.* Center for Reproductive Rights. https://reproductiverights.org/covid-19-resources/

CEPAL [Economic Commission for Latin America]/UN Women (2020). *Cuidados en América Latina y el Caribe en tiempos de COVID-19. Hacia sistemas integrales para fortalecer la respuesta y la recuperacíon.* July 9 2020. https://lac.unwomen.org/en/digiteca/publicaciones/2020/08/cuidados-en-america-latina-y-el-caribe-en-tiempos-de-covid-19

Chenoweth, E. (2022). Can nonviolent resistance survive COVID-19? *Journal of Human Rights, 21*(3), 304–316.

Chiozza, G., & King, J. (2022a). Introduction to a special issue on beyond complacency and acrimony: Studying human rights in a post-COVID-19 world. *Journal of Human Rights, 21*(3), 245.

Chiozza, G., & King, J. (2022b). The state of human rights in a (post) COVID-19 world. *Journal of Human Rights, 21*(3), 246–262.

Chosid, H. (2021). Overlapping crises: Gender-based violence, maternal mental health, and COVID-19. *New Security Beat.* https://www.newsecuritybeat.org/2021/03/overlapping-crises-gender-based-violence-maternal-mental-health-covid-19/?utm_source=feedburner&utm_medium=email&utm_campaign=Feed%3A+TheNewSecurityBeat+%28New+Security+Beat%29

Clay, C., et al. (2022). The effect of the COVID-19 pandemic on human rights practices: Findings from the Human Rights Measurement Initiative's 2021 Practitioner Survey. *Journal of Human Rights, 21*(3), 317–333.

Cooper, L., & Aitchison, G. (Eds.). (2020). *The dangers ahead: COVID-19, authoritarianism and democracy.* http://eprints.lse.ac.uk/105103/4/dangers_ahead.pdf

Cousins, S. (2020). 2.5 million more child marriages due to COVID-19 pandemic. *The Lancet, 396*(10257), 1059. https://doi.org/10.1016/S0140-6736(20)32112-7

Dlamini, J. (2021). Gender-based violence, twin pandemic to COVID-19. *Critical Sociology, 47*(4–5), 583–590. https://doi.org/10.1177/0896920520975465

Doepke, M., Tertilt, M., & Voena, A. (2012). The economics and politics of women's rights. *Annual Review of Economics*, *4*(1), 339–372. https://doi.org/10.1146/annurev-economics-061109-080201

Equality Now (2020). *The impact of COVID-19 on discrimination and violence against women and girls in Eurasia and the way forward.* https://d3n8a8pro7vhmx.cloudfront.net/equalitynow/pages/3362/attachments/original/1589463991/Equality_Now_Briefing_COVID-19_VAWG_Eurasia_May_2020_(1).pdf?1589463991

Farmer, P. (2005). *Pathologies of power.* University of California Press.

Farre, L., Fawaz, Y., Gonzalez, L., & Graves, J. (2020). *How the Covid-19 lockdown affected gender inequality in paid and unpaid work in Spain.* SSRN Scholarly Paper, ID 3643198, Social Science Research Network, 7 July 2020. https://papers.ssrn.com/abstract=3643198

Frayer, L. (2020, 5 June). For Bangladesh's struggling garment workers, hunger is a bigger worry than pandemic. *NPR (National Public Radio).* https://www.npr.org/2020/06/05/869486297/for-bangladeshs-struggling-garment-workers-hunger-is-a-bigger-worry-than-pandemic

Frye, J. (2020, April 23). On the frontlines on the frontlines at work and at home: The disproportionate economic effects of the coronavirus pandemic on women of color. *Center for American Progress.* https://www.american-progress.org/issues/women/reports/2020/04/23/483846/frontlines-work-home/

Garikapati, S., & Kambhampati, U. (2020, June 21). Women leaders are better at fighting the pandemic. *VOXEU CEPR.* https://voxeu.org/article/women-leaders-are-better-fighting-pandemic

Germain, S., & Yong, A. (2020). COVID-19 highlighting inequalities in access to healthcare in England: A case study of ethnic minority and migrant women. *Feminist Legal Studies*, *28*(3), 301–310. https://doi.org/10.1007/s10691-020-09437-z

Gostin, L. O., Constantin, A., & Meier, B. (2020). Global health & human rights in the age of populism. In L. O. Gostin & B. M. Meier (Eds.), *Foundations of global health & human rights* (pp. 439–458). Oxford University Press.

Graham-Harrison, E., Giuffrida, A., Smith, H., & Ford, L. (2020, March 28). Lockdowns around the world bring increase in domestic violence. *The Guardian.* https://www.theguardian.com/society/2020/mar/28/lockdowns-world-rise-domestic-violence?CMP=Share_iOSApp_Other

Greenbaum, J., Stoklosa, H., & Murphy, L. (2020). The public health impact of coronavirus disease on human trafficking. *Frontiers in Public Health*, *8*, 561184. https://doi.org/10.3389/fpubh.2020.561184

Greer, S. L., King, E. J., da Fonseca, E. M., & Peralta-Santos, A. (2021). *Coronavirus politics: The comparative politics and policy of COVID-19.* University of Michigan Press. https://doi.org/10.3998/mpub.11927713

Haradisani Gupta, A. (2020, May 9). Why some women call this recession a 'Shecession'. *The New York Times.* https://www.nytimes.com/2020/05/09/us/unemployment-coronavirus-women.html

Hassan, J., & O'Grady, S. (2020, April 20). Female world leaders hailed as voices of reason amid the coronavirus chaos. *The Washington Post.* https://www.washingtonpost.com/world/2020/04/20/female-world-leaders-hailed-voices-reason-amid-coronavirus-chaos/

Hudson, V. M., Bowen, D. L., & Nielsen, P. L. (2020). *The first political order: How sex shapes governance and national security worldwide.* Columbia University Press.

IDEA-Institute for Democracy and Electoral Assistance (2021). *Global state of democracy report 2021: Building resilience in a pandemic era.* https://www.idea.int/gsod/global-report#chapter-2-democracy-health-check:-an-overview-of-global-tre

International Labor Organization. (2020, 15 June). *Impact of the Covid-19 crisis on loss of jobs and hours among domestic workers.* https://www.ilo.org/global/topics/domestic-workers/publications/factsheets/WCMS_747961/lang–en/index.htm

ILO (2021). *ILO monitor: COVID-19 and the world of work* (7th ed.). World Employment and Social Outlook: Trends. https://www.ilo.org/wcmsp5/groups/public/—dgreports/—dcomm/documents/briefingnote/wcms_824092.pdf

Kashen, J., Glynn, S. J., & Novello, A. (2020, October 30). How COVID-19 sent women's workforce progress backwards. *Center for American Progress.* https://www.americanprogress.org/issues/women/reports/2020/10/30/492582/covid-19-sent-womens-workforce-progress-backward/

Koo, J. -W. (2022). Global perceptions of South Korea's COVID-19 policy responses: Topic modeling with tweets. *Journal of Human Rights*, *21*(3): 334–353.

Korolczuk, E., & Graff, A. (2018). Gender as "Ebola from Brussels": The anticolonial frame and the rise of illiberal populism. *Signs: Journal of Women in Culture and Society*, *43*(4), 797–821. https://doi.org/10.1086/696691

Krajewska, A. (2020, November 2). Reproductive rights and democracy in Poland. *Oxford Human Rights Hub.* https://ohrh.law.ox.ac.uk/reproductive-rights-and-democracy-in-poland/

Lawson-Remer, T. (2012, August 21). *Gender equality matters for development outcomes.* Council On Foreign Relations. https://www.cfr.org/blog/gender-equality-matters-development-outcomes

Lee, C. (2021, November 24). COVID-19 pandemic exacerbates violence against refugee women and girls. *New Security Beat.* https://www.newsecuritybeat.org/2021/11/covid-19-pandemic-exacerbates-violence-refugee-women-girls/

Lewis, H. (2020, March 19). The coronavirus is a disaster for feminism. *The Atlantic*. https://www.theatlantic.com/international/archive/2020/03/feminism-womens-rights-coronavirus-covid19/608302/

Li, N. (2020, March 6). Taiwan first in Asia in gender equality, based on UN Data. *Taipei Times*. https://www.taipeitimes.com/News/biz/archives/2020/03/06/2003732143

Londono, E., Andreoni, M., & Casado, L. (2020, June 18). Brazil, once a leader, struggles to contain virus amid political turmoil. *The New York Times*. https://www.nytimes.com/2020/05/16/world/americas/virus-brazil-deaths.html

Mariotti, I., Sadasivam, B., & Miyaoi, K. (2021, September 2021). *Investing in care: A pathway to gender-responsive COVID-19 recovery*. Global Policy Network Brief.

Mclay, M. M. (2021). When "shelter-in-place" isn't shelter that's safe: A rapid analysis of domestic violence case differences during the COVID-19 pandemic and stay-at-home orders. *Journal of Family Violence* (January 7):1-10. https://doi.org/10.1007/s10896-020-00225-6

McGovern, T., & Ahmed, A. (2020). Equity in health: Sexual and reproductive health and rights. In L. O. Gostin & B. M. Meier (Eds.), *Foundations of Global Health & Human Rights* (pp. 307–326). Oxford University Press.

Meier, B. M., & Gostin, L. O. (2018). Framing human rights in global health governance. In B. M. Meier & L. O. Gostin (Eds.), *Human rights in global health: Rights-based governance for a globalizing world* (pp. 63–85). Oxford University Press.

Migration Data Portal (2021). *Migration data relevant to the COVID-19 pandemic*. Retrieved September 7, 2021, from https://migrationdataportal.org/themes/migration-data-relevant-covid-19-pandemic

Muntaner, C., & Ng, E. (2019, 16 January). Here's why having more women in government is good for your health. *World Economic Forum*. https://www.weforum.org/agenda/2019/01/the-more-women-in-government-the-healthier-a-population/

Murdie, A. (2022). Hindsight is 2020: Lessons from the COVID-19 pandemic for future human rights research. *Journal of Human Rights*, *21*(3).

Namubiru, L., Wepukhulu, K. S., & Cullinan, K. (2020, June 4). Sex workers abandoned as COVID-19 crackdowns undo Africa's HIV efforts. *Mail and Guardian*. https://mg.co.za/africa/2020-06-04-sex-workers-abandoned-as-covid-19-crackdowns-undo-africas-hiv-efforts/

Neely, T. (2020). *Essential and expendable: Gendered labor in the Coronavirus crisis*. The Clayman Center for Gender Research, Stanford University. https://gender.stanford.edu/news-publications/gender-news/essential-and-expendable-gendered-labor-coronavirus-crisis

Organisation for Economic Co-operation and Development (2020, 19 October). What is the impact of the Covid-19 pandemic on immigrants and their children? http://www.oecd.org/coronavirus/policy-responses/what-is-the-impact-of-the-covid-19-pandemic-on-immigrants-and-their-children-e7cbb7de/

Powell, C. (2020, June 4). The color and gender of COVID: Essential workers, not disposable. *Think Global Health*. https://www.thinkglobalhealth.org/article/color-and-gender-covid-essential-workers-not-disposable-people

'Quarantined to Starvation': A Bangladeshi Sex Worker's Struggles Amid the COVID-19 Lockdown," [by "Maliha"] (2020, April 24). *The Diplomat*. https://thediplomat.com/2020/04/quarantined-to-starvation-a-bangladeshi-sex-workers-struggles-amid-the-covid-19-lockdown/

Ramji-Nogales, J., & Goldner Lang, I. (2020). Freedom of movement, migration, and borders. *Journal of Human Rights*, *19*(5), 593–602. https://doi.org/10.1080/14754835.2020.1830045

Ravindran, S., & Shah, M. (2020). *Unintended consequences of lockdowns: COVID-19 and the shadow pandemic* (working paper series, working paper no. 135). Berkeley, CA: University of California Center for Effective Global Action. https://doi.org/10.26085/C34S3K

Robertson, C., & Gebeloff, R. (2021, April 18). How millions of women became the most essential workers in America. *New York Times*. https://www.nytimes.com/2020/04/18/us/coronavirus-women-essential-workers.html

Salomon, J., & Alford, C. (2020, September 2020). Activists in Latin America battle to guarantee access to safe abortion in COVID-19 world. *Amnesty International*. https://www.amnesty.org/en/latest/news/2020/09/activists-latin-america-access-safe-abortion-covid19/

Sekalala, S., & Harrington, J. (2020). Communicable diseases, health security, and human rights: From AIDS to Ebola. In Lawrence O. Gostin & Benjamin Mason Meier (Eds.), *Foundations of global health and human rights* (pp. 221–242). Oxford University Press.

Sekalala, S., Formal, L., & Habibi, R., (2020). Health and human rights are inextricably linked in the COVID-19 response. *BMJ Global Health*, *5*(9), e003359. https://doi.org/10.1136/bmjgh-2020-003359

Smith-Ramakrishnan, V. (2021, August 4). No vaccine to end the shadow pandemic of gender-based violence. *New Security Beat*. https://www.newsecuritybeat.org/2021/08/no-vaccine-end-shadow-pandemic/

Sussman, A. L. (2020, June 8). The sexual-health supply chain is broken. *The Atlantic*.

"Taiwan No. 1 in Asia, No. 6 in World for Gender Equality." (2021, January 9). *Taipei Times*. https://www.taipeitimes.com/News/taiwan/archives/2021/01/09/2003750242

Theidon, K. (2020). A forecasted failure: Intersectionality, COVID-19, and the perfect storm. *Journal of Human Rights, 19*(5), 528–536. https://doi.org/10.1080/14754835.2020.1822156

Thompson, L., & Clement, R. (2019). Defining feminist foreign policy. *International Center for Research on Women.* https://www.icrw.org/publications/defining-feminist-foreign-policy/

United Nations Development Program. *COVID-19 global gender response policy tracker.* https://data.undp.org/gendertracker/: Fact Sheet on Arab States Region (May 21, 2021), Fact Sheet on Europe and Central Asia (December 2020).

United Nations Population Fund [UNFPA]. (2020, 27 April). *Impact of the COVID-19 pandemic on family planning and ending gender-based violence, female genital mutilation and child marriage.* Interim Technical Note. https://www.unfpa.org/resources/impact-covid-19-pandemic-family-planning-and-ending-gender-based-violence-female-genital

United Nations Human Rights Committee, general comment no. 36 (2018) on Article 6 of the International Covenant on Civil and Political Rights, on the right to life. (https://www.ohchr.org/Documents/HRBodies/CCPR/CCPR_C_GC_36.pdf).

United Nations Office of Drugs and Crime, Impact of the COVID-19 Pandemic on Trafficking in Persons, https://www.unodc.org/documents/Advocacy-Section/HTMSS_Thematic_Brief_on_COVID-19.pdf.

United Nations Human Rights. Office of the High Commissioner. (2020, 15 April). *COVID-19 and women's human rights: Guidance.* https://www.ohchr.org/EN/NewsEvents/Pages/COVID19Guidance.aspx

United Nations Office of the High Commissioner of Human Rights. Sexual and reproductive health and rights. https://www.ohchr.org/en/issues/women/wrgs/pages/healthrights.aspx

United Nations Sustainable Development Group (2020). *Shadow pandemic: UN India responds to uptick in violence against women and girls during COVID-19.* https://unsdg.un.org/latest/stories/shadow-pandemic-un-india-responds-uptick-violence-against-women-and-girls-during

UN Women (2020). *Addressing the impacts of the COVID-19 pandemic on women migrant workers.* https://www.unwomen.org/-/media/headquarters/attachments/sections/library/publications/2020/guidance-note-impacts-of-the-covid-19-pandemic-on-women-migrant-workers-en.pdf?la=en&vs=2259

UN Women (2021, 16 December). *Women and girls left behind: Glaring gaps in pandemic response..* https://data.unwomen.org/publications/women-and-girls-left-behind-glaring-gaps-pandemic-responses.

UN Women (2020, April 23), *Rapid Assessment Survey on the socio-economic consequences of COVID-19 on women's and men's economic empowerment.* https://www.unwomen.org/sites/default/files/Headquarters/Attachments/Sections/Library/Publications/2020/Guidance-note-Impacts-of-the-COVID-19-pandemic-on-women-migrant-workers-en.pdf

UN Women (2020, April 29), *Surveys show that COVID-19 has gendered effects in Asia and the Pacific.* https://data.unwomen.org/resources/surveys-show-covid-19-has-gendered-effects-asia-and-pacific

UN Women (2020, April 6). *Violence against women and girls: The Shadow Pandemic.* Statement by Statement by Phumzile Mlambo-Ngcuka, Executive Director of UN Women. https://www.unwomen.org/en/news/stories/2020/4/statement-ed-phumzile-violence-against-women-during-pandemic

Vogelstein, R. (2021, February 2). There will be another pandemic. Women can stop it. *Foreign Policy.* https://foreignpolicy.com/2021/02/02/next-pandemic-women-leadership-global-health-system-coronavirus/

Wadekar, N. (2020, May 4). The coronavirus is cutting off Africa's abortion access. *Foreign Policy.* https://foreignpolicy.com/2020/05/04/coronavirus-africa-abortion-access/?utm_source=PostUp&utm_medium=email&utm_campaign=21311&utm_term=Editors

Wenham, C., Smith, J., & Morgan, R. (2020). COVID-19: The gendered impacts of the outbreak. *Lancet (London, England), 395*(10227), 846–848. https://www.thelancet.com/journals/lancet/article/PIIS0140-6736(20)30526-2/fulltext

Wenham, C., Smith, J., Davies, S. E., Feng, H., Grépin, K. A., Harman, S., Herten-Crabb, A., & Morgan, R. (2020). Women are most affected by pandemics - lessons from past outbreaks. *Nature, 583*(7815), 194–198. https://doi.org/10.1038/d41586-020-02006-z

Wheeler, S. (2020, May 4). Sex workers struggling to survive COVID-19 pandemic. *Human Rights Watch.* https://www.hrw.org/news/2020/05/04/sex-workers-struggle-survive-covid-19-pandemic#

Whelan, D. (2010). *Indivisible human rights: A history.* University of Pennsylvania Press.

Williams, C., Getgen Kestenbaum, J., & Meier, B. M. (2020). Populist nationalism threatens health and human rights in the COVID-19 response. *American Journal of Public Health, 110*(12), 1766–1768. https://ssrn.com/abstract=3744962

Wittenberg-Cox, A. (2020, April 13). What do countries with the best coronavirus responses have in common? Women leaders. *Forbes.* https://www.forbes.com/sites/avivahwittenbergcox/2020/04/13/what-do-countries-with-the-best-coronavirus-reponses-have-in-common-women-leaders/?fbclid=IwAR3DG5Yp-_mFN_I57FVd2kP0e2gjgPJdIq1fwZj3lwNHqIMIO_bkQrNWGfs&sh=183703ac3dec

Wolfe, J. (2020, April 8). Domestic workers are at risk during the coronavirus crisis. *Working Economics Blog. Economic Policy Institute.* https://www.epi.org/blog/domestic-workers-are-at-risk-during-the-coronavirus-crisis-data-show-most-domestic-workers-are-black-hispanic-or-asian-women/

World Economic Forum (2021). *Global gender gap report.* http://www3.weforum.org/docs/WEF_GGGR_2021.pdf?utm_campaign=wp_todays_worldview&utm_medium=email&utm_source=newsletter&wpisrc=nl_todayworld

Yancey-Bragg, N. (2020, April 17). Female world leaders are handling coronavirus crisis 'in a really impressive manner,' experts say. *USA TODAY.* https://www.usatoday.com/story/news/world/2020/04/17/coronavirus-women-world-leaders-praised-handling-crisis/5144421002/

The effect of the COVID-19 pandemic on human rights practices: Findings from the Human Rights Measurement Initiative's 2021 Practitioner Survey

K. Chad Clay, Mennah Abdelwahab, Stephen Bagwell, Morgan Barney, Eduardo Burkle, Tori Hawley, Thalia Kehoe Rowden, Meridith LaVelle, Asia Parker, and Matthew Rains

ABSTRACT

Health is a human right; as such, a public health crisis is a human rights crisis. Yet the human rights impact of the 2020 COVID-19 pandemic seems to have varied widely, both across rights and across countries. How have human rights practices been affected by the pandemic so far? Which human rights were most negatively affected by the COVID-19 pandemic? Which states were most likely to experience these negative effects, and which states avoided a reduction in the enjoyment of human rights due to the pandemic? To provide some early answers to these questions, the Human Rights Measurement Initiative (HRMI) added questions to its annual practitioner survey that aimed at determining how a subset of civil, political, economic, and social rights was affected by COVID-19 in 2020 in 39 countries around the world. Using both quantitative and qualitative data from this survey, in combination with other indicators, this article provides a description of COVID-19's human rights impact as seen by practitioners on the front lines around the world, as well as insight into the larger question of which factors enabled states to maintain a high level of enjoyment of human rights just when those rights were needed the most.

Health is a human right; as such, a public health crisis, like the COVID-19 pandemic, is a human rights crisis. Yet, observations about the human rights impact of the COVID-19 pandemic seem to have varied widely across rights, time, and countries.[1] For instance, given the potential for COVID-19 to spread in prisons and jails, the earliest phase of the pandemic was marked by many countries releasing prisoners, especially those who were most vulnerable to the virus (Human Rights Watch, 2020). These releases may have temporarily reduced the number of people arbitrarily detained worldwide, albeit to a far lesser extent than recommended by human rights advocacy groups. On the other hand, by later in the pandemic, many governments had used COVID-19 as an excuse to silence critics and journalists, engaging in wide-ranging crackdowns on free expression in the name of public health and safety, ultimately leading to many arbitrary arrests around the world (Human Rights Watch, 2021). Which of these stories is more representative of the human rights effects of the pandemic? How have human rights practices been affected by COVID-19 so far?

To provide early answers to these questions, the Human Rights Measurement Initiative (HRMI) added questions to its annual practitioner survey to determine how some civil, political, economic, and social rights were affected by COVID-19 during 2020 in 39 countries and territories. This article introduces those data for use by researchers hoping to learn more about the effects of the COVID-19 pandemic on human rights. Using both quantitative and qualitative data from this survey, we describe COVID-19's human rights impact as seen by practitioners on the front lines in our sample of countries around the world. We also try to give some preliminary insight into the larger question of which factors enabled states to maintain a high level of enjoyment of human rights just when those rights were needed the most, as they were during the recent global public health crisis.

We first briefly describe HRMI and its approach to measuring human rights, both in general and during the COVID-19 pandemic. We then summarize some of the key findings from the HRMI 2021 Practitioner Survey that provide insight into the effects the COVID-19 pandemic exerted on human rights in 2020. Finally, we conduct some brief exploratory analyses that suggest some of the factors that enabled states to weather the COVID-19 pandemic with fewer ill-effects to the human rights enjoyment of the people within their borders.

Measuring human rights practices during the COVID-19 pandemic

HRMI (pronounced like the English words "her me") was founded in 2015 with the goal of producing human rights data that would be used by and useful to academics, policymakers, practitioners, activists, and everyone else (Brook et al., 2020). As a global collaborative project including human rights scholars, practitioners, and others, HRMI tries to accomplish this goal by codesigning its products with potential users and human rights experts from different backgrounds. HRMI aims to be as comprehensive as possible and thus plans to expand its reach to cover every human right listed in the core UN human rights instruments (OHCHR, 2021), as well as in other important human rights documents like the UN Declaration on the Rights of Indigenous Peoples (United Nations, 2007) and the Yogyakarta Principles (2020) including the Yogyakarta Principles plus 10). Currently, HRMI collects data on five economic and social rights; eight civil and political rights; and, in a subset of Pacific countries, additional data on cultural rights, the rights of indigenous people, the human rights implications of the climate crisis, and societal violence against women, children, people with disabilities, and LGBTQIA + people (HRMI, 2021a).

HRMI uses publicly available international datasets to produce annual country-level scores on the intensity of government fulfillment of economic and social rights obligations. However, few equivalently reliable sources exist for other human rights. Furthermore, it is often difficult to find data that provide sufficient disaggregation to understand the distribution of human rights violations and enjoyment, including economic and social rights. To overcome these limitations, HRMI conducts an annual practitioner survey in several countries around the world, adding new countries every year (Clay et al., 2021a). This survey primarily targets respondents who work for human rights international non-governmental organizations (INGOs) or non-governmental organizations (NGOs), human rights lawyers, journalists who cover human rights issues, and individuals who work for national human rights institutions (NHRIs) rated as fully compliant with the Paris Principles. In countries with populations under 120,000, government employees with high amounts of human rights knowledge and low conflicts of interest are also allowed to participate.

Every year, the survey asks questions about the prevalence of government violations of eight different civil and political rights, grouped into the two broad categories of empowerment rights (i.e., the rights to expression, political participation, and assembly and association) and "safety from the state," or physical integrity rights (i.e., the rights to be free from torture and ill-treatment, extrajudicial killing, the death penalty, disappearance, and political or arbitrary arrest and detention; see Clay et al., 2021a). For each of these rights, survey respondents also answer questions about a set of hypothetical countries. Together, these responses are used in a model to estimate the latent level of government respect for each right via the Bayesian Aldrich-McKelvey

(BAM) scaling algorithm (Clay et al., 2020; Hare et al., 2015). This approach allows HRMI to account for the facts that (1) not every response to every question, nor every individual respondent, will be equally well-informed, and (2) different respondents may interpret questions and scales differently. As a result, HRMI produces annual scores with credible intervals for the intensity of respect for each of these eight civil and political rights in every country included in the survey, as well as overarching measures of physical integrity and empowerment rights derived from a Bayesian factor model (Clay et al., 2021b).

The survey also asks who was at risk for violations of each of these eight civil and political rights, as well as who was at risk for lack of enjoyment of five different economic and social rights—that is, the rights to food, housing, work, health, and education (Clay et al., 2021a). In each case, HRMI reports the proportion of respondents who selected each preselected identifier in the survey (of which there were 39 in the 2021 survey), as well as summaries of additional qualitative information provided in open-ended follow-up questions.

The annual HRMI Practitioner Survey has been used to collect data in countries around the world since 2017. The current civil and political rights data set contains 19 countries in 2017, 33 countries in 2018, and 39 countries in 2019 and 2020. The 19 countries for which HRMI has civil and political rights data for the entire 2017–2020 time period were chosen with the aim of maximizing diversity in terms of population, geography, political institutions, income, and other factors. That sample consisted of Angola, Australia, Brazil, Democratic Republic of Congo, Fiji, Jordan, Kazakhstan, Kyrgyzstan, Liberia, Mexico, Mozambique, Nepal, New Zealand, Saudi Arabia, South Korea, the United Kingdom, the United States, Venezuela, and Vietnam. Since then, another 20 countries have been added as part of focused efforts to expand HRMI's coverage regionally in Asia and the Pacific. Those countries are American Samoa, the Cook Islands, French Polynesia, Guam, Hong Kong, Kiribati, Malaysia, the Marshall Islands, the Federated States of Micronesia, Nauru, New Caledonia, Niue, the Northern Mariana Islands, Papua New Guinea, Samoa, the Solomon Islands, Taiwan, Tonga, Tuvalu, and Vanuatu. More information on the annual survey and the data it produces can be found in Brook et al. (2020), Clay et al. (2020), and the various methodology notes found on HRMI's (2021d). Likewise, the data themselves, along with accompanying visualizations, are available at HRMI (2021a).

Although these annual data will provide a foundation on which we can build comparisons between human rights practices before and after the COVID-19 pandemic began, it may be challenging to use them to determine which changes are directly related to the pandemic. To help parse this potential attribution problem, HRMI added new questions to its 2021 survey about the effects of COVID-19 on human rights in 2020. For each category of rights covered by the practitioner survey (i.e., physical integrity, empowerment, and economic and social rights), HRMI asked a question about the effect the COVID-19 pandemic had on that set of rights in 2020, such as the following:

> During 2020 in [COUNTRY NAME], what effect did the Covid-19 pandemic have on physical integrity rights violations, including disappearance, extrajudicial killing, death penalty execution, torture or ill-treatment, and political or arbitrary arrest and detention, committed by government agents (such as soldiers, police officers, or others working for or with the government)?

The responses to this question range from the pandemic having improved respect for physical integrity rights overall to it having led to much worse practices. Of course, much as with HRMI's questions about the intensity of respect for physical integrity and empowerment rights, different respondents could understand and interpret both this scale and this question differently while trying to convey the same information. HRMI has taken this issue, known as *differential item functioning* (DIF), seriously in developing its metrics, as HRMI intends to produce data that are comparable across time and space.

Thus, as with HRMI's civil and political rights intensity measures, HRMI aggregated survey responses about the size of the effect of COVID-19 on human rights practices in 2020 by using the Hare et al. (2015) Bayesian Aldrich-McKelvey (BAM) scaling algorithm, much as described in

Clay et al. (2020). The survey asked respondents questions about the effect of COVID-19 on human rights practices in their own country, as well as questions about the pandemic's impact on human rights practices in a set of hypothetical countries, each described in a series of vignettes. These anchoring vignettes provide insight into how respondents interpret the questions and the scale of responses, as all respondents have the same information about those cases. Furthermore, these are the only cases for which every respondent provides answers. As such, they serve as bridging observations in the BAM model that ensure that the model can be effectively estimated and that the resulting metrics are comparable cross-nationally.[2]

The calculation of the COVID-19 effects metrics uses the exact same BAM model as that used for estimating HRMI's other civil and political rights metrics, with the same distributional information and priors described in Clay et al. (2020). We ran two chains for 22,000 iterations, saving the last 2,000 draws to summarize the posterior distributions of all estimated model parameters. Neither the Gelman-Rubin statistic nor visual inspection of density plots shows evidence of nonconvergence. While the initial posterior means were all between −1 and 1, we rescaled the estimated posterior distributions to range between 1 and 5 for presentation purposes. High scores imply that COVID-19 had few negative effects on that category of rights, and lower scores indicate more negative effects. All replication materials necessary to calculate these scores are available with the replication data for this article.

Beyond these questions about the overall effect of COVID-19 on these three broad categories of rights, the HRMI Practitioner Survey also asked (1) follow-up questions about which particular rights were most affected in each category, (2) open-ended questions about how COVID-19 affected the distribution of abuse and enjoyment of each right in 2020, and (3) open-ended questions that give respondents the space to provide other details about the relationship between each set of rights and the pandemic.[3] In the next section, we summarize data from the 2021 survey before providing some brief exploratory analyses that suggest some of the factors that enabled states to weather the COVID-19 pandemic with fewer ill-effects to the human rights enjoyment of the people within their borders.

Human rights in 2020: Changes and the effect of COVID-19

As with any large data set, HRMI's data covering 2020 suggest far more stories than could be contained in a single article. Some of those stories are summarized in HRMI's (2021b) report, *Human Rights During the Pandemic*, and its corresponding appendix, which contains summaries of the data collected in the COVID-19 module for each country included in the 2021 survey. Other stories can be explored using the data and visualizations at HRMI (2021a). As such, in this section, we do not attempt to provide a comprehensive overview of all of the important COVID-related information contained in HRMI's research. Instead, we provide a few high-level descriptions of patterns that appear in the data before digging deeper into the attributes of states that performed well on human rights during the pandemic according to our metrics.

In HRMI's sample, 2020 was not a good year for civil and political rights

There was some hope at the beginning of the pandemic that this crisis would open up room for improvements in human rights practices worldwide, and there was even some evidence in the first half of 2020 that maybe some positive changes were happening. However, by the end of 2020, that possibility seems to have largely faded.

Looking at HRMI's annual civil and political rights data, most changes were decreases in government respect for those rights. Indeed, there were only two positive changes in our civil and political rights data in 2020 in which the 80 percent credible interval for the 2020 estimate did not overlap with the credible interval for the 2019 estimate. Those changes corresponded to a reduction in the use of

Table 1. Percentage of countries with greater than .5 probability of worse human rights practices than observed in prior year.

	Number of countries	2019 Percentage	2020 Percentage
Arbitrary or political arrest and detention	27	59	63
Assembly and association	29	62	79
Forced disappearance	30	50	63
Extrajudicial killing	29	52	69
Opinion and expression	29	45	59
Political participation	28	43	57
Torture and ill-treatment	30	30	50

the death penalty in Saudi Arabia during 2020 and a reduction in the use of torture and ill-treatment in Venezuela. (It should also be noted that both of those states still ranked among the worst in our sample on freedom from the death penalty and freedom from torture and ill-treatment, respectively).

On the other hand, once again focusing on cases in which a country's 2020 80 percent credible interval had no overlap with the same interval for 2019, one country experienced a decrease in respect for the right to freedom from the death penalty (Taiwan), two countries experienced reductions in respect for the rights to be free from torture and ill-treatment (Jordan and Vanuatu), two experienced reductions in respect for the right to opinion and expression (Hong Kong and Malaysia), four experienced reductions in respect for the right to political participation (Angola, Hong Kong, Kyrgyzstan, and Malaysia), and eight countries experienced reductions in respect for the right to assembly and association (Angola, Fiji, Hong Kong, Malaysia, New Zealand, South Korea, the United Kingdom, and the United States).

We can also look at the likelihood of decreases in civil and political rights in 2020 by estimating the number of country-metrics with a greater than .5 probability of decreasing relative to the same country-metric in 2019. To do this, we limit the sample to only those country-metrics that we have estimates for in 2018, 2019, and 2020. We then draw 2000 estimates from the posterior distribution of each metric in each year. We then calculate the proportion of draws in each year that is less than the draw from the previous year, simulating the probability that the later metric is lower than that observed in the same country in the previous year.[4]

Using this methodology, we found that about 62 percent of our civil and political rights metrics had a greater than .5 probability of being lower in 2020 than in 2019. This compares poorly to the previous year, when approximately 51 percent of those metrics were estimated to be lower in 2019 than observed in 2018. Looking across the various rights draws an even starker picture. As shown in Table 1, our metrics indicate that, for every single civil and political right we measure, at least half of the countries in our sample were more likely to have decreased, rather than increased, respect for that right in 2020. Furthermore, the proportion of countries with a greater than .5 probability of a decrease was also higher in 2020 than in 2019 for every single right. Overall, our data indicate that most of the countries in our sample are likely to have decreased their respect for at least some civil and political rights in 2020.

According to our respondents, COVID-19 contributed to worse human rights outcomes

According to our respondents, the COVID-19 pandemic largely had the effect of making things worse for respect for civil and political rights and enjoyment of economic and social rights in 2020. On average, our respondents said COVID-19 had its largest effect on economic and social rights, followed by empowerment rights and, finally, the least effect on physical integrity rights. Nevertheless, a majority of respondents said that the COVID-19 pandemic had the effect of making things worse for respect for all three of these types of rights in 2020. Looking at the raw responses, 63 percent of expert respondents said that the COVID-19 pandemic led to worse respect for physical integrity rights in their country in 2020; 82 percent said that the COVID-19

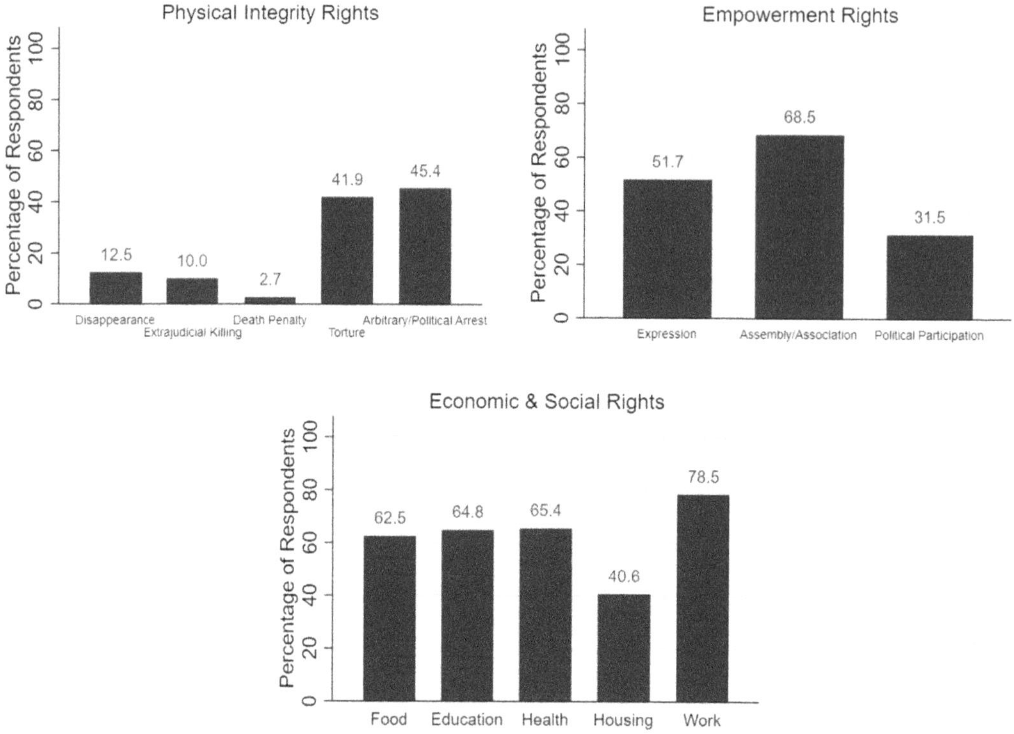

Figure 1. Percentage of expert respondents identifying each right as affected by the COVID-19 pandemic in their country.

pandemic led to worse respect for empowerment rights, and 89 percent said that COVID-19 led to lower enjoyment of economic and social rights in their country. For each set of rights, less than two percent of our respondents said that COVID-19 made human rights practices better in their country over the course of the year. As shown in Figure 1, our respondents identified some rights as far more affected by COVID-19 than others. In particular, a majority of respondents identified the rights to opinion and expression, assembly and association, food, education, health, and work as being most affected by the pandemic.

If COVID-19 worsened enjoyment of one set of rights, it likely worsened enjoyment of others

Building on the insight that COVID-19 has served to reinforce the interconnectedness and interdependence of human rights (Murdie, 2022), as well as the threat that such interdependence can lead to negative cascades when a crisis strikes at one set of rights (Goodhart, 2020), the data from our respondents indicate that countries whose human rights practices were more negatively impacted in one area often experienced negative impacts in other areas.

We asked HRMI's practitioner respondents to tell us how COVID-19 affected three overarching categories of human rights over the course of the year, with responses ranging from COVID-19 having made human rights outcomes better to having made those human rights outcomes much worse. To ensure that our metrics on the effects of COVID-19 on human rights are comparable across respondents and countries, we used the same Bayesian Aldrich-McKelvey (BAM) scaling methodology as that used on our annual civil and political rights intensity scores (Clay et al., 2020; Hare et al., 2015). The resulting estimates are shown in the three graphs displayed in Figure 2, along with labels on the *y*-axis providing our interpretation of the scores, based on reference to the practitioners' raw responses to the survey.

With some exceptions, countries that have relatively higher mean scores on one set of rights generally have higher scores on the others; likewise, countries with lower scores on one set of rights usually have lower scores on the others. Table 2 presents the Pearson correlation, the Spearman's rank correlation, and the Kendall's *tau* rank correlation between the means of the posterior distributions of the estimated effects of COVID-19 on each category of human rights. As shown, all three variables correlate positively—in most cases, highly—with all but two correlation estimates coming in above .5. Overall, it would appear that the effects of COVID-19 on empowerment rights and economic and social rights share the weakest correlation, whereas the strongest correlation unsurprisingly seems to exist between the effects of COVID-19 on the two types of civil and political rights—that is, physical integrity and empowerment rights.

Human rights practitioners in the field saw deep, often troubling connections between COVID-19 and human rights outcomes

The HRMI Practitioner Survey also contains several open-ended questions that asked respondents to tell us more specific information about who was at risk for human rights abuses and how the COVID-19 pandemic affected human rights outcomes in their countries. The qualitative data from our survey respondents offer rich insight into the plethora of ways the COVID-19 pandemic affected respect and fulfillment of human rights. General themes include the interconnectedness of rights, the tension between public health and respect and fulfillment of human rights, and the heightened vulnerability of marginalized groups.

In keeping with the findings from the quantitative data, as well as some of the expectations discussed in other literature on COVID-19 and human rights (e.g., Goodhart, 2020; Murdie, 2022), HRMI's expert respondents also often invoked the notion that all rights are interconnected and interdependent. Job loss, for example, did not just mean reduced enjoyment of the right to work; it often meant that one would experience greater difficulties enjoying the rights to food, housing, and health. In the United States, respondents stated that arbitrary arrest often resulted in violations of the right to health, as governments failed to make the necessary changes to protect detainees from COVID-19. In Jordan and Brazil, respondents said that failure to administer elections with the necessary health protocols not only resulted in violations of the right to health but also made citizens uncomfortable going to the polls, violating their right to political participation.

The pandemic also gave rise to tension between public health measures and the respect and fulfillment of human rights, invoking the "negative interdependence" discussed by Goodhart (2020) and exemplified by the discussion of human rights issues in Koo (2022). This could especially be seen with empowerment rights, as public health protocols placed restrictions on the right to participate in government, freedom of assembly and association, and freedom of opinion and expression. Those who protested peacefully, for instance, were often detained.

Furthermore, in some countries, such as the United States, respondents claimed that whether protesters were targeted by the government often depended on what they were protesting, with Black Lives Matter protestors and others on the political left more frequently targeted for limitations on assembly than those on the political right. Our respondents also stated that the government used the pandemic to impose restrictions on empowerment rights in places such as the Democratic Republic of Congo, Fiji, Hong Kong, Kazakhstan, Malaysia, Nepal, or the Solomon Islands. Overall, as suggested by Chenoweth (2022) and Badran and Turnbull (2022) in this volume, many respondents noted that these restrictions continued to be imposed even when they may have no longer been necessary.[5]

This tension also affected other rights. For example, our respondents said that lockdowns, travel restrictions, and disruptions to the transport of food limited people's access to food in places such as Australia, Nepal, and the Cook Islands. Even when governments tried to remedy this situation, the food they provided was not always culturally appropriate, such as in Australia and

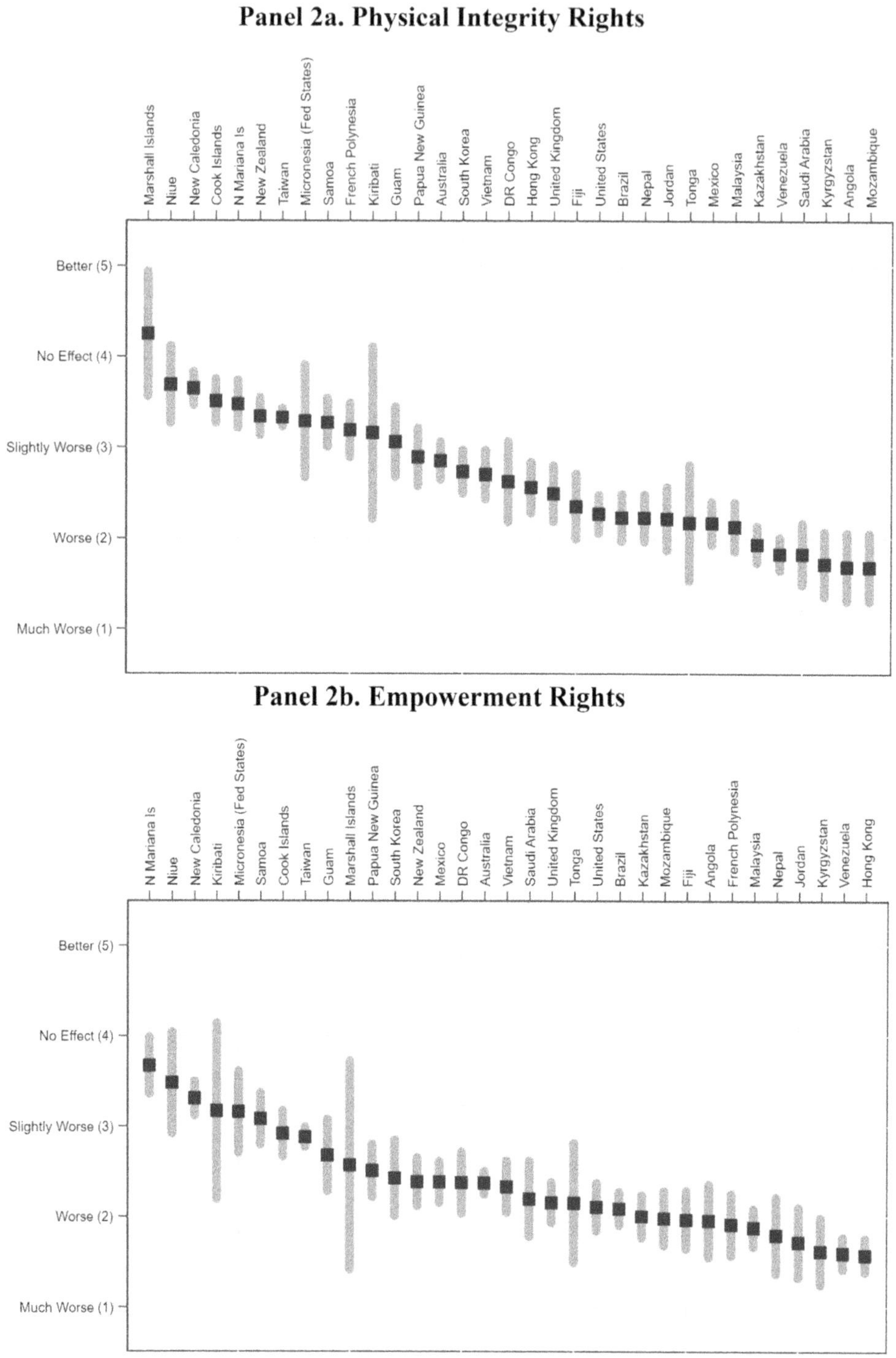

Figure 2. Estimates of the effect of COVID-19 on human rights in 2020 (80 percent credible intervals). Panel 2a: Physical integrity rights. Panel 2b: Empowerment rights. Panel 2c: Economic and social rights.

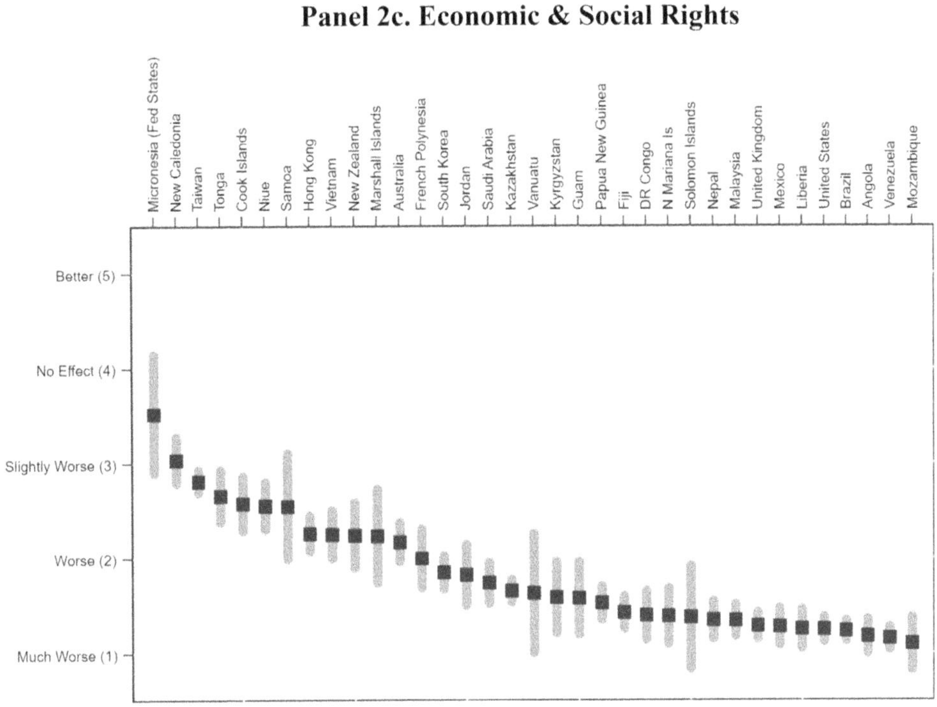

Figure 2. Continued.

Table 2. Pearson correlation between estimated mean effect of COVID-19 on types of human rights.

	Physical integrity rights	Empowerment rights	Economic and social rights
Physical integrity rights	1		
Empowerment rights	.77 (.78) [.59]	1	
Economic and social rights	.65 (.65) [.48]	.55 (.50) [.35]	1

Spearman's rank correlation in parentheses; Kendall's tau in brackets.

Hong Kong. In Malaysia and Mexico, inadequate food was provided to those in detention, and in Kyrgyzstan, Mozambique, and Liberia, the government failed to effectively distribute food to those in need. Respondents said that the enforcement of restrictions also resulted in rights violations, as security forces or police used violence against those not abiding by protocols in states such as Liberia, Mexico, and the United States. Respondents also said that those who did not comply with COVID-19 restrictions were at greater risk of being tortured or ill-treated in some places, including Angola, the Democratic Republic of Congo, Mozambique, Papua New Guinea, and Fiji.

On the other hand, respondents pointed out that some states, such as Brazil and Mexico, understated the severity of COVID-19 or outright denied its existence. In turn, they implemented few or no health protocols to mitigate the spread of the pandemic, clearly violating their populaces' right to health. In such states, governments attacked individuals who attempted to spread accurate information about safety protocols or COVID-19's death toll. In Venezuela, respondents claimed that those sharing COVID-19 statistics contrary to the government's narrative were at greater risk of extrajudicial killing. Governments also harassed or fired public officials who tried to implement safety protocols in their localities. Even in countries in which the government acknowledged COVID-19—like Jordan, Saudi Arabia, Malaysia, Nepal, and Taiwan—the government attempted to restrict individuals' ability to criticize its handling of the pandemic.

People from marginalized communities, who were already vulnerable to rights violations, were particularly vulnerable due to the pandemic, according to respondents. Indigenous people were vulnerable in a variety of ways. For example, in many countries, our respondents pointed out that indigenous people often lacked access to the internet. As schools turned to virtual learning because of the pandemic, indigenous people were thus unable to connect to the internet, reducing their ability to enjoy the right to education. In Brazil and the Democratic Republic of Congo, indigenous people were less able to access healthcare, making them especially vulnerable to dying from COVID-19. The pandemic also limited access to traditional diets or food-collecting traditions for indigenous people in French Polynesia, Guam, and New Caledonia. Furthermore, indigenous people were targeted for violating curfew or COVID-19 protocols in states such as Australia and French Polynesia.

Migrants, refugees, and those without legal status were also vulnerable. In Malaysia, for example, migrants and refugees were at particular risk of being evicted, and the government targeted and detained them in unsanitary conditions in the name of slowing the spread of the virus. The Malaysian government also used COVID-19 to restrict freedom of expression for migrants, refugees, and their advocates. Refugees, noncitizens, and others without legal status could not access government assistance and were particularly affected by job loss in places like Australia and the Northern Mariana Islands. COVID-19 public health information also was not available in migrants' or refugees' languages, putting their health at risk. In Taiwan, those without legal status struggled to purchase masks.

As discussed by Brysk (2022) in this volume, the pandemic also negatively impacted women and girls. In Liberia, for example, women and girls were restricted from accessing food markets. Furthermore, women were especially affected by unemployment triggered by the pandemic in states such as Mozambique, Nepal, and Vanuatu, among others. Mozambique also saw women's and girls' political participation decrease because of the pandemic. The pandemic also detracted from issues for which women were advocating, such as the ability to have land to build homes in Tuvalu.

Of course, there is far more detail in the qualitative responses than can be included here. Summaries of the qualitative responses can be found at HRMI (2021a) and HRMI (2021b).

Maintaining respect for rights during a crisis: The pandemic, the 'will,' and the 'way'

Whereas the data presented above allow us to provide information on the effect of the COVID-19 pandemic across several diverse contexts, we should also be able to use them to provide insight into the factors that enabled states to weather the pandemic with fewer adverse human rights effects. We hope that, as more data become available from the pandemic, researchers will be able to use these data to understand the human rights consequences of COVID-19 in 2020 and beyond. The analyses that follow should thus be used as illustrative of some of the kinds of questions one may be able to approach using our data. Although there are many possible ways of categorizing the potential factors at play here, we focus on a few that affected a state's *ability* (or opportunity) to maintain a consistent, higher level of respect for human rights and the factors that demonstrate a state's *willingness* to respect human rights (Most & Starr, 1989). As Murdie (2022) might put it, which states had the "will" and the "way" to protect human rights during the pandemic?

Two of the factors that determined whether a state could maintain (or even improve) existing human rights practices during the pandemic are its general capacity to respect the human rights of its population overall and the size of the additional challenge posed by COVID-19 to that state. The state's capacity to respect human rights has been found to have an important impact on human rights in several previous studies (Cingranelli et al., 2014; Clay & Digiuseppe, 2017; Englehart, 2009), both by delimiting the possible policy options that are available to the state and by affecting the state's ability to recruit, train, monitor, and incentivize its agents.

There are many ways to measure state capacity (e.g., Hendrix, 2010), but at the time of this writing (in mid-2021), many of those metrics are not yet available for 2020. Furthermore, because we are looking at a broad set of human rights outcomes, not all of which have been thoroughly

Table 3. Summary statistics.

	N	Mean	Std. dev.	Min	Max
COVID effect on physical integrity (mean)	33	2.68	.68	1.68	4.25
COVID effect on physical integrity (standard deviation)	33	.26	.13	.08	.74
COVID effect on empowerment (mean)	33	2.38	.56	1.57	3.67
COVID effect on empowerment (standard deviation)	33	.28	.17	.08	.90
COVID effect on economic and social rights (mean)	35	1.84	.62	1.10	3.52
COVID effect on economic and social rights (standard deviation)	35	.21	.11	.08	.49
Respect for physical integrity (2019 mean)	38	6.40	1.90	2.07	8.89
Respect for physical integrity (2019 standard deviation)	38	.88	.11	0.79	1.32
Respect for empowerment (2019 mean)	37	5.88	2.00	1.01	8.51
Respect for empowerment (2019 standard deviation)	37	.84	.05	.78	.99
Social and economic rights fulfillment (SERF) index (most recent year available)	18	78.13	17.07	42.38	96.37
GDP *per capita* PPP	26	18121.45	18450.81	752.79	56054.92
Population	27	47935280	74719720	59618	332915074
Total COVID-19 cases per million	27	8435.09	14921.05	3.18	60536.24

examined in light of state capacity, we will focus here on the overall resource base to which the government had access, in the form of GDP *per capita*, as the overall income of the country has long been found to be an important determinant of human rights outcomes (e.g. Fukuda-Parr et al., 2015; Poe et al., 1999; Richards et al., 2015).

We will also look at the effect of population, as higher populations correspond to a higher number of people whose rights the state is obligated to respect, protect, and fulfill. As such, by mere probability alone, countries with higher populations are likely to have a larger share of people whose rights are violated or not enjoyed. Furthermore, larger populations may also place more pressure on the government, especially if that population is at risk for a disease like COVID-19 (Fukuda-Parr et al., 2015). Indeed, many previous studies have found that countries with larger populations often have worse human rights outcomes, all else being equal (e.g., Henderson, 1993; Poe et al., 1999; Richards et al., 2015).

Of course, any pressures typically placed on the state to fulfill the human rights of its population under normal constraints would be exacerbated as states face the grave risk to the right to the highest attainable standard of health posed by the COVID-19 pandemic. Those states also face potential human rights costs associated with the pandemic's mitigation strategies, such as reduced access to work and pay (e.g., Fana et al., 2020), the potential loss of housing as income drops (Benfer et al., 2021), the loss of access to education as schools shut down or move online (Lorente et al., 2020), the postponement of elections (International Institute for Democracy and Electoral Assistance (International IDEA), 2021), imposed limits on expression and assembly (UN Human Rights Council, 2020), and increased contact between state agents (like police) and people who are running afoul of the state's mitigation strategist (World Organization Against Torture (OCMT), 2021; Richards & Gelleny, 2021). In general, higher numbers of COVID-19 cases serve to threaten people's health and human rights directly through the disease and its effects, and indirectly through the strategies embraced by the state to reduce transmission of that disease.[6]

In terms of state willingness, multiple factors, ranging from regime type to the salience of human rights practices, could be included. However, as a starting point, we will focus on something that is readily available to us and is perhaps the best representation of whether the state has put efforts into ensuring enjoyment of rights previously: past human rights practices. It is, of course, possible that a lack of violations of human rights in previous years could result from a lack of problems leading to worse human rights outcomes. However, that is unlikely, as the consistent fulfillment of every human right requires positive effort (and resource allocation) on the part of the state (Donnelly, 2013). As such, we posit that countries that demonstrated higher respect for human rights before the pandemic were better equipped to maintain higher practices during the pandemic, as well as less likely to use the pandemic as an excuse to engage in

Table 4. Associates of the effect of COVID on human rights practices.

	Effect of COVID on:					
	Physical integrity rights		Empowerment rights		Economic and social rights	
	Observations	Coefficient (standard Error)	Observations	Coefficient (standard error)	Observations	Coefficient (standard error)
Total COVID-19 cases per million (ln)	24	−.132*** (.048)	24	−.092** (.045)	27	−.071* (.044)
GDP *per capita* (ln)	23	.035 (.117)	23	−.008 (.096)	26	.097 (.086)
Population (ln)	24	−.163*** (.065)	24	−.019 (.092)	27	−.073 (.062)
Physical integrity rights	33	.190*** (.060)	33	.097** (.055)	35	.151*** (.057)
Empowerment rights	33	.203*** (.053)	33	.164*** (.065)	34	.134** (.057)
Economic and social rights	15	.008 (.009)	15	.004 (.009)	18	.013** (.007)

Notes: Coefficients from bivariate linear regressions combined via Rubin's rules (1987). Intercepts omitted for clearer presentation. One-tailed *t*-tests: *< .1, **<.05, ***.01.

violations and limitations of human rights for their own benefit, under the guise of concern for public health.

Data and analysis design

Table 3 provides the descriptive statistics for all of the data used in the analyses that follow. As a reminder, the variables we introduced above on the effects of COVID-19 on human rights potentially range from 1 to 5, with higher scores corresponding to generally fewer negative effects from COVID-19 and lower scores indicating that COVID-19 made human rights outcomes in that category of rights much worse. Aside from these, the various human rights data are all from the HRMI (2021c) Human Rights Dataset. The respect for physical integrity and empowerment rights indicators potentially range from 0 to 10, with higher scores representing greater state respect for that subset of rights.

Because the COVID-19 human rights data and the HRMI civil and political rights variables are based on posterior distributions of country–year estimates from Bayesian Aldrich-McKelvey models, we provide descriptive statistics on both the means and the standard deviations of those normal distributions. HRMI's economic and social rights data use the methodology created by Fukuda-Parr et al. (2015), updated and described further in Randolph et al. (2021). Their Social and Economic Rights Fulfillment (SERF) Index potentially ranges from 0 to 100, with higher scores indicating better state fulfillment of its legal economic and social rights obligations. In this particular implementation, we focus on the data from the low- and middle-income assessment standard, as we have too few observations on the high-income assessment standard to draw conclusions from those data.

Our data on the total number of 2020 COVID-19 cases, gross domestic product (GDP) *per capita* adjusted for purchasing power parity in constant 2011 dollars, and population are all taken from the *Our World in Data* COVID-19 data repository (Appel et al., 2021). The COVID-19 case data are from the COVID-19 Data Repository of the Center for Systems Science and Engineering (CSSE) at the Johns Hopkins University (Dong et al., 2020). The GDP data are from the most recent year available from the World Bank's (2020) World Development Indicators via the International Comparison Program. Population data come from the United Nations (2019) World Population Prospects. Due to skewness in the total COVID-19 case, GDP, and population data, we use the natural log of those data in the analyses below.

Our sample of states is not large. We have data on 35 countries for the effects of COVID-19 on economic and social rights, and 33 countries for the effects of COVID-19 on civil and political rights. Furthermore, many of those countries are not treated as independent states by the United Nations, the World Bank, and other international institutions. Thus, in many cases, we lack comparable data on state attributes we would like to use to understand the effects of the pandemic, even further limiting our sample size in many cases. As such, we would caution against reading the following results as causal. Instead, we will merely be attempting to establish associations that may help us gain a high-level description of the attributes of states that navigated the difficulties associated with COVID-19 without significantly worsening the enjoyment of human rights of people in that country. Furthermore, several alternative attributes should also be analyzed in future work, particularly as more data from the pandemic become available. The following results are only intended as an example of some things that can be learned from these data; we hope other work will expand on this.

Given the small sample size, we do not attempt multivariate regressions. Instead, we report the results of a series of bivariate linear regressions relating each of the state attributes of interest to our measure of COVID's effect on each type of human right. To completely use the available information about the amount of uncertainty surrounding the Bayesian estimates used in the following analyses (as represented by the standard deviations described in Table 3), we take 10 draws from each of those Bayesian posterior distributions and run 10 separate regressions, combining the results of those 10 regressions using Rubin's (1987) rules.

Results

Table 4 shows the results of the bivariate regressions described above. First, countries in our sample in which higher proportions of the population contracted COVID-19 also tended to experience more negative effects on physical integrity, empowerment, and economic and social rights due to the pandemic, according to HRMI's expert respondents. On some level, this is to be expected—but it does suggest that many states required a reasonably high level of COVID-19 transmission before using the COVID-19 pandemic as a reason for reduced respect for human rights. That is, the fact of a global pandemic may not have been enough for a state to reduce its respect for rights greatly; rather, that pandemic needed to impact the population directly.

Interestingly, our other two indicators of state ability to maintain respect for human rights during the pandemic perform worse than might be expected. Higher populations are significantly associated with larger adverse COVID-related effects on government respect for physical integrity rights; in all other cases, neither population nor GDP *per capita* attains statistical significance. However, we should not draw too many conclusions from these null findings. They could have something to do with the particular sample of countries being analyzed here, or they could be related to the fact that the standing GDP of countries before the pandemic mattered less than the effect COVID-19 had on countries' economies during 2020 (which might be captured better by the proportion of the population affected by COVID, which was found to be significantly associated with outcomes above). It will be essential to reanalyze all of this as more data become available.

As for our indicators of state willingness to respect human rights (i.e., past respect for human rights), in most cases, they were related to fewer negative effects on human rights practices due to COVID-19. Past respect for physical integrity rights and past respect for empowerment rights are both related to fewer negative COVID-related effects on physical integrity, empowerment, and economic and social rights across the board. Respect for economic and social rights, measured via the low- and middle-income assessment standard on the Social and Economic Rights Fulfillment (SERF) Index, is not significantly associated with the effect of COVID-19 on physical integrity or empowerment rights. Still, it is significantly associated with fewer negative effects of COVID-19 on economic and social rights in our sample. Overall, rather than increasing the probability that the pandemic would lead to worse human rights outcomes by leaving the state further to fall, it would seem that higher prior respect for human rights does indicate that a state was more likely to maintain those practices through the struggles of the pandemic, at least in our sample of states.

Conclusion

By most accounts, 2020 was not a good year for global human rights practices. In general, the human rights practitioners and experts who responded to HRMI's annual survey agreed, producing data that indicate that most countries likely experienced some form of decline in respect for human rights practices over the course of the year. As Chiozza and King (2022a) state in their introduction to this volume, COVID-19 has exerted a "profoundly negative" effect on human rights conditions worldwide.

However, there may still be room for optimism amid the bad outcomes of 2020. The pandemic has driven an increased awareness of the interdependence between different human rights, and thus, the necessity to ensure respect for each human right to truly guarantee respect for all human rights (Goodhart, 2020). This interdependence in outcomes appears to be supported by the data presented in this article. We hope the accumulated evidence from the pandemic will encourage states to stop approaching the list of internationally recognized human rights as a menu of options and to see it more as a necessarily connected whole that must be embraced in its entirety. Likewise, the degree to which the adverse human rights effects of COVID-19 were disproportionately experienced by marginalized groups, as noted by HRMI's respondents, has led to a wider understanding of the longstanding inequities in rights enjoyment across populations and, thus, growth in solidarity with those experiencing human rights abuses (Libal & Kashwan, 2020).

Strictly from the results presented in this article, we would encourage human rights advocates to take heart in the finding that countries with better human rights practices prior to the pandemic tended to experience fewer negative effects from the pandemic on human rights. In general, this implies that hard-fought past gains in human rights practices were not entirely lost during this period of recession. "Two steps forward, one step back" still leaves us further along the road than when we started. If these findings hold up to further scrutiny in the years to come, it provides more strength to the claim that the best way to protect human rights in times of crisis is to encourage states to adopt stronger human rights norms during calmer times (e.g., Conrad & Ritter, 2019).

Of course, it is still too early to draw firm conclusions about the long-term effects of the COVID-19 pandemic on human rights, and there is much more to learn. We hope that the metrics discussed here, combined with data produced by others, will help researchers find important patterns while aiding practitioners and policymakers in evaluating the steps they have taken so far. Through these efforts, we all may be able to work together to provide the tools and policies necessary to lessen and avoid such widespread human rights crises in the future.

Notes

1. For a review of the literature on the relationship between human rights and the COVID-19 pandemic, see Chiozza and King (2022b) in this volume.
2. See Bakker et al. (2014) for more discussion of the use of anchoring vignettes, and Clay et al. (2020) for discussion that places that use in the human rights context.
3. A paper version of HRMI's 2021 survey (which is taken in Qualtrics) can be viewed in full in Appendix 1, included with the replication data at the *Journal of Human Rights* dataverse.
4. We exclude freedom from the death penalty from this analysis, as death penalty executions occurred in only four countries in our sample over the 2019–2020 time period.
5. It may bear mentioning that there is a mechanism in international law that would allow states to derogate from some of their obligations under the International Covenant on Civil and Political Rights (ICCPR) during COVID-19 related crises. However, many more states restricted the exercise of civil and political rights than entered derogations at the United Nations (Helfer, 2021). Indeed, in our sample of states

(which includes some countries that have not ratified the ICCPR), Kyrgyzstan is the only state of which we are aware that entered formal derogations to its ICCPR obligations during 2020 (United Nations, 2020).

6. As suggested by an anonymous reviewer, all of this is further complicated by the possibility that limitations on some rights, including those permitted via legal derogation procedures, may have served to reduce the caseload in some countries. In the current study, it is possible that worse practices on some rights served to decrease the COVID-19 caseload, which may serve to attenuate the generally negative correlations we find between COVID-19 cases and change in these broad categories of human rights outcomes. Future researchers with access to more disaggregated data should evaluate this possibility further.

References

Appel, C., Belotecan, D., Gavrilov, D., Giattino, C., Hasell, J., Macdonald, B., Mathieu, E., Ortiz-Ospina, E., Ritchie, H., Rodés-Guirao, L., Roser, M. (2021). *Data on COVID-19 (Coronavirus).* Our World in Data. Retrieved October 1, 2021, from https://github.com/owid/covid-19-data/tree/master/public/data/.

Bakker, R., Jolly, S., Polk, J., & Poole, K. (2014). The European Common Space: Extending the Use of Anchoring Vignettes. *The Journal of Politics*, *76*(4), 1089–1101.

Badran, S., & Turnbull, B. (2022). The COVID-19 pandemic and authoritarian consolidation in North Africa. *Journal of Human Rights*, *21*(3), 263–282. https://doi.org/10.1080/14754835.2022.2080496

Benfer, E. A., Vlahov, D., Long, M. Y., Walker-Wells, E., Pottenger, J. L., Gonsalves, G., & Keene, D. E. (2021). Eviction, health inequity, and the spread of COVID-19: Housing policy as a primary pandemic mitigation strategy. *Journal of Urban Health*, *98*(1), 1–12. https://doi.org/10.1007/s11524-020-00502-1

Brook, A. M., Clay, K. C., & Randolph, S. (2020). Human rights data for everyone: Introducing the Human Rights Measurement Initiative (HRMI). *Journal of Human Rights, 19*(1), 67–82. https://doi.org/10.1080/14754835.2019.1671176

Brysk, A. (2022). Pandemic patriarchy: The impact of a global health crisis on women's rights. *Journal of Human Rights, 21*(3), 283–303. https://doi.org/10.1080/14754835.2022.2071105

Chenoweth, E. (2022). Can nonviolent resistance survive COVID-19? *Journal of Human Rights, 21*(3), 304–316.

Chiozza, G., & King, J. (2022a). Introduction to a special issue on beyond complacency and acrimony: Studying human rights in a post-COVID-19 world. *Journal of Human Rights, 21*(3), 245.

Chiozza, G., & King, J. (2022b). The state of human rights in a (post) COVID-19 World. *Journal of Human Rights, 21*(3), 246–262.

Cingranelli, D., Fajardo-Heyward, P., & Filippov, M. (2014). Principals, agents and human rights. *British Journal of Political Science, 44*(3), 605–630. https://doi.org/10.1017/S0007123413000070

Clay, K. C., Abdelwahab, M., Bakker, R., Barney, M., Brook, A. M., Hill, D. W., Jr., LaVelle, M., Murdie, A., Rains, M. (2021b). *HRMI 2021 Civil and Political Rights Methodology Handbook.* Human Rights Measurement Initiative. Version 2021.7.20. Retrieved January 31, 2022, from https://humanrightsmeasurement.org/wp-content/uploads/2021/07/HRMI-CPR-Methodology-Guide-2021.pdf.

Clay, K. C., Abdelwahab, M., Barney, M., Brook, A. M., Chong, C., Kehoe-Rowden, T., LaVelle, M., Rains, M., Randolph, S. (2021a). *HRMI 2021 Annual Survey & People Data Report.* Human Rights Measurement Initiative. Version 2021.7.24. Retrieved October 1, 2021, from https://humanrightsmeasurement.org/wp-content/uploads/2021/07/HRMI-Annual-Survey-Report-2021.pdf.

Clay, K. C., Bakker, R., Brook, A. M., Hill, D. W., Jr,., & Murdie, A. (2020). Using practitioner surveys to measure human rights: The Human Rights Measurement Initiative's civil and political rights metrics. *Journal of Peace Research, 57*(6), 715–727. https://doi.org/10.1177/0022343320959688

Clay, K. C., & Digiuseppe, M. R. (2017). The physical consequences of fiscal flexibility: Sovereign credit and physical integrity rights. *British Journal of Political Science, 47*(4), 783–807. https://doi.org/10.1017/S0007123415000502

Conrad, C. R., & Ritter, E. H. (2019). *Contentious compliance: Dissent and repression under international human rights law.* Oxford University Press.

Dong, E., Du, H., & Gardner, L. (2020). An interactive web-based dashboard to track COVID-19 in real time. *The Lancet, 20*(5), 533–534.

Donnelly, J. (2013). *Universal human rights in theory and practice.* Cornell University Press.

Englehart, N. A. (2009). State capacity, state failure, and human rights. *Journal of Peace Research, 46*(2), 163–180. https://doi.org/10.1177/0022343308100713

Fana, M., Pérez, S. T., & Fernández-Macías, E. (2020). Employment impact of Covid-19 crisis: From short term effects to long terms prospects. *Journal of Industrial and Business Economics, 47*(3), 391–410. https://doi.org/10.1007/s40812-020-00168-5

Fukuda-Parr, S., Lawson-Remer, T., & Randolph, S. (2015). *Fulfilling social and economic rights.* Oxford University Press.

Goodhart, M. (2020). Revisiting interdependence in times and terms of crisis. *Journal of Human Rights, 19*(5), 520–527. https://doi.org/10.1080/14754835.2020.1814709

Hare, C., Armstrong, D. A., Bakker, R., Carroll, R., & Poole, K. T. (2015). Using Bayesian Aldrich-McKelvey scaling to study citizens' ideological preferences and perceptions. *American Journal of Political Science, 59*(3), 759–774. https://doi.org/10.1111/ajps.12151

Helfer, L. R. (2021). Rethinking derogations from human rights treaties. *American Journal of International Law, 115*(1), 20–40. https://doi.org/10.1017/ajil.2020.92

Henderson, C. W. (1993). Population pressures and political repression. *Social Science Quarterly, 74*(2), 322–333.

Hendrix, C. S. (2010). Measuring state capacity: Theoretical and empirical implications for the study of civil conflict. *Journal of Peace Research, 47*(3), 273–285. https://doi.org/10.1177/0022343310361838

Human Rights Measurement Initiative (HRMI) (2021a). *HRMI Rights Tracker.* Retrieved October 1, 2021, from https://rightstracker.org/en.

Human Rights Measurement Initiative (HRMI). (2021b). *Human Rights during the Pandemic.* June 24. Retrieved January 31, 2022, from https://humanrightsmeasurement.org/human-rights-during-the-pandemic/.

Human Rights Measurement Initiative (HRMI). (2021c). *HRMI Human Rights Dataset.* Retrieved October 1, 2021, from https://humanrightsmeasurement.org/. Version 2020.6.23.

Human Rights Measurement Initiative (HRMI). (2021d). "Methodology Handbook." Retrieved June 19, 2022, from https://humanrightsmeasurement.org/methodology-handbook/.

Human Rights Watch. (2020, May 27). *Covid-19 prisoner releases too few, too slow.* Retrieved October 1, 2021, from https://www.hrw.org/news/2020/05/27/covid-19-prisoner-releases-too-few-too-slow#

Human Rights Watch. (2021, February 11). *Covid-19 triggers wave of free speech abuse.* Retrieved October 1, 2021, from https://www.hrw.org/news/2021/02/11/covid-19-triggers-wave-free-speech-abuse.

International Institute for Democracy and Electoral Assistance (International IDEA). (2021, September 27). *Global overview of Covid-19 impact on elections*. Retrieved October 1, 2021, from https://www.idea.int/news-media/multimedia-reports/global-overview-covid-19-impact-elections

Koo, J.-W. (2022). Global perceptions of South Korea's COVID-19 policy responses: Topic modeling with tweets. *Journal of Human Rights, 21*(3), 334–353.

Libal, K., & Kashwan, P. (2020). Solidarity in times of crisis. *Journal of Human Rights, 19*(5), 537–546. https://doi.org/10.1080/14754835.2020.1830046

Lorente, L. M. L., Arrabal, A. A., & Pulido-Montes, C. (2020). The right to education and ICT during covid-19: An international perspective. *Sustainability, 12*(21), 9091. https://doi.org/10.3390/su12219091

Most, B. A., & Starr, H. (1989). *Inquiry, logic, and international politics*. Univ of South Carolina Press.

Murdie, A. (2022). Hindsight is 2020: Lessons from the COVID-19 pandemic for future human rights research. *Journal of Human Rights, 21*(3), 354–364.

Office of the High Commissioner for Human Rights (OHCHR). (2021). *The Core International Human Rights Instruments and their monitoring bodies*. Retrieved September 13, 2021, from https://www.ohchr.org/en/professionalinterest/pages/coreinstruments.aspx

Poe, S. C., Tate, C. N., & Keith, L. C. (1999). Repression of the human right to personal integrity revisited: A global cross-national study covering the years 1976–1993. *International Studies Quarterly, 43*(2), 291–313. doi:10.1111/0020-8833.00121

Randolph, S., Stewart, J., Fukuda-Parr, S., Lawson-Remer, T. (2021). *HRMI Economic and Social Rights Scores 2020 Technical Note*. Retrieved October 3, 2021, from https://humanrightsmeasurement.org/wp-content/uploads/2021/06/HRMI-ESR-Methodology-Handbook-2021.pdf

Richards, D. L., Gelleny, R. (2021). Torture in the time of COVID-19. Retrieved October 1, 2021, from https://ssrn.com/abstract=3914295.

Richards, D. L., Webb, A., & Clay, K. C. (2015). Respect for physical-integrity rights in the twenty-first century: Evaluating Poe and Tate's model 20 years later. *Journal of Human Rights, 14*(3), 291–311. https://doi.org/10.1080/14754835.2015.1061423

Rubin, D. B. (1987). *Multiple imputation for nonresponse in surveys*. Wiley.

Simmons, B. A. (2009). *Mobilizing for human rights: International law in domestic politics*. Cambridge University Press.

Smith-Cannoy, H. (2012). *Insincere Commitments: Human Rights Treaties, Abusive States, and Citizen Activism*. Georgetown University Press.

The Yogyakarta Principles. (2022). Retrieved June 19, 2022, from https://yogyakartaprinciples.org

United Nations. (2007). *United Nations Declaration on the Rights of Indigenous Peoples*. A/RES/61/295. Retrieved October 1, 2021, from https://undocs.org/A/RES/61/295.

United Nations. (2019). *World Population Prospects 2019*. Retrieved October 1, 2021, from https://population.un.org/wpp/Download/Standard/Population/

United Nations. (2020). C.N.129.2020.TREATIES-IV.4. *International Covenant on Civil and Political Rights. Notification under Article, 4*(3). Retrieved October 1, 2021, from https://treaties.un.org/Pages/CNs.aspx?cnTab=tab1

United Nations Human Rights Council. (2020, April 23). *Report of the Special Rapporteur on the promotion and protection of the right to freedom of opinion and expression*. (David Kaye). UN Doc A/HRC/44/49. Retrieved October 1, 2021, from https://undocs.org/A/HRC/44/49

Walker, P. G. T., Whittaker, C., Watson, O. J., Baguelin, M., Winskill, P., Hamlet, A., Djafaara, B. A., Cucunubá, Z., Olivera Mesa, D., Green, W., Thompson, H., Nayagam, S., Ainslie, K. E. C., Bhatia, S., Bhatt, S., Boonyasiri, A., Boyd, O., Brazeau, N. F., Cattarino, L., … Ghani, A. C. (2020). The impact of COVID-19 and strategies for mitigation and suppression in low-and middle-income countries. *Science, 369*(6502), 413–422.

World Bank. (2020). *World Development Indicators*. Retrieved October 1, 2021, from https://datatopics.worldbank.org/world-development-indicators/

World Organisation Against Torture (OMCT). (2021, March 17). *Police brutality reaches torture levels during the Covid-19 pandemic*. Retrieved October 1, 2021, from https://www.omct.org/en/resources/reports/police-brutality-reaches-torture-levels-during-the-covid-19-pandemic

OPEN ACCESS

Global perceptions of South Korea's COVID-19 policy responses: Topic modeling with tweets

Jeong-Woo Koo

ABSTRACT

This article focuses on South Korea as a case, analyzes a collection of 87,487 tweets referencing both COVID-19 and South Korea during the period of the pandemic, and examines global users' understandings and/or assessments of South Korean responses to the health crisis. This article uses Pseudo-document-based Topic Model (PTM) as an advanced machine learning technique for classifying short texts into viable topics or themes. In the PTM results, human rights-related topics received much less attention than other topics on government responses, health measures, vaccines, and economic issues. Furthermore, discussions on surveillance, restrictions on assembly, and stigmatization of religious groups tended to emerge rather briefly and soon subsided. Rights protection in the South Korean context appeared at odds with the larger target of protecting public health and the safety of society. The analyses demonstrate a tradeoff between implementing public health imperatives and respecting human rights in South Korea.

Introduction

Governments worldwide have struggled to respond to the COVID-19 pandemic, an unprecedented global health crisis, with vulnerable groups at risk of infection, devastation, cynicism, and depression (Forman & Kohler, 2020; Hatcher, 2020; Kavanagh & Singh, 2020; Travaglino & Moon, 2020). In tandem with governments' measures to control its spread (e.g., tracking and testing, lockdowns, and closure of public places), individuals and group members did their part by practicing personal hygiene and social distancing, although they also coped with psychological depression (Lee et al., 2020).

As time and this parallel movement advanced, scholars began to address citizens' public discussions of the pandemic on different social media platforms such as Twitter, Instagram, and Reddit (Ordun et al., 2020). This scholarly interest stemmed from indications that online platforms are invaluable venues for citizens to respond to health policy measures, express their feelings and thoughts, and share their views with other users. Public opinion of this sort characterizes the collective voices on social media and, thus, analyzing and understanding these opinions as expressed in these forums are critical. As Murdie (2022) emphasizes in this volume, public opinion related to human rights merits attention for future scholarship of human rights. Added to this is the value of social media postings in providing policy implications as well as highlighting the connections between policymaking, public opinion, and media coverage (Wicke & Bolognesi, 2020).

Analyses of COVID-19 postings in general have provided insights into how citizens in many parts of the world felt about and reacted to the unfolding health crisis, but they often lack analytical power because they were not focused on a particular country or specific policy response (Yin et al., 2020). Although COVID-19 was a global pandemic, the cases, deaths, and responses were all decidedly particular to individual nations. As Chiozza and King (2022) report in this volume, from the initial phase of the pandemic, we witnessed a great deal of variation in government responses and learned the salience of the regime type. With an emphasis on individual attitudes, Chilton et al. (2020) show that national public opinions vary greatly about the legitimacy of liberty restrictions designed to combat COVID-19. Against this backdrop, I focus on South Korea as a case, analyzing a collection of 87,487 tweets referencing both COVID-19 and South Korea during the period of the pandemic, January 2020 to August 2021, and examining global users' understandings and assessments of South Korean responses to the health crisis.

South Korea serves as an excellent laboratory for such a study because its case demonstrates both the achievements and limits of a national response from a human rights perspective. The South Korean strategy called the "K-quarantine" was once hailed as a model for other countries, involving, as it did, using extensive testing, tracking, and treatment to keep the cases low and encouraging social distancing and wearing masks as daily practices. The K-quarantine appeared to have worked in halting a large outbreak without shutting down the country's borders or locking down towns (Kim et al., 2020). Although the strategy aimed at sustaining a fragile balance between using government power to protect public health and not infringing on civil liberties, critics challenged the K-quarantine from the perspectives of civil liberty and basic human rights (Ryan, 2020; Yamin & Habibi, 2020). Therefore, I examined how much attention human rights issues received from global Twitter users and what specific topics were of most interest to users who appeared to care about human rights.

For this article, I used Pseudo-document-based Topic Model (PTM) as an unsupervised machine learning technique for classifying short texts into viable topics or themes (Zuo et al., 2016). PTM shares the topic model advantages of automatically providing a mixture of topics from a document and data *corpus* but mitigates its disadvantages of not effectively handling short texts that lack sufficient word co-occurrence information. The use of a topic model fits with the key empirical focus of this article: the themes in the public discussion on Twitter regarding South Korean responses to the pandemic. The technique allowed for gauging the value online users attached to public health, foreign responses, patients' rights, and human rights in general in the response to the COVID-19 pandemic.

The rise of the K-quarantine

A pandemic triggers national health authorities and other government entities to mobilize to contain the infecting virus, treat the infected, and alert citizens (You, 2020). In response to COVID-19, countries' preparedness, experiences, resources, and support from citizens varied greatly, and governments thus appeared to be responding differently to the crisis (Spadaro, 2020). The severity of infections and associated mortality rates also contributed to differences in national responses related to, for instance, lockdowns, travel bans, the use of personal equipment like masks, and privacy restrictions (Duic & Sudar, 2021).

Nonetheless, countries do respond to infectious disease outbreaks in strikingly similar ways: They immediately implement emergency management policies that involve readying health facilities and professionals, tracking and tracing the spread of the virus, ensuring proper individual hygiene, and, if need be, restricting normal activities of individuals and communities. Proper coordination and collaboration with health agencies and professionals are imperative for containing the spread of viruses.

The South Korean response was no exception. The COVID-19 pandemic ushered in unprecedented policy measures to bring the spread under control that had been chosen and implemented with consideration for the country's handling of previous infectious diseases, such as the Middle East respiratory syndrome (MERS) outbreak of 2015. In the aftermath of its flawed MERS response, the South Korean government made four dozen reforms to strengthen public health emergency preparedness including ensuring effective testing, tracing, and treatment (You, 2020).

A South Korean white paper summarized the government's response in three policy strategies: (1) swift action; (2) the "3Ts" of widespread and rigorous testing, contact tracing, and treatment; and (3) public–private partnerships and civic awareness (ROK, 2020). Scholars have emphasized the country's democratic unitary political system coupled with strong public trust in healthcare professionals as the key conditions that enabled speedy implementation of policy decisions at the local level (Chung & Choe, 2008; You, 2020). The implementation was further buttressed by a well-coordinated national plan aided by governing bodies, including the Korean Ministry of Health and Welfare and the Korean Center for Disease Control and Prevention. The government's and communities' efforts halted a large outbreak without shutting Korea's borders or locking down towns (Kim et al., 2020).

These efforts are why the South Korean path to COVID-19 containment was hailed as a successful case. International society praised the country's readiness associated with the efficient 3Ts, timely provision of personal protective equipment (PPE), effective treatment of patients, and invoking civic conscience for the shared goal of fighting the virus (Lee & Lee, 2020). The K-quarantine, a rhetorical nod to the global popularity of K-pop, was also praised for allowing the government and the nation to pursue the two-pronged strategy of containing the spread of the virus while keeping the economy running (Yi & Lee, 2020).

Rights debates

Just as policy responses elsewhere inevitably involved legal and policy measures restricting various rights of citizens, and traded off certain rights in favor of health-related entitlements (Brysk, 2022; Chenoweth, 2022; Chiozza & King, 2022), South Korea also implemented and consolidated measures that limited basic civil rights as well as restricting economic activities (e.g., restaurants, bars, and shops; Botto, 2020). Following the path of other countries—including China, Hong Kong, and Singapore—South Korea also turned to surveillance as a means of containing and removing the virus and brought back policies that severely limited citizens' right to association and assembly (Cha, 2020). To ensure effective surveillance, the country relied heavily on IT-based epidemic containment strategies used for documentation, modeling, and contact tracing (Park et al., 2020). South Korea took part in the global response that 34 countries worldwide, including 22 democracies adopted, employing some type of digital programs immediately after the pandemic began (Chiozza & King, 2022; Eck & Hatz, 2020).

Surveillance

In March 2021, the South Korean government launched the COVID-19 Epidemiological Investigation Support System (EISS), a new computer network designed to support epidemiological investigations of confirmed cases (Ryan, 2020). It targeted confirmed patients with remarkable speed and accuracy of information acquisition aided by an AI-driven smart city technology system. EISS allows investigators to combine the results of interviews with medical records, credit card transactions, transportation card details, and CCTV footage by automatically identifying a confirmed person's location and movements over time. The system was updated with data added from overseas immigration and healthcare facility records.

What made all these surveillance strategies possible was a legal breakthrough triggered by the flawed response to the 2015 MERS outbreak. One of the four dozen legal reforms after 2015 included amending the Contagious Disease Prevention and Control Act and this amendment permitted health authorities to override certain provisions in the Personal Information Protection Act, which initially banned the collection, use, and disclosure of personal data without consent from infected individuals and those suspected to be infected. All of these developments raised concerns from various sectors of society over privacy and personal information protection. As Brysk (2022) points out in this volume, health-related international jurisprudence established responsibilities of medical professionals and government agencies relative not only to patients' access to essential medicines but also to their privacy.

Several months after the first confirmed case in South Korea in January, 2020 international media and human rights groups began to criticize that personal information released by the South Korean government disrupted private lives and invoked social stigma and warned of human rights infringements caused by the IT-based system, including mobile apps designed to collect users' geolocated movement data. During the earlier phase of the emergency in 2020, the public decried the authorities' handling and sharing of intimate personal details on infected and potential patients, such as their location, age, and sex and the names of the restaurants, shops, and other business premises they had visited. Public disclosures of the travel paths and contacts of confirmed cases increasingly raised concerns about privacy invasion (Park et al., 2020).

On March 9, 2020, the National Human Rights Commission of Korea issued a recommendation warning that excessive public disclosures could undermine public health by dissuading those suspected of infection from cooperating voluntarily and causing public disdain or social stigma. This intervention served as an impetus for the health authority to go through a serious of revisions on the disclosure guidelines ranging from limiting the scope of disclosures, through excluding a confirmed patient's personal details, to making route disclosures nearly anonymized in late 2020. The subsequently decreased privacy concerns coupled with a high level of public support for contact tracing led to the intrusive surveillance structure being sustained and deployed.

From June 2020, the contact tracing method evolved into the QR code-based system through which the managers at restaurants, cafes, fitness centers, and other public places asked visitors to produce an ephemeral QR code and have the QR code scanned. To alleviate private concerns, the authority ensured that ephemeral and pseudonymized QR codes are separated from personally identifiable data, the pieces of the data are combined only when a visitor is confirmed positive, and the collected data are removed from the server after four weeks (Park et al., 2020). Nonetheless, public anxiety remains about the potential leakage of the personal data collected through the QR code, and concerns remain about the lack of legal basis for how long the information needs to be kept and when it should be removed.

Stigmatization

From the beginning of the pandemic, South Koreans received flurries of emergency text messages from authorities, alerting them to be wary of the movements of citizens with COVID-19 infections. A typical alert contained the infected person's age, gender, and area of residence and a detailed log of his or her movements to the minute; the names of businesses he or she had visited and at what times were also released. Singapore followed suit, but the alerts there never reached the detail of those in South Korea. South Korean authorities released details such as when people left for work, whether they wore masks on the subway, the stations where they changed trains, and the massage bars they visited for leisure.

The specificity of the released public data about infected persons raised inevitable concerns about privacy because the data could be identifiable, and one problem was, expectedly, social stigmatization. In many multicultural societies, certain specific groups were stigmatized in efforts to blame the coronavirus pandemic on those associated as carriers of the virus (Roberto et al., 2020). In South Korea, infected patients and those who were suspected were perceived as responsible for the spread of the virus. They were often ignored or treated as criminals when they had no possible individual responsibility (Oh et al., 2020). Infected citizens who violated health authority mandates were considered candidates for the same electronic monitoring anklets worn by sex offenders.

After cases were confirmed at the Itaewon club, local newspapers explicitly named the club as a gay bar and ran articles stigmatizing sexual minorities and holding them responsible for the virus's spread. The government's monitoring technology and standardized tracing methods all escalated the atmosphere for demonizing the LGBTQ community. Visitors to the club were pressured to hide their identity, and a private education institution instructor was accused of causing further infection by hiding his job and movements; he was eventually arrested and sentenced to six months in jail. Scholars assert that the government's overconfidence in the K-quarantine and their quarantine-first strategy inevitably resulted in targeting the groups that contracted the virus, and it tarnished the impacts of the government regimen. These groups included religious groups, foreigners, and participants in public protests (Oh et al., 2020).

The right of assembly at a crossroads

As the country was consumed in the second and third waves of the pandemic during the period of 2020–2021, government authorities, including President Moon, became increasingly strident, promising to use the blunt force of the law to punish those who betrayed the government's epidemiological efforts. "No freedom of religion, assembly, or expression can be asserted at the cost of such damage," Moon stressed, accusing religious group members and protesters of spreading the virus and thus risking the public safety by attending weekly services or occupying the streets. As Badran and Turnbull (2022) show in this volume, such a policy direction needs to be viewed in the larger global context in which many governments began to use the pandemic as a reason for consolidating power, using excessive force and legal measures such as declaring states of emergency *vis-à-vis* controlling civil society. The government rightfully imposed certain restrictions on public gatherings to curb the spread of the virus but also wrongly used its enhanced power to demonize public demonstrations and crush dissent.

During 2020–2021, rallies of more than 10 protesters were mostly banned in South Korea, and most rallies were prohibited from several key avenues in downtown Seoul. In the summer of 2021, when the country was grappling with a fourth wave of infection fueled by the Delta variant, the police took even more stringent measures to ban and punish one-person rallies in consideration of virus outbreaks from antigovernment rallies in the summer of the previous year and as a caution against the possibility of small rallies growing larger. The police used the repressive tactic of erecting so-called bus walls, using parked police buses along main avenues and around the central square in downtown Seoul to seal off the entire area. The police also set up more than 80 checkpoints to block vehicles that were suspected of carrying protesters and equipment to check pedestrians to ensure that they would not join the protests. This suppression of public rallies was often juxtaposed on TV screens with images of thousands of shoppers gathered in packed retail stores without any intervention from enforcement officers.

South Korea's imperfect balancing efforts between protecting the public health and protecting human rights could serve as a reminder of the economy-first mentality that pervaded the country under authoritarian governments in the 1970s and 1980s (Koo & Choi, 2019). Protesters defying COVID-19 warnings were easily stigmatized and criminalized and in the aftermath, the country witnessed the erosion of the democratic foundation that had buttressed the country and often garnered the nation praise for having achieved both economic growth and democracy. As Chenoweth (2022) asserts in this volume, protesters who were wearing masks and social distancing outdoors seized the opportunities to accommodate the public health interests with their right to peaceful assembly. South Korean protesters demanding labor reforms, religious rights, and freedom of expression were no exception.

The anticipated rights discussion online

The South Korean response to the pandemic and the rights debate provide a larger context in which citizens made sense of and discussed the COVID-19 pandemic both on and offline. Researchers have recognized Twitter as a cyber public sphere that permits netizens to address their perceptions of and attitudes toward government policies shaping collective life. I hypothesize that global Twitter users paid attention to different aspects of the rights debate even if their attention was relatively marginal compared with the degree of attention paid to public health issues. I further hypothesize that Twitter users' discussions of rights issues might have centered around the surveillance, stigmatization, and right of assembly issues that received notable attention from the media and past studies.

Data collection

I collected Twitter data using the Twitter API v1 accessed through the Academic Research product track and constructed a text *corpus* of 87,487 tweets from January 20, 2020, when the first COVID-19 patient was reported in South Korea, to August 31, 2021, the end of the observation period for this article. Using searchtweets (a Python library) to extract Twitter data, I queried the Academic Research product track on several combinations of terms, such as *covid + south korea*, *pandemic + south korea*, and *pandemic + korea*, to create the dataset of COVID-19 tweets focused on South Korea.

For topic modeling, I only focused on non-retweets, which decreased the *corpus* from 120,000 to 87,487 tweets. In other words, I had to preprocess the *corpus* only on the "text" field without duplication, removing retweets that would inflate the number of texts unnecessary for the analyses. With the information accessed through the API, I had to remove all the metadata, including the https hyperlink, and short words of fewer than three characters. Hashtags were also removed, because these features could cause strong influence over classification of latent topics. I next conducted standard preprocessing to prepare the Twitter data for topic modeling. I processed each tweet text to remove all punctuation marks, numbers, stopwords, and web addresses, and further implemented lower-casing, stemming, and tokenization. I needed to reduce the complexity of the data *corpus* in order to effectively identify the patterns that emerged from the public discussions.

Topic models

Topic models refer to a suite of algorithms for discovering the hidden semantic structures in large collections of documents (Blei, 2012; Park et al., 2019). Using vast amounts of documents as input, a topic model produces a set of interpretable topics and assesses the extent to which each document exhibits those topics. These individual documents with different weights of topics are often aggregated alongside a time unit (e.g., year), and this aggregation reveals which topics show higher probabilities than others within that time window. This powerful approach of topic models has been applied in many different fields, such as marketing, sociology, political science, digital humanities, and human rights (Boyd-Graber et al., 2017; Lynam, 2016).

The most popular technique of topic modeling is Latent Dirichlet Allocation (LDA) as the simplest model of the kind. LDA posits that the documents themselves are observed, whereas the topic structure—the topics, topic distributions in a document, and topic assignment of a word in a document—is hidden (DiMaggio et al., 2013). The key computation problem of LDA, a family of Bayesian probabilistic approaches, is inferring the hidden topic structure—that is, posterior distribution, using the observed document (Bagozzi & Berliner, 2018).

Although LDA is a powerful tool and has been used widely, it suffers from several technical problems, and there is an ongoing debate on the nature of and solutions for these limits (Dieng et al., 2019). One stream involves its low performance when LDA is applied to a set of short texts, including tweets. The problem stems from the lack of information on word co-occurrence in each short text relative to conventional documents that comprise longer sections of text. Short texts make it difficult for algorithms to discern a meaningful number of topics in different proportions, which in turn decreases the number of topics a researcher has available for extracting semantic meanings from large documents. Efforts were made to aggregate short texts into regular-sized pseudo-documents using auxiliary contextual information— such as authorship, hashtags, time, and locations (Hong & Davison 2010).

Among the aggregation solutions, I used PTM, which uses implicit aggregation of short texts against data sparsity. In this way, the topic distribution modeling of a vast number of short texts is transformed into the topic modeling of many fewer pseudo-documents, which in turn are much more beneficial for parameter estimation. PTM assumes a high volume of extremely short texts are generated from much less yet regular-sized pseudo-documents (Zuo et al., 2016), and does not require the use of auxiliary information, which is not always available or is too costly for deployment (Zuo et al., 2016).

I provide the algorithm describing the generative process for topic modeling with PTM. From Steps 1–3, I first consider three multinomial distributions that follow Dirichlet Allocations (ψ, θ_l, Φ_z) with the corresponding hyperparameters (λ, α, β). In Step 4(a), a multinomial distribution ψ is introduced to model the distribution of short texts over pseudo-documents. I assume each short text belongs to one and only one pseudo-document. Then, in step 4(b), each word in a short text is generated by first sampling a topic z from topic distribution θ_l of its pseudo document, and then sampling a word from word distribution Φ_z (Zuo et al., 2016).

1. Sample $\psi \sim Dir(\lambda)$
2. For each topic z:
   a. Sample $\Phi_z \sim Dir(\beta)$
3. For each pseudo document d'_l:
   a. Sample $\theta_l \sim Dir(\alpha)$
4. For each short text d_s:
   a. Sample a pseudo document $l \sim Multi(\psi)$:
   b. For each word w_i in d_s:
      i. Sample a topic $z \sim Multi(\theta_l)$:
      ii. Sample the ith word $w_i \sim Multi(\Phi_z)$

I used the Tomotopy package in Python to perform the PTM using the PTModel functions whose implementation was based on the algorithms used in this article.

Topic modeling requires the number of topics to be specified. I ran several different experiments varying the number of topics from 15 to 45, with 5 as the step unit, and selected the final model in consideration of both the highest coherence values measuring semantic similarity between high scoring words in the topic and the lowest perplexity values measuring how well the selected model predicts a sample. I settled with a solution that generated 35 topics with a coherence value score of 3,529.99 and a perplexity value score of .73, a best fitting model characterizing interpretability of the identified topics as well as predictability of the model (Bagozzi and Berliner, 2018; Syed and Spruit, 2017).

Analyses

Table 1 shows the 35-topic solution, listing the 20 highest-ranked terms for each topic, the labels corresponding to the terms of each topic and the topic's reference number. These 35 topics from the final model are the best characterizations of the collected *corpus* of COVID-19 tweets. They are presented in clusters around broader themes and appear in order from the themes with more attention to those with less. Within each theme, the corresponding topics are displayed in the order of their probability scores or the degree of attention. The themes constructed from the topics were (1) countries' responses and records; (2) infections, testing, tracing, treatment, and social distancing; (3) vaccine and vaccination; (4) economic issues; (5) US military base in Korea and US forces; (6) human rights; (7) youth and culture; and (8) technology.

Countries' responses and records topics

Seven of the 35 topics that emerged from the tweet *corpus* reflected the theme of countries' responses and records with the highest probability scores. These tweets discussed countries' responses to the pandemic and their records of infection and death under the following topics: successful models (Topic 1), fatalities in the United States (Topic 3), government responses (Topic 7), death tolls in different countries (Topic 10), assessment of K-quarantine (Topic 14), COVID-19 deaths in South Korea and the United States (Topic 15), records in the Asia-Pacific region (Topic 26), and infections in East Asia (Topic 35). The topics in this cluster reflect Twitter users' concerns about and interest in how countries, including their own, responded to the pandemic and how their performances might have been compared with the South Korean response (see Figure 1).

The topic of fatalities in the United States, for example, included the words *population*, *country*, *Trump*, *United States*, *president*, *test*, *world*, *China*, *Germany*, *Italy*, and *fatality*. These terms reflect a clear concern about COVID-related fatalities in countries around the world, including the United States. One tweet with the largest topic score under this topic went as follows: "South Korea, population 51 million. South Korea has had 2,073 covid deaths. The US, in reality, has around 800,000. How do you explain this?" Another states, "Just having a look at the case fatality rates in different countries. Apparently, you want to live in New Zealand, Sweden, or South Korea."

Although several topics under the category of countries' responses and records reflected some understanding of governments' responses compared with South Korea as a reference, Topic 14, assessment of K-quarantine, refers exclusively to the South Korean strategy, with terms such as *response*, *system*, *great*, *effort*, *quarantine*, *safe*, *privacy*, *and strategy*. The tweet that reflected Topic 14 with the highest probability stated, "Why does South Korea have a better COVID response? Because they have a better government system and a better economic system. Why is our country not doing well?" By contrast, under Topic 35, infections in East Asia, Twitter users were alarmed by the recent surges in South Korea and other Asian countries during the third and fourth waves of the pandemic. These tweets criticized the once-touted Asian collectivist model with representative messages such as, "Once a model in fighting the pandemic, the country has been slow to vaccinate its people, even as it is being hit by its worst-ever wave of infections"

Infections, testing, tracing, treatment, and social distancing topics

Topics 4, 5, 19, and 25 captured issues concerning the theme of infections, testing, tracing, treatment, and social distancing. Topic 4, waves of infection, comprised the terms *infection*, *wave*,

Table 1. Topic keywords and labeling.

No	Top words	Label
Topic 1	country, mask, china, japan, taiwan, singapore, success, public, pandemic, curve, life, contact, successful, model, control, lesson, face, germany, vietnam, new_zealand	successful models
Topic 2	smell, loss, sense, symptom, concert, british, taste, confirmed, china, vaccine, system, patient, efficient, double, outbreak, offline, public, italy, novavax, prison	patients and symptoms
Topic 3	population, country, trump, united_states, america, state, president, test, leader, world, fatality, china, caput, germany, italy, life, entire, border, donald, florida	fatality in the US
Topic 4	infection, wave, second, virus, country, disease, third, cluster, surge, patient, control, church, seoul, outbreak, curb, record, prevention, health, official, high	waves of infections
Topic 5	test, virus, positive, patient, testing, news, expert, india, result, hospital, free, rapid, health, symptom, negative, trace, recovered, medical, report,	testing, tracing, and treatment
Topic 6	online, group, event, food, korean, pandemic, concert, trip, friend, safety, video, university, business, army, park, music, march, english, tour, sport	youth culture and pandemic
Topic 7	virus, world, government, outbreak, china, good, lockdown, health, testing, fight, work, story, policy, situation, part, expert, pandemic, next, early, mass	government responses
Topic 8	student, island, contact, college, airport, exam, jeju, blockchain, international, tracing, code, tourist, private, outbreak, surge, technology, religious, hotspot, entrance	youth vaccination and Jeju island
Topic 9	member, positive, service, arrival, usfk, quarantine, military, anyone, force, community, local, united_states, mandatory, korea, individual, american, soldier, travel, task, isolation	infections in US Forces Korea and the military
Topic 10	death, virus, italy, iran, china, spain, toll, report, france, germany, virusupdate, country, breaking, japan, recovery, march, confirmed, switzerland, update, korea	death tolls in different countries
Topic 11	korea, pandemic, south, economic, crisis, global, virus, korean, economy, recovery, country, article, north_korea, research, post, asia, first, impact, digital, cooperation	economic crisis and recovery in the two Koreas
Topic 12	korea, south, fight, episode, amid, podcast, technology, surveillance, credit, casino, ai, tech, startups, look, dollar, busan, success, serious, successful, security	use of technology
Topic 13	cafe, change, outbreak, climate, masks, response, blackpink, spared, italy, france, starbucks, mask, restriction, bloomberg, show, safe, concert, leadership, competent, trope	outbreak and safety in cafe
Topic 14	response, spread, system, great, effort, quarantine, healthcare, place, india, risk, different, technology, safe, privacy, rest, approach, idea, strategy, state, study	assessments of K-quarantine
Topic 15	death, korea, first, south, trump, virus, dead, january, response, pandemic, deaths, united_states, infection, testing, march, population, toll, fact, administration, mortality	covid deaths in South Korea and US
Topic 16	international, religious, movement, concern, oppression, religion, raise, samsung, minor, scholars, call, ngos, human_rights, stop, destruction, program, leaders, remote, work, wall	protest, oppression, and human rights
Topic 17	south, north_korea, sudan, turkmenistan, tajikistan, samoa, islands, lesotho, micronesia, tonga, comoros, yemen, kiribati, country, solomon_islands, vanuatu, tuvalu, palau, marshall, nauru	authoritarian and developing countries
Topic 18	church, virus, religious, shincheonji, outbreak, world, leader, member, sect, health, jesus, news, risk, group, trump, doctor, baseball, cult, pride	church outbreaks
Topic 19	seoul, virus, school, korea, restriction, spike, outbreak, city, measure, area, level, capital, health, south, daegu, home, government, travel, public, club	new spikes in Seoul and schools

(*continued*)

Table 1. Continued.

No	Top words	Label
Topic 20	chloroquine, music, virus, news, drug, rule, hydroxychloroquine, india, viral, bitcoin, enforce, treatment, expert, trending, zinc, internet, anti-hiv, china, anti-malaria, like	use of drugs
Topic 21	military, booth, mask, trade, immunity, business, joint, free, office, store, herd, news, phone, summer, exercise, drill, united_states, loss, glove, strategy	US-South Korea military exercise
Topic 22	vaccine, korea, vaccination, country, treatment, seoul, minister, north_korea, health, company, virus, government, plan, president, emergency, ministry, drug, south, official	vaccination
Topic 23	golf, treatment, fintech, hand, steel, cure, golfing, challenge, coffee, robot, corporation, riots, murder, instagolf, koreangolfnews, corruption, staff, sanitizer, development, virus	golf and golfing during pandemic
Topic 24	election, north_korea, president, party, pandemic, home, outbreak, moon, care, world, news, general, national, leader, response, military, ship, victory, moon_jae-in	election, party, and politics
Topic 25	social, distancing, study, virus, spread, detail, status, visit, show, dashboard, patient, rule, foot, contact, lack, explosion, music, child, measure, restaurant	covid statistics and social distancing
Topic 26	japan, china, australia, singapore, india, country, taiwan, germany, italy, canada, new_zealand, travel, vietnam, thailand, hong_kong, france, malaysia, iran, indonesia, russia	records in the Asia-Pacific region
Topic 27	income, basic, virus, universal, support, seoul, home, factory, music, outbreak, online, festival, samsung, gain, demand, new, news, style, kerala, apartment	support and regulations
Topic 28	test, maryland, state, governor, hogan, trump, larry_hogan, virus, first, deal, lady, national, guard, wife, government, help, yumi, president, worker, federal	Maryland governor
Topic 29	market, impact, china, news, japan, stock, economy, global, asia, economic, growth, pandemic, source, airline, trade, asian, india, export, indonesia, payment	economic growth and market in Asia
Topic 30	vaccine, astrazeneca, pfizer, trial, first, shot, news, drug, israel, moderna, deal, clinical, johnson, celltrion, approval, phase, antibody, mrna, inovio, novavax	different vaccines
Topic 31	hyundai, world, china, italy, india, power, company, aware, refuse, supreme, motor, true, complete, thewiderwiserview, diagnostic, virus, canend, santrampalji, virusourtbreak, rampal	motor companies
Topic 32	virus, intelligence, ai, expert, sonn, artificial, jung, lockdown, answer, popular, tech, fast, kore, park, diplomat, ml, drive-thrus, attack, machinelearning	AI and fight against covid
Topic 33	plasma, church, donation, shincheonji, development, vaccine, facilitates, cure, recovered, virus, worth, declare, billion, shincheonjichurch, virusoutbreak, shincheonjipress, korea, south, member, factcheck	plasma donation from church members
Topic 34	relief, japan, vaccine, president, kpop, expert, grant, govt, attack, niger, model, army, fund, happy, album, lazarus, birthday, criticized, crypto, delivery	Olympics and K-pop
Topic 35	virus, report, news, infection, outbreak, china, record, pandemic, live, update, world, spread, global, lockdown, first, virusoutbreak, korea, spike, india, high	infections in East Asia

second, *virus*, *country*, *disease*, *third*, *surge*, *outbreak*, and *record*, reflecting the later spread of the virus in South Korea in contrast with the country's impeccable initial record. The topic terms in this tweet dominated the word assignment: "Once a COVID success story, South Korea sweats through summer of Delta surge." Topic 19, new spikes in Seoul and schools, reflected the

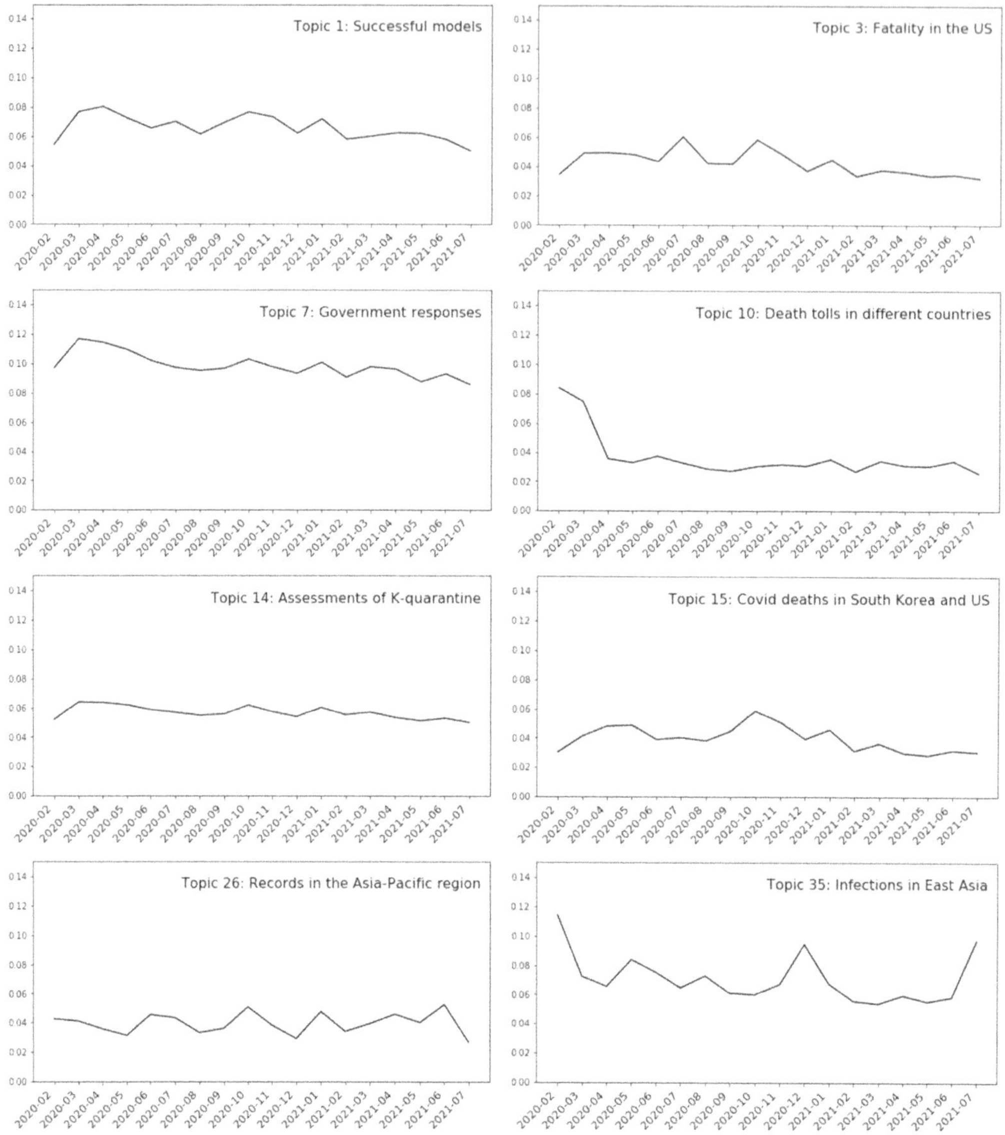

Figure 1. The average trend of "countries' responses and records" topics.

ongoing spread and related anxiety and new restrictions with a focus on metropolitan Seoul and in schools. One user posted a tweet wondering if the South Korean government had really banned public music events with music above 180 bpm due to COVID-19, and another was critical of the unprecedented new measures banning playing music faster than 120 bpm in Seoul gyms to curb rising COVID-19 cases (see Figure 2).

Vaccines and vaccination topics

Undoubtedly, vaccines and vaccination received tremendous attention from global Twitter users who mentioned both COVID and South Korea. Topics 20, 22, and 30 constituted the vaccine theme, and these comprised discussions of the availability and efficiency of certain drugs, vaccination in North

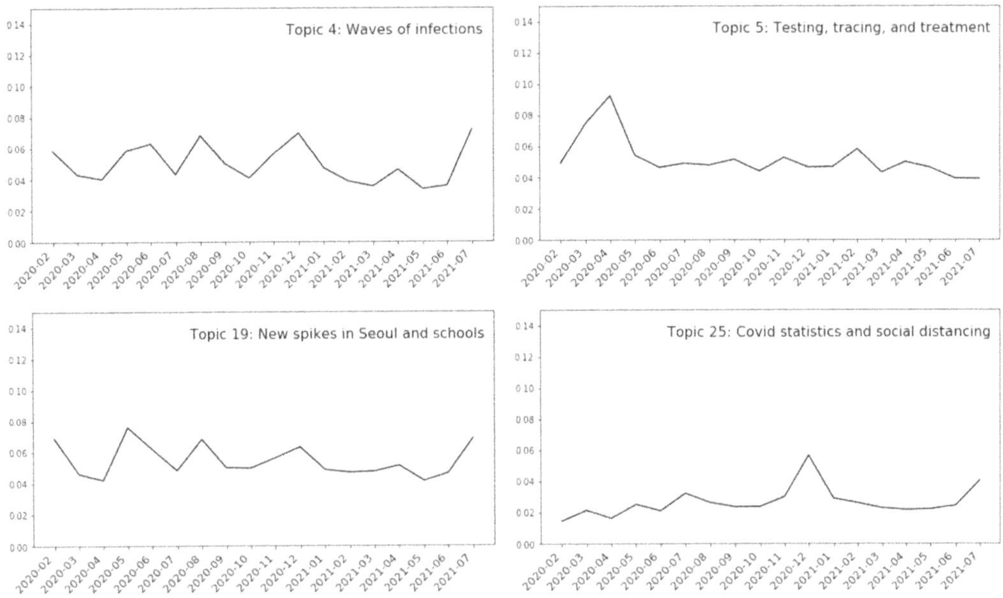

Figure 2. The average trend of "infections, testing, tracing, and treatment, social distancing" topics.

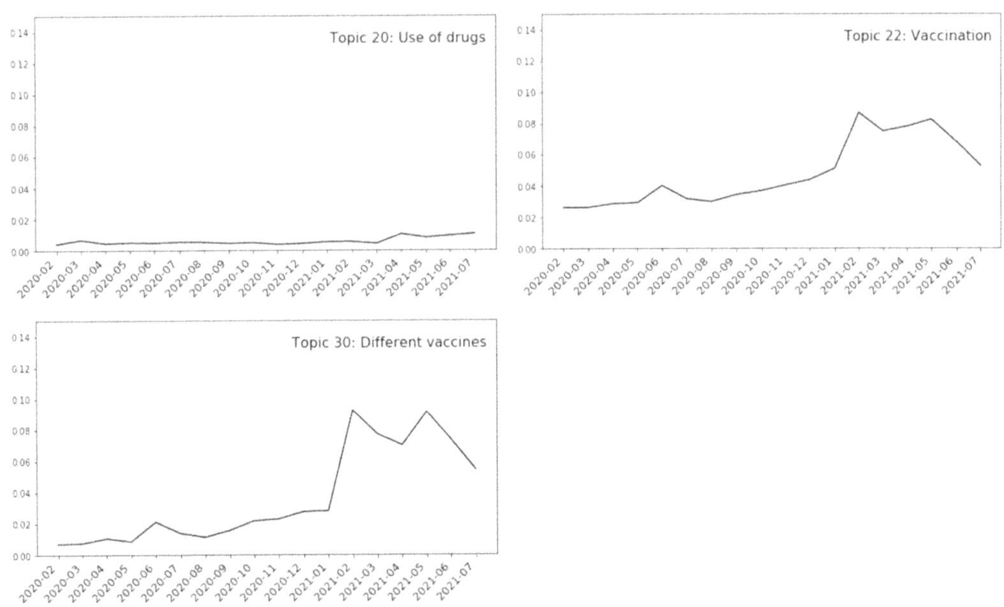

Figure 3. The average trend of "vaccines and vaccination" topics.

Korea, users' concerns about the delayed vaccine rollout, and South Korea's online vaccination reservation system. The top words under Topic 22, vaccination, were *vaccine*, *vaccination*, *treatment*, *North Korea*, *company*, and *emergency*. A tweet exhibiting this topic with the highest probability criticized the country's low vaccination record: "South Korea currently ranks second-to-last among OECD member countries, with only 13.49 percent of its population fully vaccinated, and critics have argued that the government dragged its feet in rolling out the national vaccination campaign" (see Figure 3).

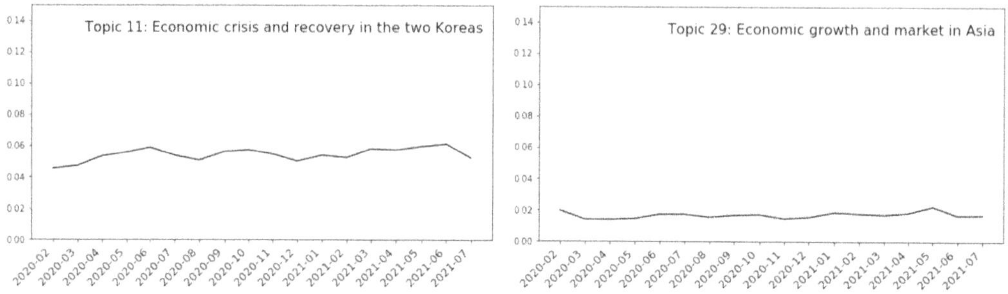

Figure 4. The average trend of "economic issues" topics.

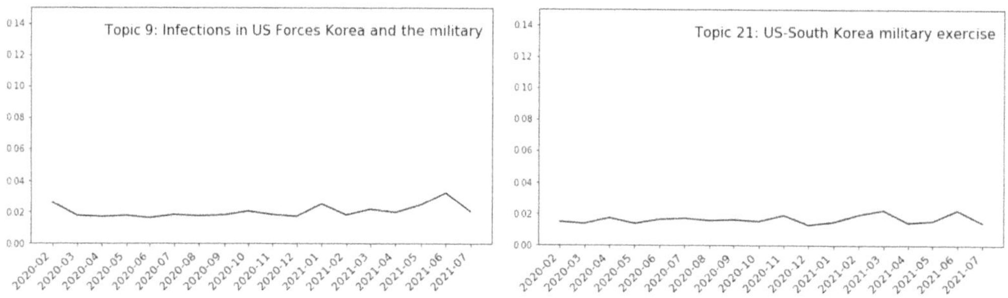

Figure 5. The average trend of "US camp and the military" topics.

Economic issues topics

Topics 11 and 29 were the most straightforward to interpret because these involved the impacts of COVID-19 on national and global economies. Topic 11, economic crisis and recovery in the two Koreas, contrasted South Korea's relatively quick recovery from the economic downturn to North Korea's experience of one of its worse economic crises in two or three decades. A tweet from this topic with high word assignment observed, "North Korea's economy took its biggest hit in 23 years in 2020 because of continued UN sanctions, COVID-19 lockdowns and bad weather." Whereas Topic 11 depicted economic difficulties and recovery in the context of the two Koreas, Topic 29 focused on what occurred in Asian countries such as China, Japan, and India during the pandemic. The most highly ranked terms include *market, impact, China, Japan, stock, economy, global, Asia, economic, growth,* and *pandemic* (see Figure 4).

US camp and the military

Two topics related to infections in the military, particularly on bases such as US Forces Korea (USFK) and in the Korean military, which was known as a major cluster of COVID-19 infections. Topic 9, infections in US Forces Korea and the military, encompassed the terms *member, positive, service, arrival, USFK, quarantine, military,* and *soldier.* Tweets under this topic referred to USFK-affiliated individuals who had tested positive for COVID-19 after arriving in South Korea and delivered information on the vaccination statuses of the people associated with USFK, from US service members to South Korean employees. This topic also comprised episodes of infections within the military, including the scandalous infection of the Cheonghae Unit. By contrast, Topic 21, US–South Korea military exercise, reflects controversies on the proper scale for US–South Korea joint drills in the middle of the pandemic, with the highest-ranked terms being *military booth, mask, trade, immunity, joint, free, office, herd, exercise, drill,* and *United States* (see Figure 5).

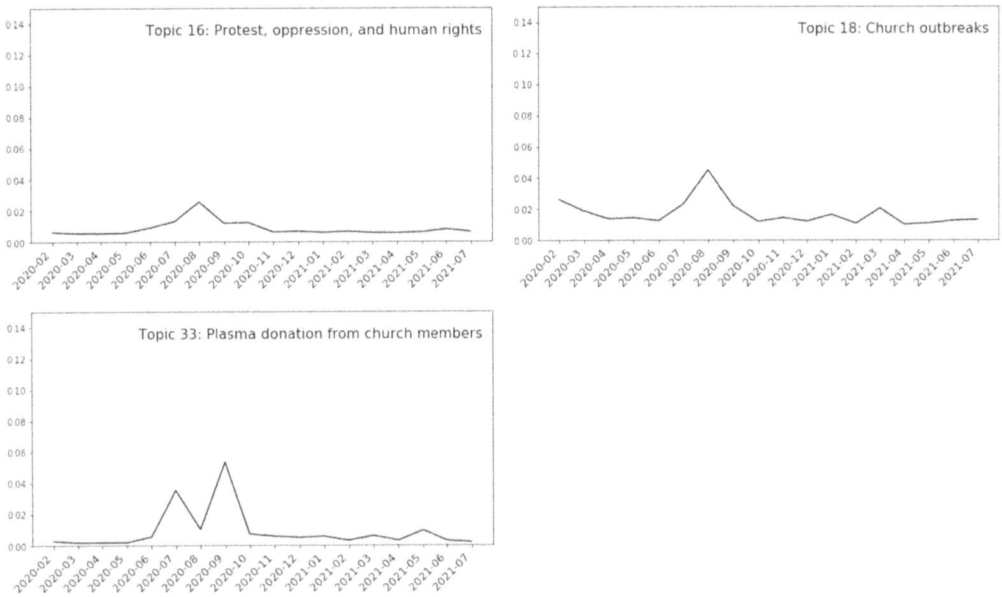

Figure 6. The average trend of "broadly human rights related" topics.

Human rights-related topics

Given my priority of noting to what extent Twitter users attended to human rights issues compared with more general health-related issues, the PTM results show that even though the human rights-related topics (Topics 16, 18, and 33) were clearly meaningful, they received much less attention than other topics that dealt with government responses, health measures, vaccines, and economic issues. Furthermore, the discussion on surveillance, restrictions on assembly, and stigmatization of religious groups tended to appear rather briefly and soon subside, as shown in Topics 16, 18, and 33 in Figure 1. All of this suggests that rights issues remained largely parochial in South Korea-focused COVID-19 tweets and in public discussions of COVID-19 and South Korea (see Figure 6).

Nevertheless, these topics are highly important ones for this study, because they represent the public discussion of South Korean government measures toward religious groups, political dissidents, and protesters, Twitter users' assessments of those measures, and how international society—including the United Nations—responded to the measures. The top words under Topic 16, protest, oppression, and human rights, included *international*, *religious*, *movement*, *concern*, *oppression*, *religion*, *raise*, *call*, *NGOs*, *human rights*, *stop*, and *destruction*, not only specifying key actors and issues with *movement*, *religion*, and *NGOs*, but also negatively portrayed what occurred with words such as *oppression*, *stop*, and *destruction*. A representative tweet whose terms contained the highest probability of this topic urged that "international leaders and human rights NGOs call on South Korea to stop oppression of minor religion for COVID-19."

Topic 33, plasma donation from church members, included terms related to plasma donation from *Shincheonji*, a church group that was largely responsible for the first wave of the pandemic in South Korea and thus became the target of public disdain—such as *plasma*, *church*, *donation*, *shincheonji*, *cure*, *recovered*, and *factcheck*. Challenging the public's view that this church group was resistant to blood donation, a tweet with the highest probability of this topic called attention to "third plasma donation drive of 4,000 church members who have fully recovered from COVID-19" using the hashtag #StopFakeNews.

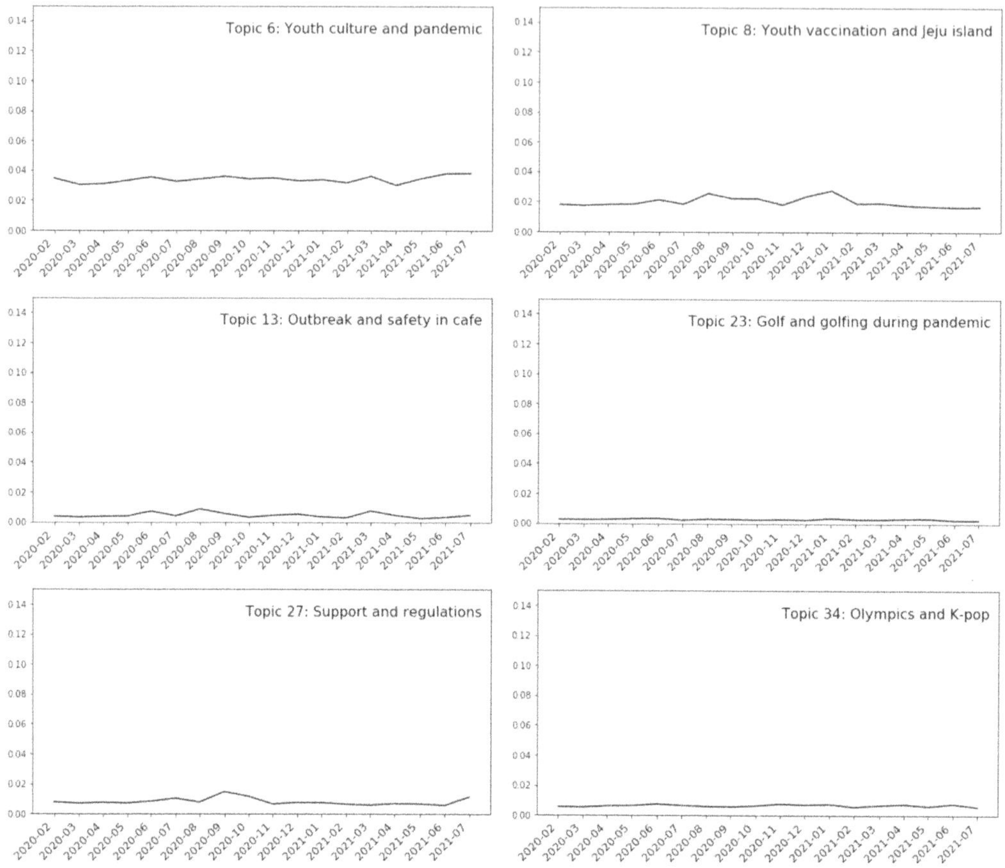

Figure 7. The average trend of "youth and culture" topic.

Youth and culture

Several topics were associated with the spread of the virus and its impacts on everyday life (Topics 6, 8, 13, 23, 27, 34) with relatively lower probability scores. Topic 6, youth culture and the pandemic—with top words such as *online*, *group*, *event*, *food*, *pandemic*, *concert*, *trip*, *friend*, *video*, *university*, *music*, and *sport*—focused on the rapid spread of the virus among youth, with their low vaccination rates, and its impacts on schooling, jobs, businesses, sports, and other cultural activities. One tweet expressed concerns about small businesses that were hard hit by semi-shutdowns and other restrictive measures: "Small business owners in South Korea are being driven out of business as the country has gone into the toughest." Another representative tweet discussed young people's economic difficulties: "Koreans in 20s and 30s give up job search amid prolonged COVID-19 crisis" (see Figure 7).

Topic 13, outbreak and safety in cafes—with top words such as *café*, *outbreak*, *masks*, *response*, *Blackpink*, and *Starbucks*—highlighted episodes of the infection that occurred in cafés as popular public gathering locations where people enjoy K-pop artists such as Blackpink; this topic warned of the dangers of not wearing masks in such indoor settings. Topic 23, golf and golfing during the pandemic, highlighted the increasing popularity of golf among young people during the pandemic. Topic 27, support and regulations, lamented the absurd regulations that were put into place, including the ban on outdoor cultural festivals as well as the ban on playing loud music in gyms. One representative tweet complained, "No music over 120 BPM allowed in gyms in South Korea? Mimicking their neighbours to the North." Topic 34, the Olympics and K-pop, touched

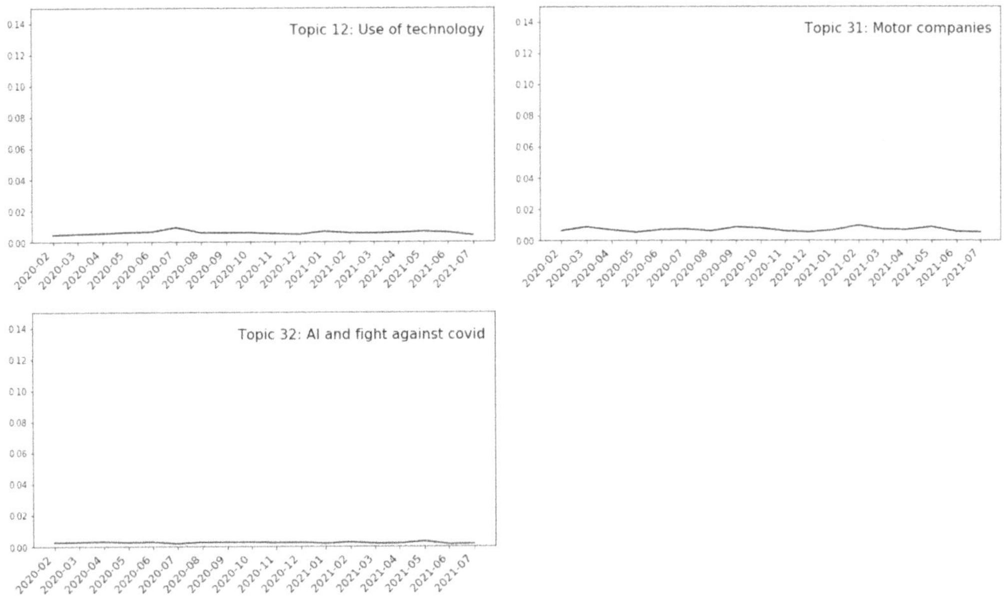

Figure 8. The average trend of "technology" topic.

on Japan's response to the pandemic during the summer Olympic games with a negative tone and discussed the popularity of K-pop despite the unprecedented pandemic crisis.

The use of technology

The final meaningful category of topics concerned technology, which has some relation to human rights issues—for instance, privacy. It is worth noting, however, that the topic scores and overall probabilities assigned to these topics were the lowest for topics in any other categories. Two topics related to technology: the use of technology by motor companies and AI and the fight against COVID-19 (see Figure 8).

Topic 12, use of technology, had the top words *podcast*, *technology*, *surveillance*, *credit*, *casino*, *αι*, *tech*, *startups*, *success*, and *security* and highlighted the potential uses of technology for surveillance in the context of successful containment of the virus during a pandemic. The tweet with the highest probability for this topic remarked, "Only South Korea used app-based contact tracing right. Benchmark for a successful COVID-19 contact-tracing operation is to trace and quarantine 80% of close contacts within 3 days of a case being confirmed." However, criticizing unbearable workloads, one Twitter user posted, "South Korea's delivery workers go on strike against overwork amid COVID-19."

Topic 32, artificial intelligence (AI) and the fight against COVID, brought to the fore the use of AI-assisted technologies in fighting the spread of the COVID-19 in South Korea; terms included *virus, intelligence, AI, expert, sonn, artificial, jung, lockdown, answer, popular, tech, fast, kore, park, diplomat, ml, drive-thrus, attack,* and *machine learning.* A tweet in which this topic dominated succinctly summarizes the country's winning strategy: "South Korea Winning the Fight Against Corona Virus Using #BigData And #AI by Go to #MachineLearning #Artificialintelligence." Topic 31 was motor companies and referred to automobile companies such as Hyundai as well as disruptions to the global supply chain.

Tweeter users' discussion of human rights in a nutshell

Here I asked whether Twitter users' attention to human rights topics corresponded with or could be predicted by my discussion of the rights debate that occurred in South Korea. The results from the PTM largely confirmed my expectations of global Twitter users' discussion of central human rights issues, such as surveillance, stigmatization, and the right of assembly. First, stigmatization was a significant concern, as indicated by the prevalence of several topics (16, 18, and 33) that consisted of terms associated with religious groups—for example, *shincheonji*, *church members*, *the youth*, *gym users*, *participants of cultural events*, and *COVID patients*.

Second, surveillance was a key issue across different topics regarding privacy in the context of the K-quarantine (Topic 14) and was viewed as an inevitable concern once technology was being used to trace the spread of the disease. Contrary to my expectation, however, Twitter users paid relatively little attention to the government's suppression of the right of assembly. Nonetheless, government's control over rights to assembly and association could be inferred from some of the dynamics of topic shifts; consider, for example, the apex of Topic 18, church outbreak in August 2021, when the government sought to crack down on protesters linked to religious groups and churches, using COVID-19 as an excuse to control peaceful protesters. This episode is consistent with what Badran and Turnbull (2022) report in this volume, regarding how the state could use the pandemic to crush dissent using public health emergencies. The conservative church groups critical of President Moon's tough stance on religious freedom insisted on maintaining a street presence, but that invited a convenient pretext to shut down ongoing dissent.

With the topic model approach revealing unexpected patterns or semantic meanings of the texts, the analyses permitted reflecting on newer, unanticipated forms of rights infringements. The findings from the PTM indicated that existential threats stemming from the pandemic prompted newer forms of government intervention in civic life. When South Korea set another new high during the second and third waves, for example, the Ministry of Health and Welfare announced the unprecedented new measures of banning playing music faster than 120 bpm in gyms in Seoul and prohibiting music events with music above 180 bpm. These measures might be understood as extending regulations that were already placed on public spaces, such as the restricted maximum capacities and hours of operation for cafes, bars, and restaurants. Yet global Twitter users often ridiculed and fiercely criticized these government measures as actively encroaching on civic life.

Other unforeseen examples of abuses were linked to workers' rights and rights with economic activities. Although they did not rise to the frequency of a formal topic or theme and did not emerge as one of the economic issues identified by PTM, the worsening working conditions of delivery workers received sizable attention from Twitter users. A sizable number of tweets expressed empathy toward platform workers who went on strike against overwork amid COVID-19 and sympathized with members of the Korean Confederation of Trade Unions who marched in major cities amid police blocks; these workers were marching for safe employment and better working conditions. The other notable theme I identified that did not fall under a topic cluster concerned what was happening to owners of restaurants, cafes, and other small businesses who were most negatively affected by government restrictions on operating hours and curfews. Alarmed by the impacts of government measures that severely hampered economic activity for small business owners, citizens began to be wary of the unfairness of government mandates on operating hours and their consequences for economic freedom.

Conclusion

South Korea's battle against COVID-19 has been triumphant, as attested to by global Twitter users' opinions of the country's efficient responses and the corresponding topics that emerged in a text analysis by algorithm. In fact, the country has maintained an enviable track record of many fewer cases of infection and deaths than in other high-income countries. Furthermore, South Korea experienced only minimal damage to its economy (only a −1 percent GDP growth rate) in 2020, a feat achieved by no OECD countries. The question arises then of whether South Korea's public health measures for achieving this success were consistent with international human rights norms.

If one prioritizes such paramount rights as the right to life and the right to health, the answer is clearly positive: many lives were saved and individuals protected from the novel coronavirus with the government's strict measures. Compared, however, with how other interconnected yet competing rights are prioritized—such as freedom of expression, assembly rights and privacy protection—the answer is not necessarily positive. My findings from the PTM of 87,487 tweets concerning COVID-19 and South Korea indicate that COVID-19-related issues of human dignity, personal information protection, and assembly rights remain parochial compared with what users considered the more important issues of public health policies: testing and tracing, vaccinations, economic issues, and the youth. Rights protection appeared at odds with the seemingly larger target of protecting the public's health and safety (Roberto et al., 2020).

Persons who were infected with COVID-19 and those who were suspected of infection were stigmatized to inform the public of the danger of the disease, but this tactic indiscriminately targeted religious groups, young people, protesters, and citizens who refused vaccination. In addition, the South Korean government actively employed surveillance to collect personal information on the public using its advanced AI technologies. Contrary to our conventional understanding of universal human rights as interconnected and indivisible, we undoubtedly witnessed tradeoffs among different kinds of rights in the case of South Korea. In this volume, Chiozza and King (2022) make the case that, in the face of global health emergencies, governments have restricted some rights to protect other types of rights.

We are not equipped with tools to measure how South Korea's handling of a myriad of human rights might compares with other high-income countries. Considering that savvy governments in most countries—autocratic and democratic—used the pandemic as an excuse to restrict civil liberties and rights, we simply cannot know where South Korea lands on the spectrum. The impacts of restricting a set of rights for the sake of protecting other prioritized rights can be only gauged through future research (Eck and Hatz, 2020). What I found, however, were concerned voices, feelings, and judgments from tens of thousands of Twitter users worldwide about the ways in which South Korea—often celebrated as a model country for the battle against the coronavirus—responded to this unprecedented project of humanity, and the collective opinion was consistent with my own evaluation of the strengths and weaknesses of this Asian country's path to managing COVID-19.

As Murdie (2022) points out in this volume, it is crucial for a country to take rights-consistent public health measures because it could make citizens less likely to see the right to health as a counter to other civil and political rights. The will of the state then would spur the will of people, a launchpad for improved human rights.

References

Badran, S., & Turnbull, B. (2022). The COVID-19 pandemic and authoritarian consolidation in North Africa. *Journal of Human Rights*, *21*(3), 263–282.

Bagozzi, B. E., & Berliner, D. (2018). The politics of scrutiny in human rights monitoring: evidence from structural topic models of US State Department Human Rights Reports. *Political Science Research and Methods*, *6*(4), 661–677. doi:10.1017/psrm.2016.44

Blei, D. M. (2012). Probabilistic topic models. *Communications of the ACM*, *55*(4), 77–84. doi:10.1145/2133806.2133826

Botto, K. (2020). *The coronavirus pandemic and South Korea's global leadership potential. [white paper].* Washington, DC: Carnegie Endowment for International Peace.

Boyd-Graber, J., Hu., & Mimno, D. (2017). Applications of topic models. *Foundations and Trends® in Information Retrieval*, *11*(2–3), 143–296. doi:10.1561/1500000030

Brysk, A. (2022). Pandemic patriarchy: The impact of a global health crisis on women's rights. *Journal of Human Rights*, *21*(3), 283–303. doi:10.1080/14754835.2022.2030209

Cha, V. (2020). Asia's COVID-19 lessons for the West: Public goods, privacy, and social tagging. *The Washington Quarterly*, *43*(2), 1–18. doi:10.1080/0163660X.2020.1770959

Chenoweth, E. (2022). Can nonviolent resistance survive COVID-19? *Journal of Human Rights*, *21*(3), 304–316.

Chilton, A., Cope, K. L., Crabtree, C., & Versteeg, M. (2020). The normative force of higher-order law: Evidence from six countries during the COVID-19 pandemic. Available at SSRN 3591270.

Chiozza, G., & King, J. (2022). The state of human rights in a (post) COVID-19 world. *Journal of Human Rights*, *21*(3), 246–262.

Chung, K., & Choe, H. (2008). South Korean national pride: Determinants, changes, and suggestions. *Asian Perspective*, *32*(1), 99–127. doi:10.1353/apr.2008.0032

Dieng, A. B., & Ruiz, F. J., & Blei, D. M. (2019). The dynamic embedded topic model. Cornell University. *arXiv preprint arXiv:1907.05545*: 1–17.

DiMaggio, P., Nag, M., & Blei, D. M. (2013). Exploiting affinities between topic modeling and the sociological perspective on culture: Application to newspaper coverage of US Government Arts Funding. *Poetics*, *41*(6), 570–606. doi:10.1016/j.poetic.2013.08.004

Duić, D., & Sudar, V. (2021). The impact of COVID-19 on the free movement of persons in the EU. *EU and Comparative Law Issues and Challenges Series (ECLIC)*, *5*, 30–56.

Eck, K., & Hatz, S. (2020). State surveillance and the COVID-19 crisis. *Journal of Human Rights*, *19*(5), 603–612. doi:10.1080/14754835.2020.1816163

Forman, L., & Kohler, J. C. (2020). Global health and human rights in the time of COVID-19: Response, restrictions, and legitimacy. *Journal of Human Rights*, *19*(5), 547–556. doi:10.1080/14754835.2020.1818556

Government of the Republic of Korea (ROK) (2020, 31 March). Tackling COVID-19: Health, Quarantine, and Economic Measures: Korean experience. https://ecck.or.kr/wp-content/uploads/2020/03/Tackling-COVID-19-Health-Quarantine-and-Economic-Measures-of-South-Korea.pdf

Hatcher, W. (2020). A failure of political communication not a failure of bureaucracy: The danger of presidential misinformation during the COVID-19 pandemic. *The American Review of Public Administration*, *50*(6-7), 614–620. doi:10.1177/0275074020941734

Hong, L., & Davison, B. D. (2010). Emperical study of topic modeling in Twitter. In *Proceedings of the first workshop on social media analytics*. ACM. https://doi.org/10.1145/1964858.1964870

Kavanagh, M. M., & Singh, R. (2020). Democracy, capacity, and coercion in pandemic response: COVID-19 in comparative political perspective. *Journal of Health Politics, Policy and Law*, *45*(6), 997–1012. doi:10.1215/03616878-8641530

Kim, M.-H., Cho, W., Choi, H., & Hur, J.-Y. (2020). Assessing the South Korean Model of emergency management during the COVID-19 pandemic. *Asian Studies Review*, *44*(4), 567–578. doi:10.1080/10357823.2020.1779658

Koo, J.-W., & Choi, J. (2019). Polarized embrace: South Korean Media Coverage of Human Rights, 1990–2016. *Journal of Human Rights*, *18*(4), 455–473. doi:10.1080/14754835.2019.1629888

Lee, H., Noh, E. B., Choi, S. H., Zhao, B., & Nam, E. W. (2020). Determining public opinion of the COVID-19 pandemic in South Korea and Japan: Social network mining on Twitter. *Healthcare Informatics Research*, *26*(4), 335–343.

Lee, S. M., & Lee, D. H. (2020). Lessons learned from battling COVID-19: The Korean experience. *International Journal of Environmental Research and Public Health*, *17*(20), 7548. doi:10.3390/ijerph17207548

Lynam, T. (2016). Exploring social representations of adapting to climate change using Topic modeling and Bayesian networks. *Ecology and Society*, *21*(4), 16. doi:10.5751/ES-08778-210416

Murdie, A. (2022). Hindsight is 2020: Lessons from the COVID-19 pandemic for future human rights research. *Journal of Human Rights*, *21*(3), 354–364.

Oh, B. -I., Chang, Y., & Jeong, S. (2020). *COVID-19 and the right to privacy: An analysis of South Korean Experiences* [White Paper]. Korean Progressive Network Jinbonet and Institute for Digital Rights.

Ordun, C., Purushotham, S., & Rraff, E. (2020). Exploratory analysis of COVID-19 tweets using topic modeling, umap, and digraphs. Cornell University. *arXiv preprint arXiv:2005.03082*: 1–19.

Park, B., Murdie, A., & Davis, D. R. (2019). The (co) evolution of human rights advocacy: Understanding human rights issue emergence over time. *Cooperation and Conflict, 54*(3), 313–334. doi:10.1177/0010836718808315

Park, S., Choi, G. J., & Ko, H. (2020). Information technology-based tracing strategy in response to COVID-19 in South Korea-privacy controversies. *JAMA, 323*(21), 2129–2130.

Roberto, K. J., Johnson, A. F., & Rauhaus, B. M. (2020). Stigmatization and prejudice during the COVID-19 pandemic. *Administrative Theory & Praxis, 42*(3), 364–378. doi:10.1080/10841806.2020.1782128

Ryan, M. (2020). In defense of digital contact-tracing: Human rights, South Korea and COVID-19. *International Journal of Pervasive Computing and Communications, 16*(4), 383–407. doi:10.1108/IJPCC-07-2020-0081

Spadaro, A. (2020). COVID-19: Testing the limits of human rights. *European Journal of Risk Regulation, 11*(2), 317–325. doi:10.1017/err.2020.27

Syed, S., & Spruit, M. (2017). Full-text or abstract? Examining topic coherence scores using latent dirichlet allocation. In *2017 IEEE International Conference on Data Science and Advanced Analytics (DSAA)* (pp. 165–174). doi:10.1109/DSAA.2017.61

Travaglino, G., & Moon, C. (2020, May 26). Explaining compliance with social distancing norms during the COVID-19 pandemic: The roles of cultural orientations, trust and self-conscious emotions in the US, Italy, and South Korea. *PsyArXiv*.

Wicke, P., & Bolognesi, M. F. (2020). Framing COVID-19: How we conceptualize and discuss the pandemic on Twitter. *PloS One, 15*(9), e0240010.

Yamin, A. E., & Habibi, R. (2020). Human rights and coronavirus: What's at stake for truth, trust, and democracy. *Health and Human Rights Journal*.

Yi, J., & Lee, W. (2020). Pandemic nationalism in South Korea. *Society, 57*(4), 446–451. doi:10.1007/s12115-020-00509-z

Yin, H., Yang, S., & Li, J. (2020). Detecting topic and sentiment dynamics due to COVID-19 pandemic using social media. In *International conference on advanced data mining and applications* (pp. 610–623). Springer.

You, J. (2020). Lessons from South Korea's COVID-19 policy response. *The American Review of Public Administration, 50*(6–7), 801–808. doi:10.1177/0275074020943708

Zuo, Y., Wu, J., Zhang, H., Lin, H., Wang, F., Xu, K., & Xiong, H. (2016). Topic modeling of short texts: A pseudo-document view. In *Proceedings of the 22nd ACM SIGKDD International Conference on Knowledge Discovery and Data Mining* (pp. 2105–2114). ACM.

Lessons learned for the future

Hindsight is 2020: Lessons from the COVID-19 pandemic for future human rights research

Amanda Murdie

ABSTRACT

The global COVID-19 pandemic affected much of the world's human rights for 2020 and 2021 and will continue to have human rights ramifications for years to come. While many things have fundamentally changed due to the pandemic, COVID-19 has also shined a spotlight on certain realities about the existing international human rights regime that may have been missed before. This concluding article to the special issue focuses on four realities that have become evident during the COVID-19 pandemic and discusses the implications of these realities on the next generation of human rights research. Understanding the future of global human rights, including the right to health, requires the holistic and long-term approach suggested by Chiozza and King, incorporating lessons learned from the current pandemic in ways that will help us predict and solve future human rights challenges.

Although the world today seems drastically different from the world in early 2019, many public health scientists predicted the 2020 global health emergency for years before it occurred. "Disease X" was often anticipated to be a Severe Acute Respiratory Syndrome coronavirus (SARS-CoV), very similar to what we now know as COVID-19. For example, in 2007, one prophetic article in the journal *Clinical Microbiology Reviews* reported that: "[th]e presence of a large reservoir of SARS-CoV-like viruses in horseshoe bats, together with the culture of eating exotic animals in southern China, is a *time bomb*" that "should not be ignored" (Cheng et al., 2007, p. 683, emphasis added). Other scholars noted that a similar disease could have begun almost anywhere in the world (Cizmar, 2020). The COVID-19 virus that started a global health emergency in 2020 was not unforeseen; its existence was not a question of "if" but "when" (Pascoe, 2006).

As I write this in 2021, I have the luxury of hindsight and the ability to say "*see, we should have known.*" The public health warning signs, global indifference, partisan fervor, and lack of capacity were all evident in the months and years leading up to our current crisis. And yet, as is so often the case, the global disaster occurred anyway, with repercussions affecting much of the world's human rights for 2020, 2021, and many years to come. Health is a human right, but, as the articles in this special issue show (Chiozza & King, 2022a), COVID-19 has altered the nature and intensity of many of the rights listed in the United Nations' Universal Declaration of Human Rights (UDHR) and related legal instruments. With the benefit of hindsight, the current pandemic allows me to focus on many realities about the existing international human rights regime that I did not fully appreciate before the crisis. Understanding the future of global human rights, including the right to health, requires the holistic and long-term approach suggested by Chiozza and King (2022b), incorporating lessons learned from the current pandemic in ways that will help us predict and solve future human rights challenges.

COVID-19 evident human rights reality #1: For improved human rights performance, countries need both the "will" and the "way"

COVID-19 has highlighted how the enjoyment of the right to health may be lacking in even the most highly capable states when a country's population or leaders lack the willingness to act. As Kavanagh and Singh (2020) point out, "some of the countries considered to be the most prepared… have failed to respond effectively to the pandemic" (p. 997). Many high-income countries have had problems providing the "testing, tracing, and treatment" needed to control the pandemic (Forman & Kohler, 2020, p. 547). Although many countries have the bureaucratic capacity to handle the pandemic, political will and "failures of communication" have exacerbated the pandemic's toll on human life (Hatcher, 2020, p. 614). Focusing on bureaucratic or state capacity alone may cause us to miss the political factors which lead a capable country to fail to combat an outbreak and protect public health (Kavanagh & Singh, 2020, pp. 997–998).

At the same time, we have seen some low-income countries willing to take action to protect against the virus still have widespread outbreaks because of a lack of state and bureaucratic capacity.[1] Global differences in state capacity, inequality, and a lack of international cooperation have also complicated vaccine roll-out, ultimately leading to an increase in deaths in countries without the state capacity necessary to individually produce and provide a COVID-19 vaccine (Hafner et al., 2020; Nhamo et al., 2021). Increased suffering in countries without the capacity to produce their own vaccine often coincided with growing vaccine hesitancy in individuals in high-capacity countries with widespread vaccine access (Abbas, 2020; Santoro & Shanklin, 2020; Rutschman, 2021). While these countries had the capacity for vaccine-induced herd immunity, their political leaders often lacked the political will to encourage vaccination and speak out again vaccine misinformation (Hornsey et al., 2021; Muric et al., 2021; Rutschman, 2021). Like in other areas of human rights, it appears that both the "will" and the "way" are jointly necessary for improved human rights performance. Neither state capacity nor state willingness is sufficient on its own to control the spread of the pandemic and protect the right to health.

We have known for many years that state capacity is often associated with improved human rights performance (Cingranelli et al., 2014; Englehart, 2009; Mitchell, 2009). At the same time, signals of a country's willingness to abide by human rights norms, like their ratification of human rights treaties, are often associated with improved human rights outcomes (Hill, 2010; Fariss, 2014). Rarely, however, have the levers of government capacity and willingness been studied in tandem.[2]

The pandemic has also raised an issue sometimes forgotten in the push for improved human rights: the will of the people to take action to improve human rights cannot be taken for granted. If human rights scholarship looked at popular will, it often assumed that the average person was supportive of human rights ideals, especially ideals related to basic human rights like bodily integrity (Keck & Sikkink, 1998, p. 195). The focus was often not on convincing individuals that human rights are important but convincing powerful elites to share power or allocate resources to improve human rights (Gerber & Mendelson, 2002, p. 272; Roth, 2015, np). Unfortunately, in this era of populism and nationalistic backlash, the fallacy of this assumption has become clear. Solidarity around human rights ideals can vary, and a lack of solidarity may undermine advocacy attempts before they even start (Libal & Kashwan, 2020). We can no longer assume that the average person supports improved human rights, especially the right to health. When the costs of human rights improvement are presented as coming at the expense of economic rights or mobility, citizens in many countries around the world have shown little willingness to support even minor human rights-consistent policies designed to protect health.

Implication of this reality for future research: We need future scholarship to focus more on (a) public opinion related to human rights and (b) principal-agent dynamics with respect to potential abusers

The importance of both the "will" and the "way" in jointly influencing human rights performance suggests many avenues for future research. First, we need to problematize support for human rights ideals and examine what characteristics influence individual-level support for various human rights. Are there certain rights that we can still assume the public generally supports? Are there specific personal or societal characteristics that make it more likely to defend the human rights of others? Many innovative scholars are already using surveys and survey experiments to examine how specific characteristics affect individual-level support for torture and other physical integrity rights abuses (Allendoerfer, 2017; Conrad et al., 2018; Edwards & Arnon, 2021; Koo, 2017; Lupu & Wallace, 2019; McEntire et al., 2015; Wallace, 2013, 2014; Zvobgo, 2019). Future work in this vein needs to extend to other human rights and examine the ways in which the potential costs for the full enjoyment of human rights could influence public willingness to act in support of certain human rights policies.

Further, Chiozza and King (2022b) point out how frequently the right to health has been portrayed as inconsistent with physical integrity rights. The current pandemic shows a critical need for more public opinion research concerning when and under what conditions individuals see a tradeoff between various rights. When rights are in conflict, what rights are seen as paramount? Can certain government policies counter this tradeoff? For example, if a country is taking rights-consistent public health measures, are individuals less likely to see the right to health as a counter to physical integrity rights? While there has been a growth in public opinion studies regarding COVID-19 and public health, there is a need for more human rights-specific research in this area.[3] As Koo (2022) shows in this volume, there is much variation in individual opinions and social media posts about rights-consistent public health actions concerning COVID-19. More research that specifically examines public opinion about public health and human rights in tandem is necessary.

Second, the current reality also reminds us that human rights performance depends on the actions and duties of bureaucrats, state delegates, non-state actors, and individuals. We need more focus on the process by which human rights-related policies are delegated and enforced, paying particular attention to how individual actors are motivated to either follow orders to abuse others or push back against state directives (DeMeritt, 2015). When do regional and local leaders, for example, push back against misinformation campaigns or limited public health responses? In the United States, for example, partisanship was the "most important predictor" for when state governors instituted their own social distancing policies (Adolph et al., 2021, p. 215). In a similar vein, we need to understand how individual actors are motivated to either support the human rights of others or to take actions, like that of not wearing a mask during a pandemic, which could endanger their neighbor's full enjoyment of their human rights. The political processes underlying the underinvestment in both national and international public health measures deserve future attention (Stasavage, 2020).

COVID-19 evident human rights reality #2: Human rights are interconnected across rights and across borders

The United Nations (UN) General Assembly resolution that created the UN Human Rights Council stated that "all human rights are universal, indivisible, interrelated, interdependent and mutually reinforcing, and that all human rights must be treated in a fair and equal manner, on the same footing and with the same emphasis" (UN General Assembly, 2006). The current pandemic has made the interconnected nature of human rights painfully clear. For example, in the

United States, racial and ethnic minority populations, those who have been historically denied their full enjoyment of many human rights, have been contracting and dying of COVID-19 at a much higher rate than the white population (Keating et al., 2020). Even in a rich, democratic country like the United States, poor individuals have limited access to health care, but often work in industries where there were limited work-from-home options (Patel et al., 2020). COVID-19 has exacerbated the "justice gap" (Dhital & Walton, 2020, p. 582).

Goodhart (2020) talks about this phenomenon as "negative interdependence," where "crises can trigger chain reactions of right violations and deprivations that disproportionately affect oppressed and vulnerable people" more (p. 320). For example, in mid-2020, the organization Refugees International reported that COVID-19 is more than just a health crisis for refugees; it is also a "socio-economic crisis" and a "protection crisis," which further limited the inclusion of refugees into the economic system and increased discrimination and xenophobia (Dempster et al., 2020, np, see also Cheri, 2021; Ramji-Nogales & Goldner Lang, 2020). Likewise, prisoners have disproportionately experienced the negative interdependence of human rights abuses because of the pandemic, in addition to many abuses already felt by those in the criminal justice system (Fassin, 2020; Muntingh, 2020). Women are also experiencing more abuses as a result of the pandemic, a phenomenon that Brysk (2022) referred to as the "pandemic patriarchy" in this volume; these abuses are heightened as gender intersects with race and ethnicity, class, and citizenship status. Toxic masculinity heightens abuses and could influence poor public health decision-making, although the connection requires further research (Theidon, 2020; Windsor et al., 2020). Negative interdependence of human rights is also visible as we examine how the virus has diffused across borders; a lack of rights-based public health measures in Country X may limit the realization of human rights in Country Y.

A related reality visible during COVID-19 is how various human rights can appear at odds or may even be fully in conflict. For example, freedom from gender-based violence is a human right that has been more at risk due to the public health measures taken to protect our health (UN Women, 2020). Similarly, school closures to combat the spread of COVID-19 have significantly reduced the enjoyment of the rights to education for over one billion students around the globe (UNESCO, 2021). The ability to travel freely, including even travel to meet up with children or family members, has been severely restricted in some countries during the pandemic (Bachelor, 2021; Ramji-Nogales & Goldner Lang, 2020). In addition, COVID-19 related health measures are estimated to increase child, early, and forced marriage by over 13 million girls in this decade, ultimately influencing the full enjoyment of many additional human rights for years to come (Affoum & Recavarren, 2020, np). As Chiozza and King (2022b) outline in the introductory article of this volume, there are "practical realities" that have in many countries created a tradeoff of "certain rights in favor of the right to health" (p. 14).

Further, as the UN Special Rapporteur on Opinion and Expression said, COVID-19 is a "pathogen of repression" (UN Human Rights Council, 2020). Opportunistic governments have used the pandemic as an excuse to restrict wide swaths of rights concerning the freedom of opinion and expression (Clay, 2022; Eck & Hatz, 2020). Assembly rights have been harmed (Chenoweth, 2022). Wong and Wong (2020) go as far as to argue that population-level public health measures are fundamentally at odds with individual human rights, although others, like Spadaro (2020) disagree, and see rights-based public health measures as an "obligation" under human rights law (p. 324). Any restrictions to derogable civil and political rights for public health emergencies can and must be legal and legitimate, justified by necessity and proportionality, and closely monitored for potential overreach (Bennoune, 2020; Lebret, 2020; Mykhalovskiy et al., 2020; Ponta, 2020). Unfortunately, as Badran and Turnbull (2022) show in this volume, for many individuals in 2020 and 2021, governments relied on rhetoric concerning public health to rationalize abusive policies inconsistent with international human rights law.

Implication of this reality for future research: We need future scholarship to focus on how rights abuses diffuse across rights and across countries. We also need to stop our overwhelming focus on physical integrity rights in IR (mainly quantitative) human rights scholarship

My undergraduate human rights course starts with the idea that human rights are interdependent and interconnected. However, in my own research, I often ignore that fact and focus only on a specific set of rights, overlooking how the enjoyment of these rights may be dependent on the enjoyment of other rights across space and across time. The negative interdependence observed between rights during the pandemic reminds me that I must extend my own focus beyond a narrow subset of rights. I need to stop automatically setting my dependent variable to physical integrity rights indicators like CIRI's Physical Integrity Rights Index (Cingranelli et al., 2014), the Political Terror Scale (Gibney et al., 2020), or Fariss (2014)'s latent human rights score. For quantitative human rights scholars, our focus on physical integrity rights may be driven by a desire to connect to the repression and conflict literatures more broadly; it may simply be path dependence. However, like Cope et al. (2018) and others point out, restricting our focus to physical integrity rights has significantly limited our ability to understand the myriad of ways that governments often try to control their population.[4] Further investigations into violations of empowerment rights, also called "oppression," and the fulfillment of social rights are "ripe for academic inquiry" and better reflect the reality for the billions living without the full enjoyment of their human rights (Cope et al., 2018, p. 196). In particular, abuses that could be labeled oppression or violations of empowerment rights have been particularly affected by the pandemic, as many governments have used contact tracing and public health concerns as an excuse to increase surveillance and restrict freedom of movement (Duić & Sudar, 2021; Eck & Hatz, 2020). We must work to understand the ways in which these abuses are applied and the effects these COVID-justified abuses have on the future human rights trajectory of affected countries.

We need future human rights scholarship to take the investigation of all human rights seriously and seek to understand why certain rights have been largely ignored by the scholarly and advocacy communities.[5] Michelle Jurkovich's work on the right to food is an excellent example of the knowledge that can be gained by looking outside of a limited set of often-studied rights (2019). Moreover, future human rights research must engage more with authors and scholarship from the Global South, realizing that these perspectives and insights will significantly help our collective understanding of lived experiences and the post-pandemic state of the human rights regime (Hertel et al., 2020).

Further, the current reality of the pandemic implies that we need to understand how a country's performance on one subset of rights diffuses to other rights and other countries. There is existing work that examines the spatial diffusion of abuse and human rights mobilization (Bell et al., 2012; Bracic, 2016; Danneman & Ritter, 2014; Greenhill, 2010), as well as some work that examines the interconnected nature of human rights (Fariss & Schnakenberg, 2014). However, more work is necessary, especially concerning whether and when the protection of some human rights really comes at the expense of other rights.

COVID-19 evident human rights reality #3: We never observe the full nature of human rights abuses within a country

A lack of transparency, misinformation, and disinformation has been rampant in many countries during the current pandemic (Cuillier, 2020; Eck & Hatz, 2020). Some countries have criticized the Chinese government for their lack of transparency during the early days of the pandemic, even going as far as to argue that the pandemic could have been limited if China had shared information sooner (Gan 2021; Wong et al., 2020). Individuals have been imprisoned not to prevent the spread of the disease but to prevent the spread of information about the danger of the disease; censorship is widespread (Kuo, 2020). Government actors have denied the true extent of the pandemic within their borders, even hiding information from other government actors within their same country (Wong et al., 2020).

Further, due to capacity issues and variation in information flows, we know more about the virus's spread in certain countries than others, leading some leaders to claim that high infection rates are due to better testing as opposed to the actual spread of the virus (Dale, 2020). Leaders have peddled inaccurate scientific information about the virus and possible remedies (*BBC*, 2020). Governments have been accused of hiding the true extent of COVID monitoring software and technology and falsely imprisoning dissidents under the guise of public health concerns (Roth, 2020; Singer, 2020; Stojanovic, 2020).

These tragic examples show how information manipulation and bias can influence our observations of a variety of different human rights abuses, including abuses related to the right to health. Our current data on human rights abuses may be colored by what Clark and Sikkink (2013) call "information effects," where the "process of information collection and interpretation" influences the levels of abuses observed rather than the "process that actually gives rise to human rights violations or their mitigation" (p. 540). The information environment is not static over time and space (Fariss, 2014). We are always operating in a situation where governments may want to hide the spotlight and manipulate information in ways that confound our abilities to observe abuses and take action to improve human rights.

Implication of this reality for future research: Transparency and information effects are key considerations in the study of human rights abuses

The reality of the information environment around human rights has recently been a subject of much debate and innovation in the scholarly literature (Cingranelli & Filippov, 2018; Eck & Fariss, 2018; Fariss, 2019; Park et al., 2020; Richards, 2016). Understanding the factors that could distort the information we see is just as important as understanding the factors that lead to human rights abuse. One lesson from the current pandemic is that we need better theoretical insights into when governments have increased interest and capacity to hide or distort reality from the public. Similarly, we need to continue to research the role of journalists and press freedom in thwarting government attempts to manipulate information. As Gohdes and Carey (2017) found, journalist killings are "canaries in a coal-mine," signaling future increases in government human rights abuses (p. 157). Censorship and government manipulation of the internet is another potentially important line of inquiry for human rights scholars (Han, 2018). Finally, we need to increase our focus on information distortion as human rights abuse itself and as a way to hide information about other abuses, including abuses related to the right to health (Wingfield, 2019).

COVID-19 evident human rights reality #4: Human rights rhetoric can be a powerful strategic tool for political and personal gain

Finally, one of the most interesting and yet disheartening phenomena this year has been the use of rights-based language to push back against masks and other public health measures taken to stop the pandemic. As mentioned, some of this language is wholly justified; we know authoritarian leaders have used the pandemic as an opportunity to restrict human rights and consolidate power (Badran & Turnbull, 2022; Chenoweth, 2022; Clay, 2022). However, masks and other public health measures can go "hand-in-glove" with the international human rights regime (UN Human Rights Council, 2020, p. 4). Some of the rhetoric that pushes back against masks and other public health measures uses rights-based language in ways inconsistent with human rights norms and law. There are multiple viral videos of anti-maskers claiming that masks violate international and domestic human rights law (Morandin, 2020; Rivas & Bernabe, 2020). Rights-based claims may have helped make basic public health measures politically charged. Several US political candidates made use of this rhetoric and pandemic misinformation as a way to garner political support (Hatcher, 2020). The strategic misuse of human rights rhetoric is not new, but the scope of the issue is large, including both citizens and leaders from a host of different countries.

Implication of this reality for future research: we need more systematic examinations of when rights-based language is used and its effects across individuals, countries, and time

Scholars are currently studying how the lexicon of human rights has changed among advocates over time (Park et al., 2019, 2020). The current reality suggests that we must extend our examination to the use of rights-based language in political rhetoric and everyday speech. When is rights-based language invoked consistently and inconsistently with international law? How does the use of rights-based language affect public opinion? Studies on whether the general public largely follows the use of such language by leaders would also be necessary, perhaps focusing on changes in terminology over Twitter. Does a focus on human rights education help diminish the misuse of rights-based rhetoric? For example, could informing individuals of Article 29 of the UDHR (concerning the duty to community) change individual opinion about rights-based language and political rhetoric? New research could help inform future human rights education efforts and provide new tools for how to best respond when rights-based language is invoked.

Conclusion

In my own life, hindsight is a funny thing. The most powerful lessons have often come from reminders of painfully obvious realities that I somehow missed the first time. COVID-19 has harmed a tremendous number of individuals, eliminating the human rights of millions. COVID-19 will continue to have both short-term and long-term effects on the human rights reality for many across the world (Chiozza & King, 2022a, 2022b). The current pandemic is occurring in a world that is vastly different from the reality of previous pandemics. We cannot go back to the world as it was before (Goodhart, 2020). However, as I look at the situation today, I am struck by how many lessons are now visible as a result of the pandemic that I should have seen before. Focusing on these lessons in our future research may help us collectively gain insights to improve human rights in years to come.

Notes

1. See Arbogast et al. (2020) for an investigation into the low correlation of state capacity and COVID-19 deaths.
2. For notable exceptions, see Cole (2015) and Anaya-Muñoz (2019).
3. For a notable exception that examines public opinion and COVID-19 with a focus on human rights, see Bohler-Muller et al. (2021).
4. See also Haschke (2017), Beger and Hill (2019), Franklin (2020) for further discussions of the growing study of oppression and preventive repression as somewhat distinct from physical integrity rights abuses.
5. See Roth (2004) for some additional discussion on why the advocacy community has focused primarily on a narrow subset of human rights.

ORCID

Amanda Murdie http://orcid.org/0000-0002-6459-0594

References

Abbas, M. Z. (2020). *Practical implications of "vaccine nationalism": A short-sighted and risky approach in response to COVID-19*. https://www.econstor.eu/bitstream/10419/232250/1/south-centre-rp-124.pdf

Adolph, C., Amano, K., Bang-Jensen, B., Fullman, N., & Wilkerson, J. (2021). Pandemic politics: Timing state-level social distancing responses to COVID-19. *Journal of Health Politics, Policy and Law*, *46*(2), 211–233.

Affoum, N., Recavarren, I. S. (2020). *Child marriage: The unspoken consequence of COVID-19*. World Bank Blogs: Let's Talk Development. https://blogs.worldbank.org/developmenttalk/child-marriage-unspoken-consequence-covid-19

Allendoerfer, M. G. (2017). Who cares about human rights? Public opinion about human rights foreign policy. *Journal of Human Rights*, *16*(4), 428–451. doi:10.1080/14754835.2015.1129603

Anaya-Muñoz, A. (2019). Bringing willingness back in: State capacities and the human rights compliance deficit in Mexico. *Human Rights Quarterly*, *41*(2), 441–464. doi:10.1353/hrq.2019.0033

Arbogast, I., Reinbold, B., & Wen, Y. (2020). Anecdotal evidence suggests state capacity unrelated to COVID-19 spread. *The Regional Economist*, *28*(4). https://www.stlouisfed.org/publications/regional-economist/fourth-quarter-2020/anecdotal-evidence-suggests-state-capacity-unrelated-covid-spread.

Bachelor, B. (2021). *The desperate families still torn apart by COVID rules*. Retrieved May 4, 2021, from https://www.cnn.com/travel/article/families-torn-apart-covid-rules/index.html

Badran, S. Z., & Turnbull, B. (2022). The COVID-19 pandemic and authoritarian consolidation in North Africa. *Journal of Human Rights*, *21*(3), 263–282.

BBC (2020, March 31). Coronavirus: World leaders' posts deleted over fake news. *BBC*. https://www.bbc.com/news/technology-52106321

Beger, A., & Hill Jr, D. (2019). Examining repressive and oppressive state violence using the Ill-Treatment and Torture data. *Conflict Management and Peace Science*, *36*(6), 626–644.

Bell, S. R., Clay, K. C., & Murdie, A. (2012). Neighborhood watch: Spatial effects of human rights INGOs. *The Journal of Politics*, *74*(2), 354–368. doi:10.1017/S0022381611001642

Bennoune, K. (2020). "Lest we should sleep": COVID-19 and human rights. *American Journal of International Law*, *114*(4), 666–676. doi:10.1017/ajil.2020.68

Bohler-Muller, N., Roberts, B., Davids, Y.D., Gordon, S., & Majikijela, Y. (2021). COVID-19 and human rights limitations: Taking public opinion into account. http://www.hsrc.ac.za/uploads/pageContent/1045407/COVID-19%20and%20human%20rights%20limitations%20-%20Taking%20public%20opinion%20into%20account%20(1).pdf

Bracic, A. (2016). Keeping up with the Joneses: Spatial diffusion of physical integrity rights practices.

Brysk, A. (2022). Pandemic patriarchy: The impact of a global health crisis on women's rights. *Journal of Human Rights*, *21*(3), 283–303.

Cheng, V. C., Lau, S. K., Woo, P. C., & Yuen, K. Y. (2007). Severe acute respiratory syndrome coronavirus as an agent of emerging and reemerging infection. *Clinical Microbiology Reviews*, *20*(4), 660–694.

Chenoweth, E. (2022). Can nonviolent resistance survive COVID-19? *Journal of Human Rights*, *21*(3), 304–316.

Cheri, L. (2021). Perceived impact of border closure due to Covid-19 of intending Nigerian migrants. *Social Inclusion*, *9*(1), 207–215. doi:10.17645/si.v9i1.3671

Chiozza, G., & King, J. (2022a). Introduction to a special issue on beyond complacency and acrimony: Studying human rights in a post-COVID-19 world. *Journal of Human Rights*, *21*(3), 245.

Chiozza, G., & King, J. (2022b). The state of human rights in a (post) COVID-19 world. *Journal of Human Rights*, *21*(3), 246–262.

Cingranelli, D. L., Richards, D. L., & Clay, K. C. (2014). *The CIRI human rights dataset*. CIRI human rights data project. http://www.humanrightsdata.com

Cingranelli, D., & Filippov, M. (2018). Are human rights practices improving? *American Political Science Review*, *112*(4), 1083–1089. doi:10.1017/S0003055418000254

Cingranelli, D., Fajardo-Heyward, P., & Filippov, M. (2014). Principals, agents and human rights. *British Journal of Political Science*, *44*(3), 605–630. doi:10.1017/S0007123413000070

Cizmar, M. (2020). *A coronavirus expert from KU predicted this pandemic—here's what he says will happen next*. Retrieved March 20, 2020, from https://www.kansascitymag.com/heres-what-could-have-stopped-the-covid-19-epidemic-according-to-a-kansas-coronavirus-expert/

Clark, A. M., & Sikkink, K. (2013). Information effects and human rights data: Is the good news about increased human rights information bad news for human rights measures? *Human Rights Quarterly, 35*(3), 539–568. doi: 10.1353/hrq.2013.0046

Clay, K. C. (2022). The effect of the COVID-19 pandemic on human rights practices: Findings from the Human Rights Measurement Initiative's 2021 Practitioner Survey. *Journal of Human Rights, 21*(3), 317–333.

Cole, W. M. (2015). Mind the gap: State capacity and the implementation of human rights treaties. *International Organization, 69*(2), 405–441. doi:10.1017/S002081831400040X

Conrad, C. R., Croco, S. E., Gomez, B. T., & Moore, W. H. (2018). Threat perception and American support for torture. *Political Behavior, 40*(4), 989–1009. doi:10.1007/s11109-017-9433-5

Cope, K. L., Crabtree, C., & Lupu, Y. (2018). Beyond physical integrity. *Law & Contemporary Problems, 81*, 185.

Cuillier, D. (2020). Governments are using the coronavirus to hide information from reporters and citizens. *Nieman Lab.*

Dale, D. (2020, October 26). Fact check: Trump continues to falsely claim that spike in coronavirus cases is due to heightened testing. *CNN.* https://www.cnn.com/2020/10/26/politics/fact-check-testing-cases-october/index.html

Danneman, N., & Ritter, E. H. (2014). Contagious rebellion and preemptive repression. *Journal of Conflict Resolution, 58*(2), 254–279. doi:10.1177/0022002712468720

DeMeritt, J. H. (2015). Delegating death: Military intervention and government killing. *Journal of Conflict Resolution, 59*(3), 428–454. doi:10.1177/0022002713515406

Dempster, H., Ginn, T., Graham, J., Ble, M. G., Jayasinghe, D., & Shorey, B. (2020). *Locked down and left behind: The impact of COVID-19 on refugees' economic inclusion.* Center for Global Development, Refugees International, and International Rescue Committee. https://www.refugeesinternational.org/reports/2020/7/6/locked-down-and-left-behind-the-impact-of-covid-19-on-refugees-economic-inclusion

Dhital, S., & Walton, T. (2020). Legal empowerment approaches in the context of COVID-19. *Journal of Human Rights, 19*(5), 582–592. doi:10.1080/14754835.2020.1816164

Duić, D., & Sudar, V. (2021). The impact of COVID-19 on the free movement of persons in the EU. *EU and Comparative Law Issues and Challenges Series (ECLIC), 5*, 30–56.

Eck, K., & Fariss, C. J. (2018). Ill treatment and torture in Sweden: A critique of cross-case comparisons. *Human Rights Quarterly, 40*(3), 591–604. doi:10.1353/hrq.2018.0033

Eck, K., & Hatz, S. (2020). State surveillance and the COVID-19 crisis. *Journal of Human Rights, 19*(5), 603–612. doi:10.1080/14754835.2020.1816163

Edwards, P., & Arnon, D. (2021). Violence on many sides: Framing effects on protest and support for repression. *British Journal of Political Science, 51*(2), 488–506. doi:10.1017/S0007123419000413

Englehart, N. A. (2009). State capacity, state failure, and human rights. *Journal of Peace Research, 46*(2), 163–180. doi:10.1177/0022343308100713

Fariss, C. J. (2014). Respect for human rights has improved over time: Modeling the changing standard of accountability. *American Political Science Review, 108*(2), 297–318. doi:10.1017/S0003055414000070

Fariss, C. J. (2019). Yes, human rights practices are improving over time. *American Political Science Review, 113*(3), 868–881. doi:10.1017/S000305541900025X

Fariss, C. J., & Schnakenberg, K. E. (2014). Measuring mutual dependence between state repressive actions. *Journal of Conflict Resolution, 58*(6), 1003–1032. doi:10.1177/0022002713487314

Fassin, D. (2020). Hazardous confinement during the COVID-19 pandemic: The fate of migrants detained yet non-deportable. *Journal of Human Rights, 19*(5), 613–623. doi:10.1080/14754835.2020.1822155

Forman, L., & Kohler, J. C. (2020). Global health and human rights in the time of COVID-19: Response, restrictions, and legitimacy. *Journal of Human Rights, 19*(5), 547–556. doi:10.1080/14754835.2020.1818556

Franklin, J. C. (2020). Human rights on the march: Repression, oppression, and protest in Latin America. *International Studies Quarterly, 64*(1), 97–110.

Gan, N. (2021, March 3). 14 countries and WHO chief accuse China of withholding data from pandemic origins investigation. *CNN News.* https://www.cnn.com/2021/03/31/asia/who-report-criticism-intl-hnk/index.html

Gerber, T. P., & Mendelson, S. E. (2002). Russian public opinion on human rights and the war in Chechnya. *Post-Soviet Affairs, 18*(4), 271–305. doi:10.2747/1060-586X.18.4.271

Gibney, M., Cornett, L., Wood, R., Haschke, P., Arnon, D., Pisano, A., Barrett, G., & Park, B. (2020). *The political terror scale 1976–2019.* Date Retrieved, from the Political Terror Scale Website, http://www.politicalterrorscale.org.

Gohdes, A. R., & Carey, S. C. (2017). Canaries in a coal-mine? What the killings of journalists tell us about future repression. *Journal of Peace Research, 54*(2), 157–174. doi:10.1177/0022343316680859

Goodhart, M. (2020). Revisiting interdependence in times and terms of crisis. *Journal of Human Rights, 19*(5), 520–527. doi:10.1080/14754835.2020.1814709

Greenhill, B. (2010). The company you keep: International socialization and the diffusion of human rights norms. *International Studies Quarterly, 54*(1), 127–145. doi:10.1111/j.1468-2478.2009.00580.x

Hafner, M., Yerushalmi, E., Fays, C., Dufresne, E., & Van Stolk, C. (2020). *COVID-19 and the cost of vaccine nationalism*. RAND.

Han, R. (2018). *Contesting cyberspace in China*. Columbia University Press.

Haschke, P. (2017). *Human rights in democracies*. Routledge.

Hatcher, W. (2020). A failure of political communication not a failure of bureaucracy: The danger of presidential misinformation during the COVID-19 pandemic. *The American Review of Public Administration, 50*(6–7), 614–620. doi:10.1177/0275074020941734

Hertel, S., Buerger, C., & Carbonetti, B. (2020). Introduction to a special issue on human rights in the time of COVID-19. *Journal of Human Rights, 19*(5), 519–519. doi:10.1080/14754835.2020.1830615

Hill, D. W. Jr. (2010). Estimating the effects of human rights treaties on state behavior. *The Journal of Politics, 72*(4), 1161–1174. doi:10.1017/S0022381610000599

Hornsey, M. J., Chapman, C. M., Alvarez, B., Bentley, S., Salvador Casara, B. G., Crimston, C. R., Ionescu, O., Krug, H., Preya Selvanathan, H., Steffens, N. K., & Jetten, J. (2021). To what extent are conspiracy theorists concerned for self versus others? A COVID-19 test case. *European Journal of Social Psychology, 51*(2), 285–293. doi: 10.1002/ejsp.2737

Kavanagh, M. M., & Singh, R. (2020). Democracy, capacity, and coercion in pandemic response: COVID-19 in comparative political perspective. *Journal of Health Politics, Policy and Law, 45*(6), 997–1012.

Keating, D., Cha, A. E., Florit, G. (2020, November 20). "I just pray God will help me": Racial, ethnic minorities reel from higher covid-19 death rates. *The Washington Post*. https://www.washingtonpost.com/graphics/2020/health/covid-race-mortality-rate/

Keck, M. E., & Sikkink, K. (1998). *Activists beyond borders*. Cornell University Press.

Koo, J. W. (2017). The construction of human rights actorhood: Findings from the Korean General Social Survey. *Journal of Human Rights, 16*(3), 261–275. doi:10.1080/14754835.2016.1236330

Koo, J. -W. (2022). Global perceptions of South Korea's COVID-19 policy responses: Topic modeling with tweets. *Journal of Human Rights, 21*(3), 334–353.

Kuo, L. (2020). *China sentences citizen journalist to four years in prison for Wuhan lockdown reports. The Washington Post*. Retrieved December 28, 2020, from https://www.washingtonpost.com/world/asia_pacific/china-wuhan-journalist-trial-coronavirus/2020/12/28/01fac40c-48b7-11eb-97b6-4eb9f72ff46b_story.html

Lebret, A. (2020). COVID-19 pandemic and derogation to human rights. *Journal of Law and the Biosciences, 7*(1). doi:10.1093/jlb/lsaa015

Libal, K., & Kashwan, P. (2020). Solidarity in times of crisis. *Journal of Human Rights, 19*(5), 537–546. doi:10.1080/14754835.2020.1830046

Lupu, Y., & Wallace, G. P. (2019). Violence, nonviolence, and the effects of international human rights law. *American Journal of Political Science, 63*(2), 411–426. doi:10.1111/ajps.12416

McEntire, K. J., Leiby, M., & Krain, M. (2015). Human rights organizations as agents of change: An experimental examination of framing and micromobilization. *American Political Science Review, 109*(3), 407–426. doi:10.1017/S0003055415000295

Mitchell, N. J. (2009). *Agents of atrocity: Leaders, followers, and the violation of human rights in civil war*. Macmillan.

Morandin, P. (2020). Does a face mask requirement infringe on human rights? *Lexology*. https://www.lexology.com/library/detail.aspx?g=08c971b3-faa4-4bf7-a993-121775c77fe3.

Muntingh, L. M. (2020). Africa, prisons and COVID-19. *Journal of Human Rights Practice, 12*(2), 284–292. doi:10.1093/jhuman/huaa031

Muric, G., Wu, Y., & Ferrara, E. (2021). COVID-19 vaccine hesitancy on social media: Building a public Twitter dataset of anti-vaccine content, vaccine misinformation and conspiracies. *JMIR Public Health and Surveillance, 7*(11). doi:10.2196/30642.

Mykhalovskiy, E., Kazatchkine, C., Foreman-Mackey, A., McClelland, A., Peck, R., Hastings, C., & Elliott, R. (2020). Human rights, public health and COVID-19 in Canada. *Canadian Journal of Public Health/Revue Canadienne de sante publique, 111*(6), 975–979. doi:10.17269/s41997-020-00408-0

Nhamo, G., Chikodzi, D., Kunene, H. P., & Mashula, N. (2021). COVID-19 vaccines and treatments nationalism: Challenges for low-income countries and the attainment of the SDGs. *Global Public Health, 16*(3), 319–339.

Park, B., Greene, K., & Colaresi, M. (2020). Human rights are (increasingly) plural: Learning the changing taxonomy of human rights from large-scale text reveals information effects. *American Political Science Review, 114*(3), 888–910. doi:10.1017/S0003055420000258

Park, B., Murdie, A., & Davis, D. R. (2019). The (co) evolution of human rights advocacy: Understanding human rights issue emergence over time. *Cooperation and Conflict, 54*(3), 313–334. doi:10.1177/0010836718808315

Pascoe, N. (2006). A pandemic flu: Not if, but when. SARS was the wake-up call we slept through. *Texas Nursing, 80*(1), 6–10.

Patel, J. A., Nielsen, F. B. H., Badiani, A. A., Assi, S., Unadkat, V. A., Patel, B., Ravindrane, R., & Wardle, H. (2020). Poverty, inequality and COVID-19: The forgotten vulnerable. *Public Health, 183*(June), 110–111. doi:10.1016/j.puhe.2020.05.006

Ponta, A. (2020). Human rights law in the time of the coronavirus. *American Society of International Law Insights, 24*(5). https://www.asil.org/insights/volume/24/issue/5/human-rights-law-time-coronavirus

Ramji-Nogales, J., & Goldner Lang, I. (2020). Freedom of movement, migration, and borders. *Journal of Human Rights, 19*(5), 593–602. doi:10.1080/14754835.2020.1830045

Richards, D. L. (2016). The myth of information effects in human rights data: Response to Ann Marie Clark and Kathryn Sikkink. *Human Rights Quarterly, 38*(2), 477–492. doi:10.1353/hrq.2016.0033

Rivas, K., & Bernabe, A. J. (2020, June 29). Video of woman's tirade after refusing to wear a mask in Trader Joe's goes viral. *ABC News*. https://abcnews.go.com/GMA/News/video-womans-tirade-refusing-wear-mask-trader-joes/story?id=71505060

Roth, K. (2004). Defending economic social and cultural rights: Practical issues faced by an international human rights organization. *Human Rights Quarterly, 26*(1), 63–73. doi:10.1353/hrq.2004.0010

Roth, K. (2015, September 15). For human rights, majority opinion isn't always important. *Open Democracy*. https://www.opendemocracy.net/en/openglobalrights-openpage/for-human-rights-majority-opinion-isnt-always-important/

Roth, K. (2020). How authoritarians are exploiting the Covid-19 crisis to grab power. *Human Rights Watch*. https://www.hrw.org/news/2020/04/03/how-authoritarians-are-exploiting-covid-19-crisis-grab-power

Rutschman, A. S. (2021). The COVID-19 vaccine race: Intellectual property, collaboration (s), nationalism and misinformation. *Washington University Journal of Law & Policy, 64*, 167.

Santoro, M., & Shanklin, R. (2020). Human rights obligations of drug companies. *Journal of Human Rights, 19*(5), 557–567. doi:10.1080/14754835.2020.1820315

Singer, N. (2020, July 20). Virus-tracing apps are rife with problems. Governments are rushing to fix them. *The New York Times*. https://nyti.ms/2VZ8vzb

Spadaro, A. (2020). COVID-19: Testing the limits of human rights. *European Journal of Risk Regulation, 11*(2), 317–325. doi:10.1017/err.2020.27

Stasavage, D. (2020). Democracy, autocracy, and emergency threats: Lessons for COVID-19 from the last thousand years. *International Organization, 74*(S1), E1–E17.

Stojanovic, D. (2020). *Dismantling democracy? Virus used as excuse to quell dissent*. Associated Press. https://abcnews.go.com/International/wireStory/countries-crack-basic-rights-amid-virus-pandemic-69884721

Theidon, K. (2020). A forecasted failure: Intersectionality, COVID-19, and the perfect storm. *Journal of Human Rights, 19*(5), 528–536. doi:10.1080/14754835.2020.1822156

UN Human Rights Council (2020, April 23). Disease pandemics and the freedom of opinion and expression Report of the Special Rapporteur on the promotion and protection of the right to freedom of opinion and expression. https://undocs.org/A/HRC/44/49

UN General Assembly (2006). *Resolution adopted by the General Assembly on 15 March 2006*. https://documents-dds-ny.un.org/doc/UNDOC/GEN/N05/502/66/PDF/N0550266.pdf?OpenElement.

UN Women (2020). *The shadow pandemic: Violence against women during COVID-19*. https://www.unwomen.org/en/news/in-focus/in-focus-gender-equality-in-covid-19-response/violence-against-women-during-covid-19

United Nations Educational, Scientific and Cultural Organization (UNESCO) (2021). *Education: From disruption to recovery*. https://en.unesco.org/covid19/educationresponse

Wallace, G. P. (2013). International law and public attitudes toward torture: An experimental study. *International Organization, 67*(1), 105–140. doi:10.1017/S0020818312000343

Wallace, G. P. (2014). Martial law? Military experience, international law, and support for torture. *International Studies Quarterly, 58*(3), 501–514. doi:10.1111/isqu.12092

Windsor, L. C., Yannitell Reinhardt, G., Windsor, A. J., Ostergard, R., Allen, S., Burns, C., Giger, J., & Wood, R. (2020). Gender in the time of COVID-19: Evaluating national leadership and COVID-19 fatalities. *PloS One, 15*(12), e0244531. doi:10.1371/journal.pone.0244531

Wingfield, R. (2019, October 15). A human rights-based approach to disinformation. *Global Partners Digital*. https://www.gp-digital.org/a-human-rights-based-approach-to-disinformation/

Wong, E., Barnes, J. E., & Kanno-Youngs, Z. (2020, September 17). Local officials in China hid coronavirus dangers from Beijing, U.S. Agencies Find. *New York Times*. https://nyti.ms/2EbxVnr

Wong, W. H., & Wong, E. A. (2020). What COVID-19 revealed about health, human rights, and the WHO. *Journal of Human Rights, 19*(5), 568–581. doi:10.1080/14754835.2020.1819778

Zvobgo, K. (2019). Human rights versus national interests: Shifting US public attitudes on the international criminal court. *International Studies Quarterly, 63*(4), 1065–1078. doi:10.1093/isq/sqz056

Index

abortion 179, 180
abuses 37, 45, 47, 91, 92, 96, 222, 229–232
accountability 36, 55, 58, 74, 134, 138, 141, 169, 170, 173, 183
acrimony 115, 116, 127
actors 48, 50, 59, 232
Alon, I. 149
Alrababa'h, A. 148
Alston, Philip 24, 25
anti-apartheid movements 70
anti-COVID-19 measures 83, 84
antiretrovirals 39, 43
Arab Spring 147, 148, 151, 158, 161
Argentina 69, 71, 121, 174, 182
armed insurgency 151
artificial intelligence (AI) 221, 223
Ashford, Elizabeth 7, 8
Asociación Civil por la Igualdad y la Justicia (ACIJ) 69, 71, 72
asylum seekers 24, 80–82, 85, 86, 101, 106, 111, 118
asylum system 81, 85
Australia 174, 191, 195, 198
authoritarian consolidation 128, 136, 147, 157, 158
authoritarianism 115, 121, 126, 142, 148, 160
authoritarian regimes 91, 95, 148–150, 157, 160–162
authoritarian states 22, 120, 121, 148, 157
authoritarian upgrading 148, 150
autocracies 92, 94, 95, 120, 126, 136

Badran, S. 126, 136, 195, 210, 222, 230
Bayesian Aldrich-McKelvey (BAM) scaling methodology 194
Bennoune, K. 124
Black Lives Matter movement 24, 26, 29, 121, 134
Blaydes, L. 148
Bly, Robert 16
Bond, Katherine C. 37
borders 80–83, 86, 117, 118, 120, 190, 192, 229, 230, 232
Bouchard, Johanne 9
Brook, A. M. 191
Brysk, A. 23, 25, 29, 127, 149, 198, 209, 230
business incentive structures 48
Bussmann, Margit 56

Carey, S. C. 232
censorship 90–92, 94, 95, 122, 142, 152, 232
Cepaluni, G. 120, 149, 160
Cetron, Martin S. 62
Cheibub, J. A. 120
Chenoweth, E. 25, 26, 28, 126, 137, 149, 195, 211
child marriage 174, 175
Chilton, A. 207
Chiozza, G. 149, 168, 202, 223, 227, 229–230
civic solidarity 24, 26
civil society 23, 27, 28, 149, 152, 155, 157, 162, 210; organizations 26, 156
Clark, A. M. 232
Clay, K. C. 126, 127, 149, 191, 192
Clemens, Colleen 16
communications 61, 71, 91, 92, 95, 141, 142, 154
community transmission 25
complacency 115, 127
Connell, R. W. 15
contact tracing method 209
contraception 172, 179
corporate social responsibility 47, 48, 50
corruption 33, 37, 38, 135, 138
Crenshaw, Kimberlé 14
cultural rights 6, 35, 38, 190

data collection 19, 34, 92, 101, 211
Dave, D. M. 122
Delmas, Candice 28
democracies 22, 23, 90, 92, 94, 95, 120, 121, 126, 128, 141–144, 149
Dempster, H. 118
deportations 69, 74, 75, 100, 101, 103, 105, 106
detention 83, 100, 101, 105, 106, 190, 191, 197
differential pricing 49, 50
digital activism 135, 141
digital authoritarianism 141, 142, 144
discrimination 8, 9, 61, 62, 70, 72, 74, 169, 171, 172, 175, 177, 178

displacement 169, 175
diversionary conflicts 149
domestic violence 6, 14, 18, 33, 117, 119, 170, 173
domestic workers 173–177, 182
Donaldson, Thomas 51n6
Dore, G. J. 125
drug companies 43, 44, 46–50

economic distress 174
economic insecurity 169, 180
economic issues 218, 219, 222, 223
economic sustainability 48, 50
Edgell, A. B. 120
Egypt 142, 147, 148, 150, 153, 155, 157–162
emergency 22, 35, 37, 123, 126, 151, 152, 154, 156, 157, 159, 160, 209, 210
emergency law 149–157, 159–161; structure 150
employment 5, 173, 175, 177, 183; rates 175
empowerment 70, 168, 170, 181, 182, 191, 201; rights 190, 191, 193–195, 201, 231
enforcement 155, 170, 197
essential medicines 36, 45, 46, 48, 50, 171, 178, 209
ethics 48, 57, 58, 180, 182
European Medicines Agency (EMA) 37

fair pricing 38, 39
Fariss, C. J. 231
feminist empowerment 180
feminist leadership 181
Ferrero, J. P. 121
fiduciary duties 47, 48, 50
Flood, C. M. 123
forecasted failure 13–19, 172
Forman, L. 124
Foucault, M. 110
fragile masculinity 16
Franklin, J. C. 157
freedom of movement 57, 61, 80, 123, 149, 158, 177, 231
free movement 35, 83–86
Frey, C. B. 120, 149
Fukuda-Parr, S. 200

gender-based violence 169, 173–175, 179, 180, 182, 230
gender equity 181–183
gender regimes 169, 171, 172, 177
gender violence 168, 170, 171, 173, 174, 180, 183
Giubilini, A. 125
Global Gender Gap 173
global health crisis 122, 168, 169, 171, 172, 183, 206
global health emergencies 223, 227
global lockdown 134
global pandemic 39, 43, 44, 48, 50, 127, 134–136, 138, 141, 201, 207
global perceptions 206–223
global politics 56, 63
global South 43–50, 115, 124, 128
Goemans, H. E. 149
Gohdes, A. R. 232
Goldner Lang, I. 118
Goodhart, M. 123, 126, 195, 230
grassroots movements 143
Gupta, Alisha Haridasani 18
Guterres, A. 125

Hall, S. 111
Hare, C. 191
harm, gendering 18
hazardous confinement 100–107
health 10, 33–37, 45, 46, 54–59, 122, 151, 171, 178, 195, 228
health care 8, 22–24, 35, 44, 46, 48, 57, 58, 86, 118–119, 170, 171, 173, 176–179, 182
health crises 33, 36, 37, 101, 103, 121, 127, 169, 171, 172, 180, 181
health rights 168–173, 175, 180, 181, 183
herd immunity 19, 69, 228
Heydemann, S. 148
historical corporate social responsibility 50
Hong Kong 135, 141, 147, 191, 193, 195, 197, 208
human insecurity 168
human rights 6, 23, 34, 45, 48, 55, 56, 58, 70, 115, 117, 126, 127, 161, 170, 198, 201, 202, 229, 231; consequences 80, 82, 86, 198; obligations 43, 45–48, 50, 86, 117, 125; outcomes 194, 195, 198–200; practices 76, 138, 189–192, 194, 198, 199, 201, 202; practitioners 24, 195, 202; research 227, 231
Human Rights Guidelines for Pharmaceutical Companies in Relation to Access to Medicines 45–47
Human Rights Measurement Initiative (HRMI) 189
human rights-related topics 219
human rights-sensitive approach 58

immigrants 74, 82, 119, 176, 177
imprisonment 102, 151, 152
incentivize innovation 48
India 22–29, 33, 34, 69, 73, 93, 135, 174
Indigenous people 190, 197, 198
inequalities 14, 15, 22, 23, 25, 29, 111, 115, 117, 119, 123, 126, 127
information control 91, 92, 95
information manipulation 91, 92, 94, 95, 232
innovation, incentivize 48
interdependence 5–10, 126, 127, 169, 170, 172, 183, 194, 202, 230
international actors 157, 160, 161
international organization 58, 85, 116, 123, 177
intersectionality 13–15, 127
intimate partner violence 13, 18, 172, 175
invisibility 72, 175

Joseph, S. 125
justice 26–28, 69–73, 82, 103, 104

Kavanagh, M. M. 227
Keck, M. E. 157
Kimmel, Michael 17
King, J. 149, 168, 202, 223, 227, 229, 230
Kjaerum, M. 126
Kohler, J. C. 124
Koo, J.-W. 127, 195, 229
K-quarantine 207, 208, 210, 213, 222
Künnemann, Rolf 9

labor market scarring 177
labor trafficking 174
Lange, M. 122
Leenders, R. 148
legal empowerment 69–72, 75; approaches 69–76
Leung, Tiffany 62
Lind, Dara 82
Lipman, Harvey B. 62
lockdowns 73, 85, 115, 116, 118, 119, 121, 141, 152, 156, 173–176, 179

Macron, Emmanuel 101
Maerz, S. F. 121
Malaysia 38, 191, 193, 195, 197, 198
marginalized communities 69, 70, 72, 76, 169, 197
Markel, Howard 62
masculinity 15–17
Matrajt, Laura 62
maximalist people-power movements 138
media coverage 207
medical care 34, 46, 152, 178, 179
medical countermeasures 60, 61
Mesel, Felipe 72
Metternich, N. W. 121
Meyer-Bisch, Patrice 9
Michalsen, Joseph R. 62
migrants 81, 82, 85, 100, 101, 104–106, 111, 118, 170, 173, 177, 179, 198; fate of 100–107
migration 80, 83, 85
military 142, 152–156, 159, 218
Minkler, Lanse 7
Modi, Prime Minister 23, 27–28, 140, 153, 154
Monscheuer, O. 122
Moore, Natalie 17
moral responsibilities 47, 48
Morocco 126, 147–154, 156–161
multi-stakeholder initiatives 49
Murdie, A. 127, 135, 149, 198, 206, 223

Natalucci, A. 121
national health authorities 207
Navarro, J. Alexander 62
Nazdeek 69, 72–74
negative interdependence 8–10, 123, 126, 195, 230, 231
neoliberalism 23, 25
neo-liberal political economies 175
Newton, Paul N. 37
nonpharmaceutical interventions (NPIs) 59–62
Nonviolent and Violent Campaign Outcomes (NAVCO) 135
nonviolent resistance 135–138, 142–144
North Africa 136, 147, 148

Organized Communities Against Deportation (OCAD) 69, 74, 75
Ortiz, I. 136
Oxfam 125

pandemic patriarchy 127, 168, 169, 171–173, 180–183, 230
pandemic policies 179
patent rights 43, 49
patriarchy 127, 169, 171–173
people power 134–138, 140–144; campaigns 138; movements 135–139, 142–144
pharmaceutical companies 43, 45, 46, 124
physical integrity rights 127, 190, 191, 193, 201, 229, 231
Piven, Frances Fox 25
police violence 33
policy recommendation 123
political factors 58, 228
political regimes 171
political rights 6, 36, 57, 59, 123, 124, 190–193, 195, 223, 230
political solidarity 24–26, 29
Powell, C. 176
power 70, 72, 73, 123, 140, 142, 144, 149, 151, 153–155, 157, 160, 161
proportionality 39, 48, 61, 83, 84, 230
protest movements 26, 134, 136
protest restrictions 138, 140
protests 24, 26, 105, 121, 122, 124, 135–137, 140, 141, 148, 151, 156, 158
pseudo-document-based topic model (PTM) 207, 212, 219, 222, 223
public discourse 55, 57
public health 35, 36, 38, 46, 55–58, 80, 84, 86, 148, 150, 207, 229; emergencies 22, 82, 86, 95, 136, 155, 158, 173, 222, 230; interventions 59; measures 58, 62, 74, 128, 143, 195, 223, 230, 232
public opinion 127, 128, 206, 207, 229, 233

racial justice paradox 176
Ramji-Nogales, J. 118
Randolph, S. 200
refugees 23, 24, 80, 81, 83, 85, 118, 170, 180, 198, 230
regime type 58, 120, 121, 128, 199, 207

religious groups 155, 219, 222, 223
reproductive rights 18, 127, 168–171, 177, 179, 180, 183; norms 178
rights-based approaches 55, 56, 58, 59, 169
rights-based health 58
rights-based language 232, 233
right to health 5, 34–37, 45, 46, 50, 55, 57–59, 122, 195, 223, 228, 229, 232
right-wing populism 142
Rubin, D. B. 201
Ruggie principles 45–47, 49, 50

Santoro, M. A. 124
Savulescu, J. 124, 125
Schneider, Gerald 56
Scholz, Sally J. 24, 27
scientific knowledge 57, 84
Scott, Craig 7
Sekalala, S. 123
self-conscious strategy 143
self-determination 75, 169–173, 177, 179
sex work 176, 177
shareholders 45, 47, 48, 50
Shay, C. W. 137
shecession 175
Shue, Henry 7
Sikkink, K. 22, 157, 232
Singh, R. 227
Sloan, Alexandra 62
Snowden, F. 140
social contract 45, 47
social distancing 55, 58, 61, 62, 102, 104, 116, 117, 159, 160, 162, 206, 207, 213
social pathologies 168
social rights 123, 170–172, 175, 178, 181, 190, 191, 193, 194, 200, 201
social systems 168, 182
solidarity 22–29, 103, 111, 228; and human rights 24
South Korea 207–211, 213, 215–223
Spadaro, A. 123, 149
Stahl, Aviva 18
Stanley, Maclen 18
state-of-emergency law 102
state surveillance 90–92, 121
Stern, Alexandra Minna 62
stigmatization 61, 209, 211, 219, 222
surveillance 75, 76, 90–93, 95, 121, 122, 148, 154, 208, 219, 221, 222; strategies 209
Sweeney, Shawna 7

tactical innovations 135, 136, 141
Tai, D. B. G. 119
Tamburini, F. 151
technology 34, 75, 76, 92, 93, 213, 221–223, 232
teenage-pregnancy rates 172
topic modeling/models 206, 207, 211, 212, 222
Toubon, Jacques 103
toxic masculinity 15–17
tradeoffs 126, 168–170, 173, 223
trade restrictions 38
traditional gender regimes 172
transformation 24, 25, 69–71, 74–76
translation 69–72, 76
transparency 25, 37, 39, 96, 127, 231, 232
trust 15, 69–74, 76, 94, 96, 159
Turnbull, B. 126, 136, 195, 210, 222, 230

undocumented migrants 100, 101, 103, 104, 106, 111
UN Guiding Principles on Business and Human Rights 45–47
United Nations 22, 34, 45–47, 96, 190, 200, 201, 219, 229
United States 14, 17–19, 22–25, 28, 29, 38, 46, 80–82, 86, 119, 135, 142, 213

vaccination 19, 43, 62, 116, 135, 213, 216, 217, 223, 228
vaccines 34, 36, 38, 39, 43–48, 124–126, 216, 219; access to 36–37; nationalism 38, 44, 115, 124; policies 124, 125
Vienna Declaration 6, 7, 56
violence 15, 16, 18, 118, 119, 136, 137, 168, 172–175, 177, 178, 180; domesticating 18
Von Stein, J. 126
vulnerable populations 33, 35, 39, 61, 62, 86, 119, 172, 173

Wang, Y. 122
Whelan, D. 6
WHO Fair Pricing Milestones 38
Wilder, J. M. 119
Willingham, Emily 17
women 15–18, 27, 119, 168–170, 173–181, 183, 198; empowerment 180, 181, 183; rights 127, 151, 168–173, 181–183
Wong, E. A. 230
Wong, W. H. 230
workers 6, 9, 23, 24, 120, 152, 175, 176, 221, 222
World Economic Forum Gender Gap 177
World Health Organization (WHO) 33, 34, 36, 37, 44, 46, 47, 54–62, 94, 148, 154, 155, 177

Yao, L. 120, 149

For Product Safety Concerns and Information please contact our EU
representative GPSR@taylorandfrancis.com
Taylor & Francis Verlag GmbH, Kaufingerstraße 24, 80331 München, Germany

www.ingramcontent.com/pod-product-compliance
Ingram Content Group UK Ltd.
Pitfield, Milton Keynes, MK11 3LW, UK
UKHW052052230926
475702UK00025B/1121
* 9 7 8 1 0 3 2 2 1 8 2 5 0 *